Bone Marrow Pathology

Bone Marrow Pathology

BARBARA J. BAIN
MBBS, FRACP, MRCPath
Senior Lecturer in Haematology,
St Mary's Hospital Medical School,
Imperial College of Science,
Technology and Medicine, London; and
Honorary Consultant Haematologist,
St Mary's Hospital, London

DAVID M. CLARK
MD, MRCP, MRCPath
Senior Registrar in Histopathology,
St Mary's Hospital, London

IRVIN A. LAMPERT
MB ChB, DCP, FRCPath
Consultant Histopathologist,
Ealing Hospital, London;
Honorary Senior Lecturer,
Royal Postgraduate Medical School, London;
and Honorary Consultant in Histopathology,
Hammersmith Hospital, London

OXFORD
BLACKWELL SCIENTIFIC PUBLICATIONS
LONDON EDINBURGH BOSTON
MELBOURNE PARIS BERLIN VIENNA

© 1992 by
Blackwell Scientific Publications
Editorial Offices:
Osney Mead, Oxford OX2 0EL
25 John Street, London WC1N 2BL
23 Ainslie Place, Edinburgh EH3 6AJ
238 Main Street, Cambridge
   Massachusetts 02142, USA
54 University Street, Carlton
   Victoria 3053, Australia

Other Editorial Offices:
Librairie Arnette SA
1, rue de Lille
75007 Paris
France

Blackwell Wissenschafts-Verlag GmbH
Düsseldorfer Str. 38
D-10707 Berlin
Germany

Blackwell MZV
Feldgasse 13
A-1238 Wien
Austria

First published 1992
Reprinted 1993, 1994

Set by Setrite Typesetters, Hong Kong
Printed by Vincenzo Bona srl, Turin, Italy

DISTRIBUTORS

  Marston Book Services Ltd
  PO Box 87
  Oxford OX2 0DT
  (*Orders:* Tel: 0865 791155
        Fax: 0865 791927
        Telex: 837515)

USA
  Blackwell Scientific Publications, Inc.
  238 Main Street
  Cambridge, MA 02142
  (*Orders*: Tel: 800 759-6102
        617 876-7000)

Canada
  Times Mirror Professional Publishing Ltd
  130 Flaska Drive
  Markham, Ontario L6G 1B8
  (*Orders:* Tel: 800 268-4178
        416 470-6739)

Australia
  Blackwell Scientific Publications Pty Ltd
  54 University Street
  Carlton, Victoria 3053
  (*Orders:* Tel: 03 347-5552)

A catalogue record for this book is
available from the British Library

ISBN 0-632-03401-7

Contents

Preface

In this book we have set out to provide a practical comprehensive guide to the diagnosis of bone marrow disease. We have dealt both with haematological diseases and with more generalized pathological processes which may affect the bone marrow. We have sought always to place bone marrow abnormalities within the broader context of clinical and peripheral blood features. Equal weight has been given to cytological and histological assessment with a particular emphasis on the need for an integrated approach to diagnosis. We hope that for these reasons both haematologists and histopathologists will find our work of value. We hope further that our practical approach to diagnostic problems will make this a useful laboratory handbook for both trainees and practising pathologists but that at the same time its comprehensiveness will render it useful as a reference source.

We have sought throughout to emphasize what can be learnt from routine stains of bone marrow aspirates and routine stains of paraffin-embedded as well as plastic-embedded bone marrow biopsy sections. We have dealt in less detail with more specialized procedures which although sometimes illuminating may not be so readily applicable in the routine diagnostic laboratory.

B.J.B., D.M.C., I.A.L.

Acknowledgements

We should like to thank our friends and colleagues who have lent photographs or permitted us to photograph microscopic slides from their personal collections: in particular Dr S.H. Abdalla, Professor D. Catovsky, Dr Hannah Cohen, Dr Christine Costello, Dr Sally Davies, Dr Helen Dodsworth, Dr Sue Fairhead, Dr Mary Falzon, Dr D. Gill, Dr C. Jamieson, Dr Estella Matutes, Professor J.W. Stewart, Dr S.K. Suvarna, Professor S.N. Wickramasinghe and Dr A.G. Zuiable. In addition, we should like to thank our many friends and colleagues both past and present in the departments of Haematology and Histopathology at St Mary's Hospital and the Royal Postgraduate Medical School, Hammersmith Hospital, for the help they have given; particular mention is due to Dr R.D. Goldin who has critically reviewed the entire manuscript. Finally, we should like to record our debt of gratitude to Professor David Galton, who has not only read the entire manuscript and commented in great detail, but has also taught us and countless other haematologists and histopathologists a great deal over many years.

B.J.B., D.M.C., I.A.L.

Abbreviations

AIDS	Acquired immune deficiency syndrome
AILD	Angio-immunoblastic lymphadenopathy (with dysproteinaemia)
ALIP	Abnormal localization of immature precursors
ALL	Acute lymphoblastic leukaemia
AML	Acute myeloid leukaemia
ATLL	Adult T-cell leukaemia/lymphoma
BM	Bone marrow
BMG	Benign monoclonal gammopathy
CDA	Congenital dyserythropoietic anaemia
CGL	Chronic granulocytic leukaemia
CHAD	Cold haemagglutinin disease
CLL	Chronic lymphocytic leukaemia
CML	Chronic myeloid leukaemia
CMML	Chronic myelomonocytic leukaemia
CMV	Cytomegalovirus
CT	Computerized tomography
CyIg	Cytoplasmic immunoglobulin
DIC	Disseminated intravascular coagulation
EBV	Epstein−Barr virus
EMA	Epithelial membrane antigen
FAB	French−American−British (co-operative group)
GMS	Grocott's methenamine silver stain
GVHD	Graft-versus-host disease
H&E	Haematoxylin and eosin (stain)
Hempas	Hereditary erythroid multinuclearity with positive acidified serum test
HIV	Human immunodeficiency virus
HLA	Human leucocyte antigen
HTLV-I	Human T-cell leukaemia virus I
Ig	Immunoglobulin

LGL	Large granular lymphocyte
M : E	Myeloid : erythroid ratio
MALT	Mucosa-associated lymphoid tissue
McAb	Monoclonal antibody
MDS	Myelodysplastic syndromes
MGG	May Grünwald−Giemsa (stain)
MGUS	Monoclonal gammopathy of undetermined significance
MIC	Morphologic, immunologic, cytogenetic (classification)
MPD	Myeloproliferative disorder
MPO	Myeloperoxidase
NEC	Non-erythroid cells
NHL	Non-Hodgkin's lymphoma
PAS	Periodic acid−Schiff (stain)
PB	Peripheral blood
PLL	Prolymphocytic leukaemia
PNH	Paroxysmal nocturnal haemoglobinuria
POEMS	Polyneuropathy, organomegaly, endocrinopathy, M-protein, skin changes (syndrome)
PRV	Polycythaemia rubra vera
RA	Refractory anaemia
RAEB	Refractory anaemia with excess of blasts
RAEB-t	Refractory anaemia with excess of blasts in transformation
RARS	Refractory anaemia with ring sideroblasts
SBB	Sudan black B (stain)
SLVL	Splenic lymphoma with villous lymphocytes
SmIg	Surface membrane immunoglobulin
TAR	Thrombocytopenia-absent radii
TRAP	Tartrate-resistant acid phosphatase
WBC	White blood cell (count)

1: The Normal Bone Marrow

THE DISTRIBUTION OF HAEMOPOIETIC MARROW

During extra-uterine life haemopoiesis is normally confined to the bone marrow. Bones are composed of cortex and medulla. The cortex is a strong layer of compact bone; the medulla is a honeycomb of cancellous bone, the interstices of which are known as the medullary cavity and contain the bone marrow. Bone marrow is either red marrow containing haemopoietic cells or yellow marrow which is largely adipose tissue. The distribution of haemopoietic marrow is dependent on age. In the neonate virtually all the bone marrow cavity is fully occupied by proliferating haemopoietic cells; haemopoiesis occurs even in the phalanges. As the child ages haemopoietic marrow contracts centripetally, to be replaced by fatty marrow. By early adult life haemopoietic marrow is largely confined to the skull, vertebrae, ribs, clavicles, sternum, pelvis and the proximal half of the humeri and femora; however there is considerable variation between individuals as to the distribution of haemopoietic marrow.[1] In response to demand the volume of the marrow cavity occupied by haemopoietic tissue expands.

THE ORGANIZATION OF THE BONE MARROW

Bone

The cortex and the medulla differ functionally as well as histologically. Bone may be classified histologically in two ways. Classification may be by macroscopic appearance into: (i) compact or dense bone with only small interstices, not visible macroscopically, and (ii) cancellous (or trabecular) bone with large, readily visible interstices. Bone may also be classified histologically on the basis of whether there are well organized osteons in which a central Haversian canal is surrounded by concentric lamellae composed of parallel bundles of fibrils (lamellar bone) or, alternatively, whether the fibrils of the bone are in disorderly bundles (woven bone).

The cortex is a solid layer of compact bone which gives the bone its strength. It is composed largely of lamellar bone but contains some woven bone. The lamellar bone of the cortex is either well organized Haversian systems or angular fragments of lamellar bone which occupy the spaces between the Haversian systems; in long bones there are also inner and outer circumferential lamellae. Extending inwards from the cortex is an anastomosing network of trabeculae which partition the medullary space. The medullary bone is trabecular or cancellous bone; it contains some lamellae but the structure is less highly organized than that of the cortex. Most of the cortical bone is covered on the external surface by periosteum which has an outer fibrous layer and an inner osteogenic layer. At articular surfaces, and more extensively in younger patients, bone fuses with cartilage rather than being covered by periosteum. The bony trabeculae and the inner surface of the cortex are lined by endosteal cells including both osteogenic cells and osteoclasts. Osteocytes are found within lacunae in bony trabeculae and in cortical bone. Although osteoblasts and osteoclasts share the surface of the bone trabeculae they originate from different stem cells. Osteoblasts, and therefore osteocytes, are of mesenchymal origin being derived from the same stem cell as the chondrocyte and probably also the stromal fibroblasts. Osteoclasts, however, are derived from a haemopoietic stem cell, being formed by fusion of cells of the monocyte lineage.

The cells which give rise to bone-forming cells are designated osteoprogenitor cells; they are flattened, spindle-shaped cells which are capable of developing into either osteoblasts or chondrocytes, depending on the microenvironment. Osteoblasts synthesize glycosaminoglycans of the bone matrix and also the collagenous fibres which are embedded in the matrix, thus forming osteoid or non-calcified bone; subsequently mineralization occurs. Bone undergoes constant remodelling. In adult life remodelling of the bone takes place particularly in the subcortical regions. Osteoblasts add a new layer of bone to trabeculae (apposition) while osteoclasts resorb other areas of the bone; up to 25 per cent of the trabecular surface may be covered by osteoid. The osteo-clasts which are resorbing bone lie in shallow hollows, known as Howship's lacunae, created by the process of resorption, while osteoblasts are seen in rows on the surface of trabecular bone or on the surface of a layer of osteoid. As new bone is laid down osteoblasts become immured in bone and are converted into osteocytes. The bone which replaces osteoid is woven bone which in turn is remodelled to form lamellar bone. The difference between the two can be easily appreci-ated in polarized light. The organized fibrillar structure of lamellar bone, with bundles of par-allel fibrils running in different directions in successive lamellae gives rise to alternating light and dark layers under polarized light.

Other connective tissue elements

The haemopoietic cells of the bone marrow are embedded in a connective tissue stroma which occupies the intertrabecular spaces of the medulla. The stroma is composed of fat cells and a meshwork of blood vessels, branching fibro-blasts, macrophages, some myelinated and non-myelinated nerve fibres, and a small amount of reticulin. Stromal cells include cells which have been designated reticulum or reticular cells. This term probably includes two cell types of different origin. Phagocytic reticulum cells are macro-phages and originate from a haemopoietic pro-genitor. Non-phagocytic reticulum or reticular cells are closely related to fibroblasts, adventitial cells of sinusoids (see below) and probably also

osteoblasts and chondrocytes. They differ from phagocytic reticulum cells in that the majority are positive for alkaline phosphatase. There is close interaction between haemopoietic cells and their microenvironment with each modifying the other.

The blood supply of the marrow is derived in part from the central nutrient artery which enters long bones at mid shaft and bifurcates to two longitudinal central arteries.[2] Similar arteries penetrate flat and cuboidal bones. There is a sup-plementary blood supply from cortical capillaries which penetrate the bone from the periosteum. The branches of the central artery give rise to arterioles and capillaries which radiate towards the endosteum and mainly enter the bone, sub-sequently turning back to re-enter the marrow and open into a network of thin-walled sinusoids.[2] Only a minority of capillaries enter the sinusoids directly without first supplying the bone. The sinusoids drain into the central venous sinusoid which accompanies the nutrient artery. The sinusoids are large thin-walled vessels through which newly formed haemopoietic cells enter the circulation. They are often collapsed in histo-logical sections and are therefore not readily seen. (In the presence of marrow sclerosis these vessels are often held open and are then very obvious.) The walls of sinusoids consist of endothelial cells, forming a complete cover with overlapping junc-tions, and an incomplete basement membrane. The outer surface is clothed by adventitial cells, large broad cells which branch into the peri-vascular space and therefore provide a scaffolding for the haemopoietic cells, macrophages and mast cells. Adventitial cells are thought to be derived from fibroblasts; they are associated with a net-work of delicate extracellular fibres which can be stained with a reticulin stain. Reticulin fibres are concentrated close to the periosteum as well as around blood vessels. It is likely that both adventitial cells and fibroblasts can synthesize reticulin,[3] which is a form of collagen.

The marrow fat content varies inversely with the quantity of haemopoietic tissue. Fat content also increases as bone is lost with increasing age. Marrow fat is physiologically different from sub-cutaneous fat. The fat of yellow marrow is the last fat in the body to be lost in starvation. When haemopoietic tissue is lost very rapidly it is replaced initially by mucin. Subsequently the mucin is replaced by fat.

Haemopoietic and other cells

Haemopoietic cells lie in cords or wedges between the sinusoids. In man normal haemopoiesis, with the exception of some thrombopoiesis at extramedullary sites, is confined to the interstitium although in pathological conditions haemopoiesis can occur within sinusoids. Mature haemopoietic cells enter the circulation by passing transcellulary, through sinusoidal endothelial cells.[2] The detailed disposition of haemopoietic cells will be discussed below.

The marrow also contains lymphoid cells and small numbers of plasma cells (see below).

EXAMINATION OF THE BONE MARROW

Bone marrow was first obtained from living patients for diagnostic purposes during the first decade of this century but it was not until the introduction of sternal aspiration in the late 1920s that this became an important diagnostic procedure. Specimens of bone marrow for cytological and histological examination may be obtained by aspiration biopsy, by core biopsy using a trephine needle or an electric drill, by open biopsy and at autopsy. The two most important techniques, which are complementary, are aspiration biopsy and trephine biopsy.

Bone marrow aspiration

Aspiration biopsies are most commonly carried out on the sternum or the ilium. Aspiration from the medial surface of the tibia can yield useful diagnostic specimens up to the age of 18 months but is mainly used in neonates in whom other sites are less suitable. Aspiration from ribs and from the spinous processes of vertebrae is also possible but now little practised. Sternal aspiration should be carried out from the first part of the body of the sternum, at the level of the second intercostal space. Aspiration from any lower in the sternum increases the risks of the procedure. Aspiration from the ilium can be from either the anterior or the posterior iliac crest. Aspiration

from the anterior iliac crest is best carried out by a lateral approach a few centimetres below and posterior to the anterior superior iliac spine. Approach through the crest of the ilium with the needle in the direction of the main axis of the bone is also possible but is more difficult because of the hardness of the bone. Aspirates from the posterior iliac crest are usually taken from the posterior superior iliac spine. When aspiration is carried out at the same time as a trephine biopsy it is easiest to perform the two procedures from adjacent sites. This is facilitated by use of the ilium. If a trephine biopsy is not being carried out there is a choice between the sternum and the iliac crest. Either is suitable in adults and older children, although great care must be exercised in carrying out sternal aspirations. In a study of 100 patients in whom both techniques were applied sternal aspiration was found to be technically easier and to produce a suitable diagnostic specimen more frequently, although on average the procedure was more painful, both with regard to bone penetration and to the actual aspiration.[4] Sternal aspiration is also more dangerous. Although deaths are very rare at least 20 have been reported and we are aware of two further unreported fatalities; deaths have been consequent mainly on laceration of vessels or laceration of the heart with pericardial tamponade. Sternal aspiration is unsuitable for use in young children. Posterior iliac crest aspiration is suitable for children, infants and many neonates. Tibial aspiration is suitable for very small babies but has no advantages over iliac crest aspiration in older infants.

Bone marrow specimens yielded by aspiration are suitable for the following: wedge-spread films; films of crushed marrow fragments; study of cell markers (by flow cytometry or on films or cytospin preparations); cytogenetic study; ultrastructural examination; culture for microorganisms; culture to study haemopoietic precursors and histological sections of fragments.

Trephine biopsy of bone marrow

Trephine or needle biopsy is most easily carried out on the iliac crest, either posteriorly or anteriorly, as described above. The posterior approach appears to be now more generally preferred. If a trephine biopsy and a bone marrow aspiration are both to be carried out they can be performed through the same skin incision but with two areas of periosteum being infiltrated with local anaesthetic and with the needle being angled in different directions. Core biopsies obtained with a trephine needle are suitable for histological sections, for touch preparations (imprints) and for electron microscopy. A touch preparation is particularly important when it is not possible to obtain an aspirate since it allows cytological details to be studied. Biopsy specimens can be used for cytogenetic study but aspirates are much more suitable. Frozen sections of biopsies are possible and allow the application of a wide range of immunological markers but they are not usually very satisfactory because of technical difficulties, both in cutting sections and in keeping sections on the slides. Histological sections may be prepared from biopsies which have been decalcified and paraffin-embedded or from biopsies which have been embedded in plastic without prior decalcification.

PROCESSING OF TREPHINE BIOPSIES

The two principal methods of preparation of trephine biopsy specimens have both advantages and disadvantages. Problems are created because of the difficulty of cutting tissue composed of hard bone and soft, easily torn, bone marrow. Alternative approaches are to decalcify the specimen or to embed it in a substance which makes the bone marrow almost as hard as the bone. Decalcification and paraffin-embedding leads to considerable shrinkage and loss of cellular detail. Nuclear staining may become blurred. Some cytochemical activity is lost, for example that for chloroacetate esterase. Because sections are thicker, cellular detail is harder to appreciate. However immunological techniques are much more readily applicable on paraffin-embedded than on plastic-embedded specimens and with careful techniques very good results can be obtained. Plastic-embedding techniques are more expensive and, for laboratories which are processing only small numbers of trephine biopsies, are technically more difficult. However there is no shrinkage, preservation of cellular detail is excellent and the thinness of the sections means that fine cytological detail can be readily appreciated. Some enzyme activities, for example for chloroacetate esterase, are retained. Although immunological techniques can be applied excessive background staining is often a problem. Plastics with differing qualities are available for embedding. Methyl methacrylate requires very long processing and is therefore not very suitable for routine diagnostic laboratories. Glycol methacrylate is very satisfactory; however, when cellularity is low sections tend to tear and in this circumstance a small amount of decalcification may be useful.

RELATIVE ADVANTAGES OF ASPIRATION AND CORE BIOPSIES

Bone marrow aspiration and trephine biopsy each have both advantages and limitations. The two procedures should therefore be regarded as complementary. Bone marrow aspirates are unequalled in demonstration of fine cytological detail and permit a wider range of cytochemical stains and immunological markers than is possible with histological sections. Aspiration is particularly useful and may well be performed alone in investigating patients with suspected iron deficiency anaemia, anaemia of chronic disease, megaloblastic anaemia and acute leukaemia. Trephine biopsy is essential for diagnosis when a 'dry tap' or 'blood tap' occurs as a consequence of the marrow being fibrotic or very densely cellular and only a biopsy allows a complete assessment of marrow architecture and of the pattern of distribution of any abnormal infiltrate. This technique is particularly useful in investigating suspected aplastic or hypoplastic anaemia, lymphoma, metastatic carcinoma, myeloproliferative disorders and diseases of the bones. We have also found trephine biopsy generally much more useful than bone marrow aspiration in investigating patients with the advanced stages of HIV infection in whom hypocellular, non-diagnostic aspirates are common. It should not be forgotten, however, that trephine biopsy undoubtedly causes more pain to the patient than does aspiration.

Complications of bone marrow aspiration and trephine biopsy are very rare. Cardiac and great vessel laceration have been mentioned above.

Otherwise haemorrhage is uncommon but when procedures are carried out on patients with a haemostatic defect prolonged firm pressure is necessary to ensure that bleeding has stopped. Haemorrhage is also occasionally a problem when a biopsy is carried out on bone with an abnormal vasculature, for example in Paget's disease. Pneumothoraces have occurred and sternomanubrial separation has been observed in one patient. In patients with osteosclerosis needles may break. Infection is a rare complication.

Other techniques

It is occasionally necessary to obtain a bone marrow specimen by open biopsy under a general anaesthetic. This is usually only required when a specific lesion has been demonstrated at a relatively inaccessible site by radiology or bone scanning.

At autopsy specimens of bone marrow for histological examination are most readily obtained from the sternum and the vertebral bodies, although any bone containing red marrow can be used. Unless the autopsy is performed soon after death the cytological detail is often poor.

CELLULARITY

Bone marrow cellularity can be assessed most accurately in histological sections (Fig. 1.1) although haematologists necessarily also make assessments on aspirated bone marrow fragments in wedge-spread films (Fig. 1.2). Histological specimens which are suitable for assessment of cellularity are: sections of aspirated fragments; needle or open biopsy specimens; autopsy specimens. The cellularity of the bone marrow in health depends on the age of the subject and the site from which the marrow specimen was obtained. It is also influenced by technical factors, since decalcification and paraffin-embedding lead to some shrinkage of tissue in comparison with plastic-embedded specimens; this leads to estimates of cellularity based on the former being about five per cent lower than estimates based on the latter.[5]

The cellularity of histological sections can be assessed most accurately by computerized image analysis or, alternatively, by point-counting, using an eyepiece with a graticule; the process is known as histomorphometry. Results of the two procedures show a fairly close correlation.[5,6] Cellularity can also be assessed subjectively. Such estimates are less reproducible and may lead to some underestimation of cellularity but show a reasonable correlation with histomorphometric methods; in one study the mean cellularity was 78 per cent by histomorphometry (point-counting) and 65 per cent by visual estimation, with the correlation between the two methods being 0.78.[5] Bone marrow cellularity is expressed as the percentage of a section which is occupied by haemopoietic tissue. However, the denominator may

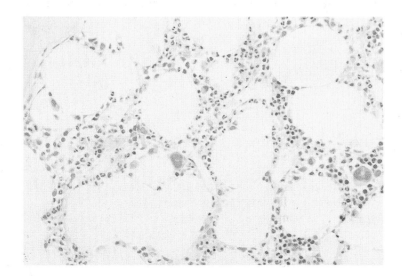

Fig. 1.1 Section of normal BM: normal distribution of all three haemopoietic lineages; note the megakaryocyte adjacent to a sinusoid. Plastic-embedded, H&E × 188.

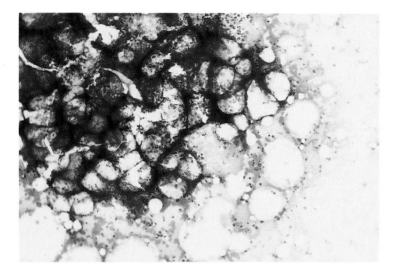

Fig. 1.2 Aspirate of normal BM: fragment showing normal cellularity. MGG × 377.

vary. The cellularity of sections of fragments is expressed in terms of haemopoietic tissue as a percentage of the total of haemopoietic and

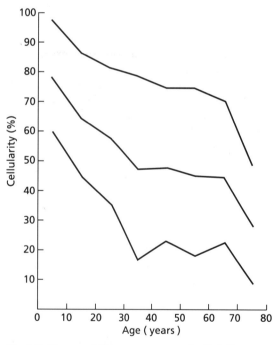

Fig. 1.3 Mean and 95 per cent range of cellularity at various ages of anterior iliac crest bone marrow which has been decalcified and paraffin-embedded. Cellularity is expressed as a percentage of the bone marrow cavity. Calculated from Hartsock.[8]

adipose tissue. In the case of a trephine biopsy, however, the cellularity may be expressed either as a percentage of the entire biopsy (including bone)[7] or as a percentage of the marrow cavity.[5,8] There are advantages in the latter approach, in which the area occupied by bone is excluded from the calculation, since the percentages obtained are then directly comparable with measurements on histological sections of aspirated fragments or estimates on fragments in bone marrow films.

The bone marrow of neonates is extremely cellular with there being negligible fat cells. Cellularity decreases fairly steadily with age with an accelerated rate of decline above the age of 70 years (Figs 1.3 and 1.4).[7-11] The decreasing percentage of the marrow cavity occupied by haemopoietic tissue is a consequence both of a true decline in the amount of haemopoietic tissue and of a loss of bone substance with age requiring adipose tissue to expand to fill the larger marrow cavity. In subjects with osteoporosis this effect can be so great that even young persons who are haematologically normal may have as little as 20 per cent of their marrow cavity occupied by haemopoietic cells.[9] In haematologically normal subjects without bone disease, typical reported rates of decline in the average marrow cellularity (expressed as a percentage of haemopoietic cells plus adipose cells) are: from 64 per cent in the second decade to 29 per cent in the eighth decade in the iliac crest;[8] from 85 per cent at age 20 to

40 per cent at age 60, also in the iliac crest;[9] and from 66 per cent at age 20 to 30 per cent at age 80 in the sternum.[11]

Bone marrow cellularity is determined also by the bone on which the assessment is made. Study of the two tissues by the same techniques has shown that the cellularity of lumbar vertebrae is, on average, about 10 per cent more than the cellularity of the iliac crest.[7] The vertebrae are also more cellular than the sternum. Because of the considerable dependence of the assessment of cellularity on methods of processing and counting, it is much more difficult to make generalizations when different tissues have not been assessed by the same techniques. Bennike et al.[4] in comparing the two sites in 100 subjects considered the sternum to be on average somewhat more cellular than the iliac crest. However, comparison of the results of histomorphometric studies by different groups show that when a single study of the sternum is compared with four studies of the iliac crest the sternum is generally found to be *less* cellular.[7-11] It should be noted that the lowest estimates of iliac crest cellularity are from a study using decalcified, paraffin-embedded bone marrow specimens[8] while the highest estimates are from a study using non-decalcified plastic-embedded specimens.[7] Some studies have been on biopsies[11] and others on autopsy specimens.[7,8,10] Because of such technical considerations it is difficult to make any generalizations about normal bone marrow cellularity. However it is possible to say that, except in extreme old age, cellularity of less than 20 per cent indicates hypoplasia and, except in those less than 20 years of age, cellularity of more than 80 per cent is likely to indicate hyperplasia.

In making a subjective assessment of the cellularity of smears prepared from aspirates the cellularity of the fragments is of more importance than the cellularity of the trails, although occasionally the presence of quite cellular trails despite hypocellular fragments suggests that the marrow cellularity is adequate. An average fragment cellularity between 25 and 75 per cent is usually taken to indicate normality, except at the extremes of age.

Because of the variability of cellularity from one intertrabecular space to the next it is not possible to assess marrow cellularity if few fragments are aspirated or if a biopsy is of inadequate size. In particular a small biopsy containing only a small amount of subcortical marrow does not allow assessment of cellularity since this area is often of low cellularity, particularly in the elderly. A biopsy containing at least five or six intertrabecular spaces is desirable (not only for an adequate assessment of cellularity but to give a reasonable probability of detecting focal bone marrow lesions). This requires a core of 20–30 mm in length.

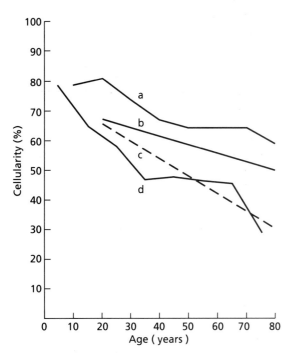

Fig. 1.4 Mean value of bone marrow cellularity at various ages expressed as percentage of bone marrow cavity: (a) iliac crest, autopsy, not decalcified (recalculated from Frisch[7]); (b) iliac crest, autopsy, not decalcified[10] (c) sternum, biopsy, not decalcified;[11] (d) ilium, autopsy, decalcified.[8]

HAEMOPOIETIC CELLS

A multipotent stem cell gives rise to all types of myeloid cell: erythrocytes and their precursors; granulocytes and their precursors; macrophages, monocytes and their precursors; mast cells; megakaryocytes and their precursors. It should be

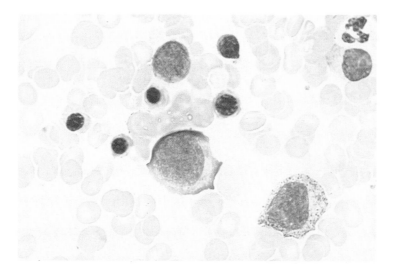

Fig. 1.5 Aspirate of normal BM: a proerythroblast, intermediate erythroblast, four late erythroblasts, a myelocyte, large and small lymphocytes and a neutrophil. MGG × 940.

mentioned that the term 'myeloid' can be used with two rather different meanings. It is used to indicate all cells derived from the common myeloid stem cell and also to indicate only the granulocytic and monocytic lineages as in the expression 'myeloid : erythroid ratio'. It is usually evident from the context which sense is intended but it is important to avoid ambiguity in using this term. The common myeloid stem cell and the stem cells committed to the specific myeloid lineages cannot be identified morphologically but it is likely that they are cells of similar size and appearance to a lymphocyte. The various myeloid lineages differ both morphologically and in their disposition in the bone marrow. The normal bone marrow contains, in addition to myeloid cells, smaller numbers of lymphoid cells (including plasma cells) and the stromal cells which have been discussed above.

Erythropoiesis

Cytology

Precursors of erythrocytes are designated erythroblasts. The term normoblast can also be used but has a narrower meaning; 'erythroblast' includes all recognizable erythroid precursors whereas 'normoblast' is applicable only when erythropoiesis is normoblastic. There are at least five generations of erythroblast between the morphologically unrecognizable erythroid stem cell and the erythrocyte. Erythroblasts develop in close proximity to a macrophage, the processes of which extend between and around the erythroblasts. Several generations of erythroblast are associated with one macrophage, the whole being known as an erythroblastic island.[12] Intact erythroblastic islands are sometimes seen in bone marrow films (see Fig. 7.4). Erythroblasts are conventionally divided on morphological grounds into four categories—proerythroblasts and early, intermediate and late erythroblasts. An alternative terminology is: proerythroblast, basophilic erythroblast, early polychromatophilic erythroblast and late polychromatophilic erythroblast. The term orthochromatic erythroblast is better avoided since the most mature erythroblasts are only orthochromatic (that is acidophilic, with the same staining characteristics as mature red cells) when erythropoiesis is abnormal.

Proerythroblasts (Fig. 1.5) are large round cells with a diameter of 12–20 μm and a large round nucleus. The cytoplasm is deeply basophilic with a perinuclear lighter-staining zone, attributable to the Golgi apparatus, sometimes being apparent. The nucleus has a finely granular or stippled appearance and contains several nucleoli.

Early erythroblasts (Fig. 1.6) are smaller than proerythroblasts and more numerous. The nucleocytoplasmic ratio is somewhat lower. They have

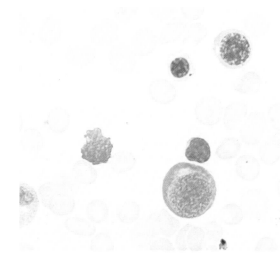

Fig. 1.6 Aspirate of normal BM: early, intermediate and late erythroblasts and a lymphocyte. MGG × 940.

strongly basophilic cytoplasm and have a granular or stippled chromatin pattern but lack visible nucleoli. A perinuclear halo which is less strongly basophilic than the rest of the cytoplasm may be apparent.

Intermediate erythroblasts (Figs 1.5 and 1.6) are smaller again, with a lower nucleo-cytoplasmic ratio than that of the early erythroblast, cytoplasm which is less basophilic, and moderate clumping of the chromatin. They are more numerous than early erythroblasts.

Late erythroblasts (Figs 1.5 and 1.6) are smaller and more numerous than intermediate erythroblasts. They are only slightly larger than mature red cells. Their nucleo-cytoplasmic ratio is lower than that of the intermediate erythroblast and the chromatin is more clumped. The cytoplasm is only weakly basophilic and in addition has a pink tinge due to the increased amount of haemoglobin. Because of the resultant pinky-blue colour the cell is described as polychromatophilic.

Late erythroblasts extrude their nuclei to form polychromatophilic erythrocytes, slightly larger than mature erythrocytes. These cells can be identified by a specific stain as reticulocytes; when haemopoiesis is normal they spend about 2 days of their 3-day life span in the bone marrow.

Small numbers of normal erythroblasts show atypical morphological features such as irregular nuclei, binuclearity and cytoplasmic bridging between adjacent erythroblasts.

Histology

Erythroblastic islands (Figs 1.7 and 1.8) are recognizable as distinctive clusters of cells in which one or more concentric circles of erythroblasts closely surround a macrophage. The erythroblasts which are closer to the macrophage are less mature than the peripheral ones. The central macrophage sends out extensive slender processes which envelop each erythroblast. The macrophage phagocytoses defective erythroblasts and extruded nuclei; nuclear and cellular debris may therefore be recognized in the cytoplasm and a Perls' stain (see page 30) may demonstrate the presence of haemosiderin. Erythropoiesis occurs relatively close to marrow sinusoids although it is probable that, as in the rat,[13] only a minority of erythroblastic islands actually abut on sinusoids.

Early erythroblasts (Fig. 1.9) are large cells; they have relatively little cytoplasm and large nuclei with dispersed chromatin and multiple small, irregular nucleoli often abutting on the nuclear membrane. More mature erythroid cells have condensed nuclear chromatin and cytoplasm which is less basophilic. The chromatin in the erythroblast nuclei is evenly distributed and as chromatin condensation occurs an even, regular pattern is retained.

There are four features which are useful in distinguishing erythroid precursors in the marrow from other cells: (i) they occur in distinctive

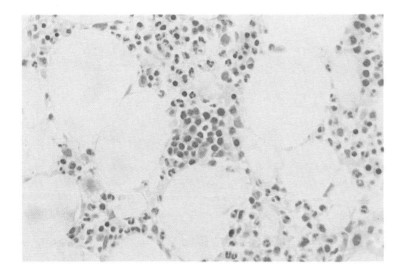

Fig. 1.7 Section of normal BM: an erythroid island (centre). Plastic-embedded, H&E × 377.

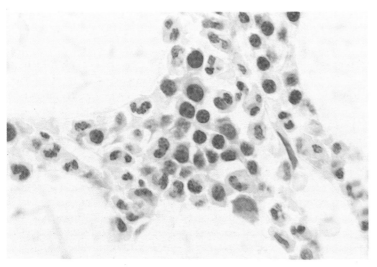

Fig. 1.8 Section of normal BM: an erythroid island containing intermediate and late erythroblasts and a haemosiderin-laden macrophage; a Golgi zone is seen in some of the intermediate erythroblasts. Plastic-embedded, H&E × 940.

erythroblastic islands containing several generations of cells of varying size and maturity (ii) erythroblasts adhere tightly to one another (iii) their nuclei are round, and (iv) in late erythroblasts the chromatin is condensed in a regular manner whereas nuclei of small lymphocytes show coarse clumping. With a Giemsa stain (Fig. 1.10) the intense cytoplasmic basophilia with a small, negatively staining Golgi zone adjacent to the nucleus is also distinctive. On paraffin-embedded specimens (Fig. 1.11) artefactual shrinking of cytoplasm of later erythroblasts can be useful in distinguishing them from lymphocytes.

When the bone marrow is regenerating rapidly, erythroid islands may be composed of cells all at the same stage of maturation. This results in some islands consisting only of immature elements. (A similar pattern is sometimes seen when erythropoiesis is abnormal, for example in myelodysplasia, but the mechanism here is different; there is intramedullary death of erythroid cells rather than a wave of synchronous development.)

The identification of abnormal erythroblasts can be more difficult than the identification of their normal equivalents, for example if well-

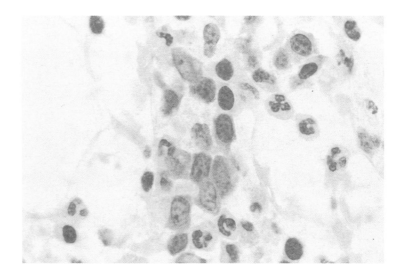

Fig. 1.9 Section of normal BM: an erythroid island containing early and intermediate erythroblasts. Plastic-embedded, Giemsa × 940.

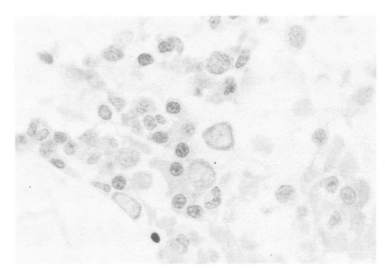

Fig. 1.10 Section of normal BM: erythroid island containing three early, one intermediate and numerous late erythroblasts; note the cytoplasmic basophilia of early erythroblasts. Plastic-embedded, Giemsa × 940.

organized erythroblastic islands are not present or if they contain only immature cells. When there is any difficulty in recognizing erythroid precursors their identity can be confirmed by cytochemical or immunocytochemical staining (see page 34).

Granulopoiesis

Cytology

There are at least four generations of cells between the morphologically unrecognizable committed granulocyte-monocyte precursor and the mature granulocyte, but cell division does not necessarily occur at the same point as maturation from one class to another. The first recognizable granulo-poietic cell is the myeloblast (Figs 1.12 and 1.13). It is similar in size to the proerythroblast, about 12–20 μm. It is more irregular in shape than a proerythroblast and its cytoplasm is moderately rather than strongly basophilic. The chromatin pattern is diffuse and there are several nucleoli. Myeloblasts are generally defined as being cells which lack granules but, in the context of the abnormal myelopoiesis of acute myeloid

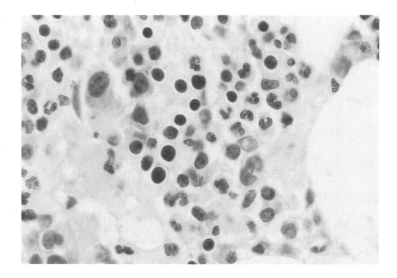

Fig. 1.11 Section of normal BM: erythroid island showing intermediate and late erythroblasts with haloes surrounding nuclei. Paraffin-embedded, H&E × 940.

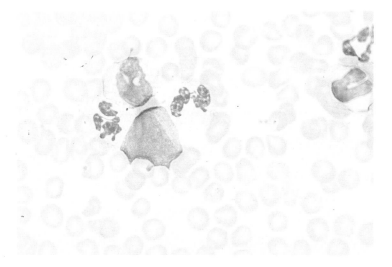

Fig. 1.12 Aspirate of normal BM: a myeloblast, three neutrophils and two monocytes; the myeloblast has a high nucleo-cytoplasmic ratio, a diffuse chromatin pattern and a nucleolus. MGG × 940.

leukaemia and the myelodysplastic syndromes, primitive cells with granules may also be accepted as myeloblasts. Myeloblasts are capable of cell division and mature to promyelocytes.

Promyelocytes (Fig. 1.13) have a nucleolated, slightly indented nucleus, a Golgi zone, and primary or azurophilic granules which are reddish-purple with a Romanowsky stain. Pro-myelocytes are larger than myeloblasts, usually 15–25 μm, and their cytoplasm is often more strongly basophilic. On light microscopy pro-myelocytes of the three granulocytic lineages cannot be distinguished but by ultrastructural

examination the distinction can be made. Pro-myelocytes are capable of cell division and mature to myelocytes.

Myelocytes (Fig. 1.13) are smaller than pro-myelocytes, and quite variable in size — from 10 to 20 μm. Their nuclei show some chromatin condensation and lack nucleoli. Their cytoplasm is less basophilic than that of a promyelocyte and specific neutrophilic, eosinophilic and basophilic granules can now be discerned, staining lilac, orange-red and purple respectively. Eosinophil myelocytes may also contain some granules which take up basic dyes and appear purple but

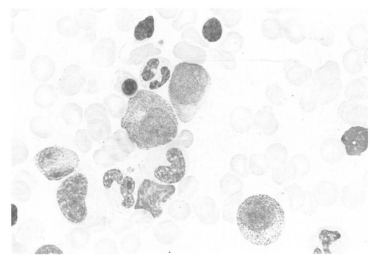

Fig. 1.13 Aspirate of normal BM: a myeloblast and a promyelocyte (centre), a myelocyte (lower right), a metamyelocyte, band forms, a neutrophil and a late erythroblast; the promyelocyte is larger than the myeloblast and is showing some chromatin condensation but with persisting nucleoli, well-developed cytoplasmic granulation and a Golgi zone. MGG × 940.

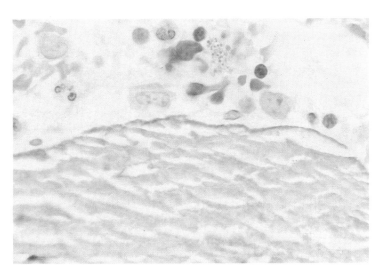

Fig. 1.14 Section of normal BM: myeloblast and promyelocyte adjacent to a bony trabecula. Plastic-embedded, H&E × 940.

these differ ultrastructurally from the granules of the basophil lineage. There are probably normally at least two generations of myelocytes so that at least some cells of this category are capable of cell division. Late myelocytes mature to metamyelocytes which are 10–12 μm in diameter and have a markedly indented or U-shaped nucleus (Fig. 1.13). The metamyelocyte is not capable of cell division but matures to a band form which has a ribbon-shaped nucleus. The band cell, in turn, matures to a polymorphonuclear granulocyte with a segmented nucleus and specific neutrophilic, eosinophilic or basophilic granules.

Histology

Myeloblasts (Fig. 1.14) are the earliest granulocyte precursors identifiable histologically; they are present in small numbers and are most frequently found adjacent to the bone marrow trabecular surfaces or adjacent to arterioles. They are fairly large cells with round to oval nuclei and one to five relatively small nucleoli. There is no chromatin clumping. They have relatively little cytoplasm. They are readily distinguished from lymphoid cells by the absence of chromatin clumping and the presence of nucleoli. Myeloblasts

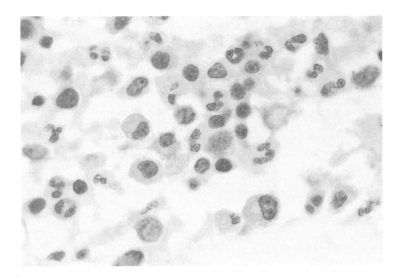

Fig. 1.15 Section of normal BM: promyelocytes, myelocytes and maturing granulocytes. Plastic-embedded, H&E × 940.

are far outnumbered in normal marrows by the promyelocytes (Figs 1.14 and 1.15) and myelocytes (Fig. 1.15) which are recognized, at least in plastic-embedded sections, by their granularity. Primary and neutrophilic granules may be seen as faintly eosinophilic granules in good quality H&E stains on plastic-embedded specimens, but they are best seen with a Giemsa stain. Eosinophilic granules are more strongly eosinophilic and are refractile and are therefore easily recognized on both H&E and Giemsa stains of either paraffin- or plastic-embedded biopsies. Basophil granules are water-soluble and basophils are therefore not often recognized in sections. As maturation occurs, granulocytic precursors are found progressively more deeply in the haemopoietic cords, but away from the sinusoids. When they reach the metamyelocyte stage they appear to move towards the sinusoids and at the polymorphonuclear granulocyte stage cross the wall to enter the circulation.

In undecalcified plastic-embedded sections the chloroacetate esterase stain is a reliable marker for neutrophil haemopoiesis from the promyelocyte stage onwards. Overnight incubation of decalcified sections in a buffer at pH 6.8 partially restores chloroacetate esterase activity. Altern-

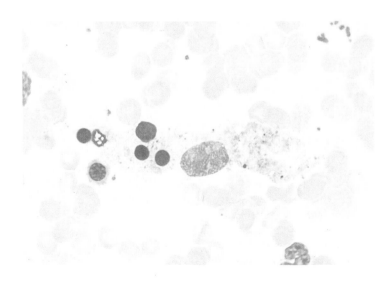

Fig. 1.16 Aspirate of normal BM: a macrophage containing granular and refractile debris and several normoblast nuclei. MGG × 940.

atively, the identity of the granulocytic lineage may be confirmed by immunocytochemistry with monoclonal antibodies (see page 34).

Monocytopoiesis

Cytology

Monocytes are derived from a morphologically unrecognizable common granulocytic-monocytic precursor. The earliest morphologically recognizable precursor is a monoblast, a cell which is larger than a myeloblast with abundant cytoplasm showing a variable degree of basophilia and with a large nucleus which may be either round or lobulated. Monoblasts are capable of division and mature into promonocytes which are similar in size to promyelocytes; they have cytoplasmic granules and usually some degree of nuclear lobulation. Promonocytes mature into monocytes which migrate rapidly into the peripheral blood. Monocytes are 12–20 µm in diameter and have a lobulated nucleus and abundant cytoplasm which is weakly basophilic. The cytoplasm may contain some fine azurophilic granules and often has a ground-glass appearance, in contrast to the clear cytoplasm of a lymphocyte.

Monocytes mature into macrophages (Fig. 1.16) in the bone marrow as well as in other tissues. These are large cells, 20–30 µm in diameter, of irregular shape, with a low nucleo-cytoplasmic ratio and voluminous weakly basophilic cytoplasm. When relatively immature they may have an oval nucleus with a fairly diffuse chromatin pattern. When mature the nucleus is smaller and more condensed and the cytoplasm may contain lipid droplets, recognizable degenerating cells and amorphous debris; an iron stain commonly shows the presence of haemosiderin. Bone marrow macrophages may develop into various storage cells which will be discussed in later chapters.

Both monocytes and their precursors are quite infrequent among marrow cells. Macrophages or histiocytes, however, are readily apparent.

Histology

Monocytes are recognized in histological sections of the marrow as cells which are larger than neutrophils with lobulated nuclei; monocyte precursors are not usually recognizable. In haematologically normal subjects only small numbers of monocytes are present. They are located preferentially near arterioles and in the centre of haemopoietic cords.

Macrophages (Fig. 1.17) are identified as irregularly scattered relatively large cells with a small nucleus and abundant cytoplasm. Some are associated with erythroblasts (erythroblastic islands), with plasma cells or with lymphoid nodules.

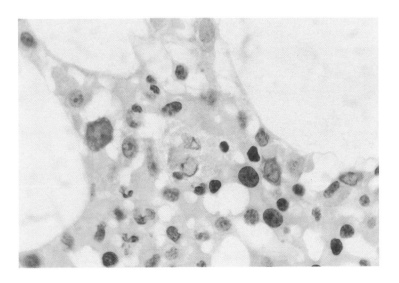

Fig. 1.17 Section of normal BM: a macrophage containing cellular debris. Plastic-embedded, H&E × 940.

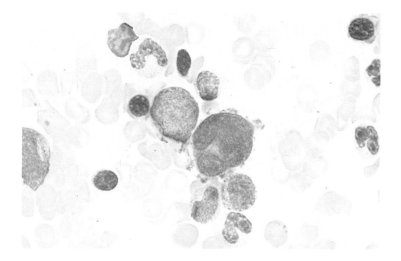

Fig. 1.18 Aspirate of normal BM: an immature megakaryocyte with a polyploid nucleus showing little chromatin condensation: cytoplasm is scanty and basophilic. MGG × 940.

Megakaryopoiesis and thrombopoiesis

Cytology

In normal marrow the earliest morphologically recognizable cell in the megakaryocyte lineage is the megakaryocyte itself, though when haemopoiesis is abnormal a megakaryocyte precursor of similar size and morphology to a myeloblast can sometimes be recognized. Megakaryocytes undergo endoreduplication as they mature, resulting in a large cell (30−160 μm) with a marked degree of heterogeneity in both nuclear DNA content (ploidy) and nuclear size. Mega-karyocytes can be classified by their ploidy level. In normal marrow they range from 4 N (tetraploid) to 32 N with the dominant ploidy category being 16 N. Megakaryocytes can also be classified on the basis of their nuclear and more particularly their cytoplasmic characteristics into three stages of maturation.[14] Group I megakaryocytes (Fig. 1.18) have strongly basophilic cytoplasm and a very high nucleo-cytoplasmic ratio. Group II megakaryocytes have a lower nucleo-cytoplasmic ratio and cytoplasm which is less basophilic and contains some azurophilic granules. Group III megakaryocytes (Fig. 1.19) have plentiful weakly basophilic cytoplasm containing abundant

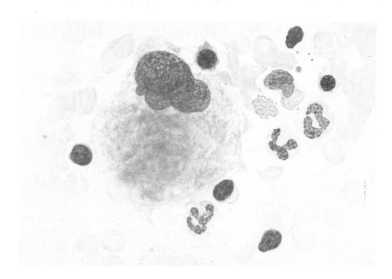

Fig. 1.19 Aspirate of normal BM: a mature megakaryocyte with a lobulated nucleus and voluminous granular cytoplasm. MGG × 940.

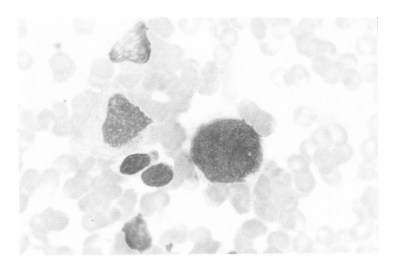

Fig. 1.20 Aspirate of normal BM: a late megakaryocyte which has shed most of its cytoplasm as platelets. MGG × 940.

azurophilic granules; the cytoplasm at the cell margins is agranular. Group III megakaryocytes are mature cells, capable of producing platelets and no longer synthesizing DNA. There is some correlation between the three stages of maturation and ploidy level. All stages of maturation include megakaryocytes which are 8 N, 16 N and 32 N but 4 N megakaryocytes are confined to group I and 32 N megakaryocytes are more numerous in group III. The nuclei of the great majority of normal polyploid megakaryocytes form irregular lobes joined by strands of chromatin. A minority have either an unlobulated nucleus or more than one nucleus. The final stage in megakaryocyte maturation is an apparently bare nucleus (actually with a thin rim of cytoplasm), the great bulk of the cytoplasm having been shed as platelets (Fig. 1.20).

An increased demand for platelets, for example due to peripheral destruction, leads to an increase in ploidy level and cell size, apparent in a bone marrow film as an increased volume of cytoplasm and a large, usually well-lobulated nucleus. It should be noted that whether or not megakaryocytes appear to be budding platelets shows little correlation with the number of platelets being produced. In patients with thrombocytosis, particularly with essential thrombocythaemia, there are often many 'budding' megakaryocytes but in auto-immune thrombocytopenia in which platelet production is also greatly increased 'budding' megakaryocytes are quite uncommon.

It is necessary to assess megakaryocyte numbers as well as morphology. In films of an aspirate this can only be a subjective assessment — that megakaryocytes are decreased, normal or increased. A more accurate assessment can be made on histological sections of aspirated fragments or on trephine biopsies. Somewhat fewer megakaryocytes are seen in sections of aspirated fragments than in trephine biopsies, presumably because these large cells are not as readily aspirated as smaller marrow cells.

Megakaryocytes may 'engulf' other haemopoietic cells (lymphocytes, erythrocytes, erythroblasts and granulocytes and their precursors), a process known as emperipolesis or pseudophagocytosis (Fig. 1.21). This process differs from phagocytosis in that the engulfed cells have entered dilated cavities in the demarcation membrane system rather than being in a phagocytic vacuole; on examination of bone marrow films the cells within the megakaryocyte are observed to be intact and morphologically normal.

Histology

Megakaryocytes are most frequently found associated with sinusoids, at some distance from bony trabeculae (Figs 1.1 and 1.22). They are found in a paratrabecular position only when haemopoiesis is abnormal. Serial sections show that in normal marrow all megakaryocytes abut on sinusoids.[15] Megakaryocytes lie directly outside the sinusoid

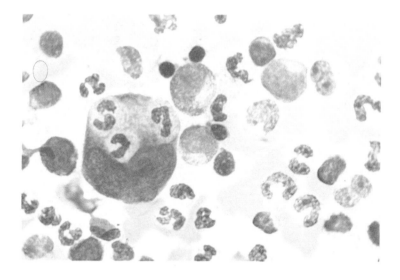

Fig. 1.21 Aspirate of non-infiltrated BM from a patient with Hodgkin's disease: a mature megakaryocyte exhibiting emperipolesis. MGG × 940.

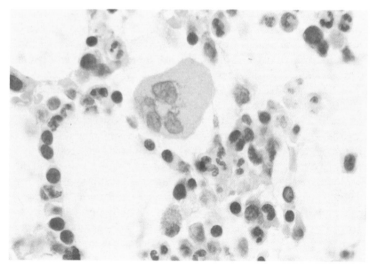

Fig. 1.22 Section of normal BM: cells of all haemopoietic lineages including a megakaryocyte with finely granular cytoplasm. Plastic-embedded, Giemsa × 940.

and discharge platelets by protruding cytoplasmic processes through endothelial cells; such processes break up into platelets. 'Bare nuclei' which have shed almost all their cytoplasm in this manner can be recognized in histological sections (Fig. 1.23) as well as in bone marrow smears. (Intact megakaryocytes and bare nuclei can also enter the circulation and are seen within vessels in histological sections of lung, spleen, liver and other organs.)

In assessing the morphology of megakaryocytes it is important to remember that the megakaryocyte is a very large cell and only a cross-section of

it is being examined. It is therefore not possible to determine the size or degree of nuclear lobulation of single megakaryocytes. However, by examining a large number of sections it is possible to form a judgement as to the average size of the megakaryocytes, the average degree of lobulation, and whether hypolobulated or micromegakaryocytes are present.

When haemopoiesis is normal megakaryocytes do not form clusters of more than four or five cells. Larger clusters of megakaryocytes are seen in regenerating marrow following chemotherapy and bone marrow transplantation, and also in

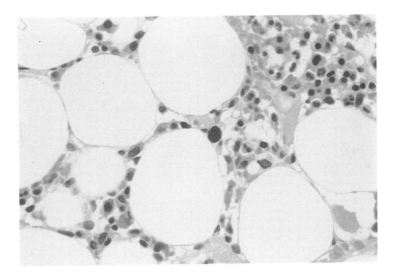

Fig. 1.23 Section of BM from patient with AIDS: 'bare' megakaryocyte nucleus. Paraffin-embedded, H&E × 390.

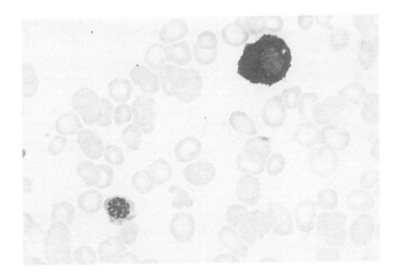

Fig. 1.24 Aspirate of normal BM: a mast cell and a normoblast; the mast cell has a round nucleus and cytoplasm packed with deeply basophilic granules. MGG × 940.

various pathological states; this feature is diagnostically useful.

Megakaryocytes can be quantified by counting their number per unit area, or a subjective impression can be formed as to whether they are present in decreased, normal or increased numbers. Depending on the processing and staining techniques employed, estimates of mean megakaryocyte number in normal marrow vary from 7 to 15/mm^2.[16] If an immunocytochemical technique is used estimates are considerably higher with the mean normal value being 25/mm^2; this is probably because more small megakaryocytes

and megakaryocyte precursors are recognized.[16]

Identification of megakaryocytes is aided by cytochemistry and immunocytochemistry (see pages 33 and 34).

Mast cells

Cytology

Mast cells (Fig. 1.24) are derived from the multipotent myeloid stem cell. In bone marrow films they appear as oval or elongated cells varying in

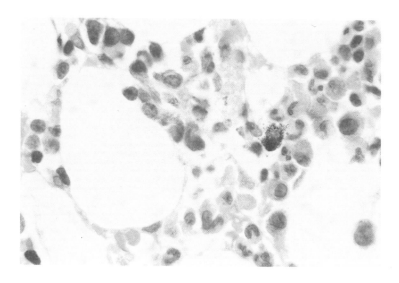

Fig. 1.25 Section of BM from a patient with renal failure: a mast cell and maturing granulocytes. Plastic-embedded, Giemsa × 940.

size from 5 to 25 μm. The nucleus is central, relatively small and either round or oval. The cytoplasm is packed with granules which stain deep purple with Romanowsky stains. Mast cells can be distinguished from basophils by the different nuclear characteristics (non-lobulated nucleus with less chromatin clumping) and by the fact that the granules do not obscure the nucleus.

Histology

Mast cells are rare in normal marrow. They are difficult to recognize in H&E-stained histological sections because the granules do not stain. They are readily recognizable in a Giemsa stain (Fig. 1.25) in which their purple-staining granules make them conspicuous. Mast cell granules also give positive reactions for chloroacetate esterase, are PAS-positive and stain metachromatically with alcian blue and toluidine blue. Mast cells are distributed irregularly in the medullary cavity but are most numerous near the endosteum, in the periosteum, in association with the adventitia of small blood vessels and at the periphery of lymphoid nodules or aggregates.[17] They appear as elliptical or elongated cells with an average diameter of 12 μm. Their cytoplasmic projections stretch out between other haemopoietic cells.

OSTEOBLASTS AND OSTEOCLASTS

Osteoblasts and osteoclasts differ in their origin but have complementary functions. Osteoblasts have a common origin with other mesenchymal cells and are responsible for bone deposition. Osteoclasts are formed by fusion of cells of monocyte lineage and are responsible for dissolution of bone.

Cytology

Osteoblasts (Fig. 1.26) are mononuclear cells with a diameter of 20–50 μm. They have an eccentric nucleus, moderately basophilic cytoplasm and a Golgi zone which is not in apposition with the nuclear membrane. The nucleus shows some chromatin condensation and may contain a small nucleolus. Osteoblasts can be distinguished from plasma cells, to which they bear a superficial resemblance, by the lesser degree of chromatin condensation and the separation of the Golgi zone from the nucleus. Osteoblasts are rarely seen in bone marrow aspirates of healthy adults but when present they often appear in small clumps. They are much more numerous in the bone marrow of children.

Osteoclasts (Fig. 1.27) are multinucleated giant cells with a diameter of 30–100 μm or more.

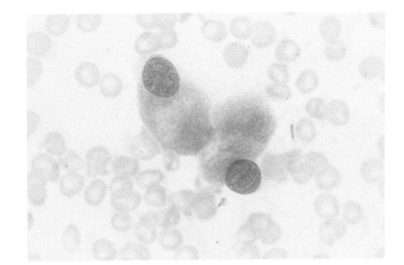

Fig. 1.26 Aspirate of normal BM: two osteoblasts; note the eccentric nucleus and basophilic cytoplasm; these cells can be distinguished from plasma cells by their larger size and the position of the Golgi zone which is not immediately adjacent to the nucleus. MGG × 940.

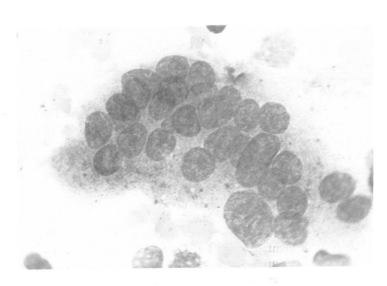

Fig. 1.27 Aspirate of normal BM: an osteoclast: note the highly granular cytoplasm and the multiple nuclei which are uniform in size and have indistinct medium-sized single nucleoli. MGG × 940.

Their nuclei tend to be clearly separate, uniform in appearance and slightly oval with a single lilac-staining nucleolus. The voluminous cytoplasm contains numerous azurophilic granules which are coarser than those of megakaryocytes. Osteoclasts are not commonly seen in marrow aspirates of healthy adults but are much more often seen in aspirates from children.

Histology

Osteocytes, osteoblasts and osteoclasts in histo-logical sections are identified by their position and their morphological features. Osteocytes (Fig. 1.28) are within bone lacunae. Osteoblasts (Fig. 1.29) appear in rows along a bone spicule or a layer of osteoid and their eccentric nuclei and prominent Golgi zones are apparent. Osteoclasts (Fig. 1.30) are likely to be found on the other side of a spicule from osteoblasts, or at some distance away. They are identified as multinucleated cells lying in hollows known as Howship's lacunae. They show tartrate-resistant acid phosphatase activity.

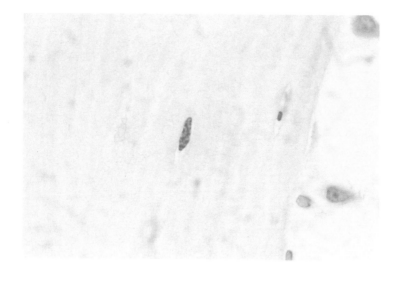

Fig. 1.28 Section of normal BM: bone spicule containing osteocyte; note myeloblasts in adjacent marrow. Plastic-embedded, H&E × 940.

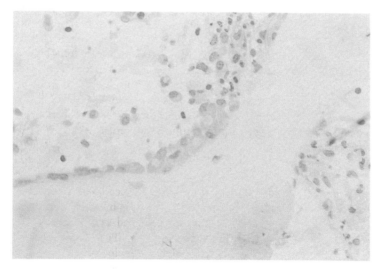

Fig. 1.29 Section of BM from a patient with Fanconi's anaemia: the trabecula is lined by osteoblasts; note the distinct Golgi zones which do not abut on the nuclear membrane. Plastic-embedded, H&E × 377.

LYMPHOPOIESIS

Lymphocytes

Both B and T lymphocytes share a common origin with myeloid cells, all of these lineages being derived from a pluripotent stem cell.

Cytology

Bone marrow lymphocytes are small cells with a high nucleo-cytoplasmic ratio and scanty, weakly basophilic cytoplasm. The nuclei show some chromatin condensation but the chromatin often appears more diffuse than that of peripheral blood lymphocytes. Lymphocytes are not very numerous in the marrow in the first few days of life but otherwise during infancy they constitute a third to a half of bone marrow nucleated cells (Table 1.1).[18] Numbers decline during childhood and in adults they are not generally more than 15–25 per cent of nucleated cells, unless the marrow aspirate has been considerably diluted with peripheral blood.

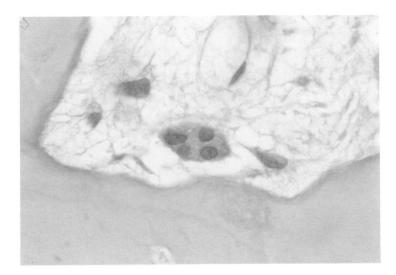

Fig. 1.30 Section of BM from a patient with renal osteodystrophy: osteoclast with four nuclei. Paraffin-embedded, H&E × 970.

Histology

Normal marrow contains scattered interstitial lymphocytes and sometimes small lymphoid nodules or follicles (Fig. 1.31). Estimates of lymphocyte numbers based on histological sections are considerably lower than those based on aspirates. In one study approximately 10 per cent of bone marrow cells were lymphocytes with the ratio of T to B cells being six to one.[19] Lymphocytes appear to concentrate about arterial vessels near the centre of the haemopoietic cords. Lymphoid follicles of normal marrow have small blood vessels at their centre and may contain a few peripheral mast cells or plasma cells. Lymphoid follicles are further discussed on page 53.

Plasma cells

Cytology

Plasma cells (Fig. 1.32) are infrequent in normal bone marrow in which they rarely constitute more than one per cent of nucleated cells. In healthy children they are even less frequent.[20] They are distinctive cells with a diameter of 15–20 μm and with an eccentric nucleus, moderately basophilic cytoplasm and a prominent paranuclear Golgi zone. The cytoplasm may contain occasional vacuoles and sometimes stains pink, consequent on the presence of carbohydrate. The nuclear chromatin shows prominent coarse clumps, although the clock-face chromatin pattern which is often discernible in histological sections is usually less apparent in films. Occasional normal plasma cells have two or more nuclei. Plasma cells may occur in small clumps and may be detected within aspirated marrow fragments and around capillaries.

Histology

Normal marrow contains scattered interstitial plasma cells but plasma cells may also be associated with macrophages and are preferentially located around capillaries (Fig. 1.33). Typical mature plasma cells in histological sections are readily identified by their eccentric nuclei and prominent Golgi zones. The chromatin is coarsely clumped and often distributed at the periphery of the nucleus with clear spaces between the chromatin clumps giving the appearance of a cartwheel or clock-face.

THE CELLULAR COMPOSITION OF BONE MARROW

Cytology

The cellular composition of aspirated bone marrow is determined by the volume of the

Table 1.1 Mean values (observed range) in healthy infants and children

	Birth[18] (n = 57)	0–24 hours[23] (n = 19)	8–10 days[23] (n = 23)	3 months[23] (n = 12)	3 months[18] (n = 24)	1 year[18] (n = 12)	18 months[18] (n = 19)	2–6 years[24] (n = 12)	2–9 years[25] (n = 13)
M : E ratio	4.4	1.2	1.35	2.4	4.9	4.8	5	5.8 (2–13)	5.3
Myeloblasts	0.3*	1 (0.5–2)	1 (0–3)	1.5 (0–4)	0.6*	0.5*	0.4*	1.0	1.3 (0.7–1.8)
Promyelocytes	0.8	1.5 (0.5–5)	2 (0.5–7)	2 (1.5–5)	0.8	0.7	0.6	0.5	2.8 (0.8–4.8)
Myelocytes	4	4 (1–9)	4 (1–11)	5 (0.5–16)	2	2	2.5	17	26.7 (18–35)†
Metamyelocytes	19	14 (4.5–25)	18 (7–35)	11 (3–33)	12	11	12	20	22 (15.7–29)
Bands	29 }	22 (10–40)	20 (11–45)	15 (2–24)	15	14	14	11	4.5 (0.9–8)
Neutrophils	7 }				3.5	6	6	10	8.3 (2.6–14)
Eosinophil series	2.7	3.5 (1–8)†	3 (0–6)†	2.5 (0–6)†	2.5	2	3	6	1.2 (0–2.5)
Basophil series	0.12	– (0–1.5)†	– (0–1)†	– (0–0.5)	0.1	0.1	0.1	–	0
Monocytes	0.9	– (0–2.5)	1 (0–3)	0.5 (0–1)	0.7	1.5	2	0.4	0
Erythroid	14.5	39.5 (23.5–70)†	7.5 (0–20.5)†	16 (3.5–33.5)†	12	8	8	13	12.5 (9.5–22.3)†
Lymphocytes	15	12 (4–22)	37 (20–62)	47 (31–81)	44	49	46	21	18.2 (8.5–28)
Plasma cells	0	0	0	0	0	0.03	0.06	–	0.13 (0.05–0.41)

* 'Unknown blasts'.
† Approximate (sum of ranges for different categories).

Fig. 1.31 Section of BM from patient with idiopathic (auto-immune) thrombocytopenic purpura: a lymphoid follicle; note the plasma cells at the periphery. Plastic-embedded, Giemsa × 377.

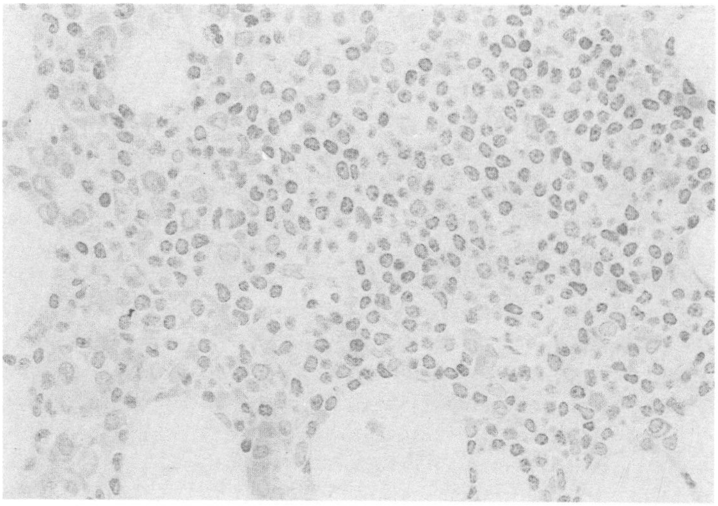

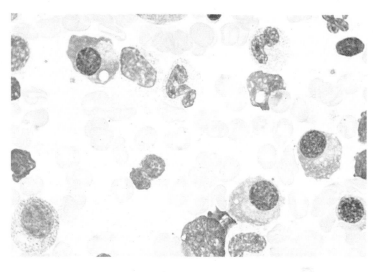

Fig. 1.32 Aspirate of BM from a patient with an inflammatory condition: three plasma cells; note the basophilic cytoplasm, eccentric nucleus and Golgi zone adjacent to the nucleus, MGG × 940.

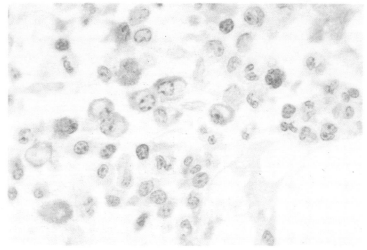

Fig. 1.33 Section of BM from patient with Hodgkin's disease (without marrow infiltration): peri-capillary plasma cells, neutrophils, eosinophils and erythroblasts. Plastic-embedded, Giemsa × 940.

aspirate since the larger the volume aspirated the more sinusoidal blood is sucked into the aspirate. Dilution of marrow with blood leads to a higher percentage of lymphocytes and mature granulo-cytes and a lower percentage of granulocyte and erythroid precursors. Dresch *et al.*[21] found, for example, that as the volume of aspirate from the sternum increased from 0.5 to 4.5 ml the total concentration of nucleated cells fell to about one-sixth; the percentage of granulocyte precursors (myeloblasts to metamyelocytes) declined from approximately 55 to approximately 30 per cent while the percentage of mature neutrophils showed a more than twofold rise. Ideally a cell count should be performed on films prepared from the first one or two drops of aspirated marrow. If large volumes are required for further tests a second syringe can be applied to the needle after the syringe containing the first few drops has been removed.

Determining the cellular composition of marrow requires that large numbers of cells be counted so that a reasonable degree of precision is achieved. This is particularly important when the cell of interest is one which is normally infre-quent, such as the myeloblast or the plasma cell. A 500-cell count provides a reasonable com-promise between what is desirable and what is practicable. The cell count should be performed in the trails behind fragments so that the cells counted represent cells which have come from fragments rather than contaminating peripheral blood cells. Alternatively the cell count can be performed on squashed bone marrow fragments. Because some cells, for example plasma cells and lymphocytes, are distributed unevenly through the marrow it is important to count the trails behind several fragments or the squashes of several fragments.

It is customary and useful to determine the myeloid:erythroid (M:E) ratio of aspirated marrow since consideration of this value together with an assessment of the overall cellularity allows an assessment of whether erythropoiesis

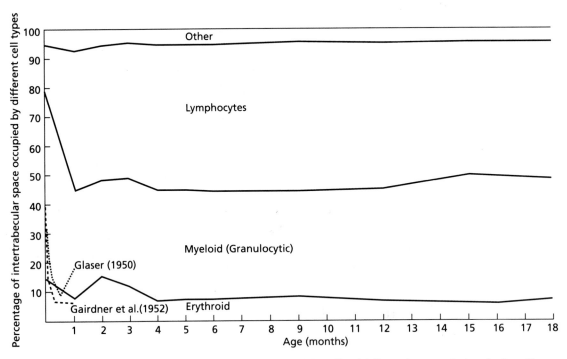

Fig. 1.34 The percentage of the intertrabecular space occupied by cells of different lineages during the first 18 months of life, derived from Rosse *et al.*;[18] the higher initial erythroid percentage and sharp fall in erythroblast number observed by Glaser *et al.*[22] and Gairdner *et al.*[23] are shown as dotted lines.

and granulopoiesis are hypoplastic, normal or hyperplastic. It is simplest to include in the myeloid component all granulocytes and their precursors and any monocytes and their precursors. However, some haematologists exclude mature neutrophils and others include neutrophils but exclude eosinophils, basophils and monocytes. These inclusions and exclusions will make a slight difference to what is regarded as a normal M : E ratio. These differences are, however, outweighed by the differences caused by different aspiration volumes. The larger the volume of aspirate the higher the M : E ratio, particularly if mature neutrophils are included in the count.

The bone marrow at birth has major erythroid and myeloid components with few lymphocytes and very few plasma cells[18,20,22,23] (Fig. 1.34). The percentage of erythroid cells declines steeply in the first weeks.[22,23] The percentage of lymphocytes increases during the first month and remains at a high level until 18 months of age.[18] In children above the age of two years the proportions of different cell types do not differ greatly from those in normal adult bone marrow. Typical values determined for the cellular composition of normal marrow at various ages are shown in Tables 1.1 and 1.2.

Histology

It is possible to perform differential counts and estimate an M : E ratio on plastic-embedded bone marrow biopsies[29,30] although this is rarely necessary in practice. Such counts have the potential to be more accurate than those on aspirates since there is no dilution with sinusoidal blood. It is also possible that larger cells or cells adjacent to trabeculae might be less likely to be aspirated. However, an element of inaccuracy is introduced by the fact that larger cells appear at more levels of the biopsy so are more likely to be counted in any given section. The lack of dilution by blood means that the estimated M : E ratio is likely to be lower than that determined from an aspirate. This is borne out by the results of a study of 13 healthy subjects which found a mean M : E ratio of 1.52 with a range of 1.36−1.61.[29]

BONE MARROW IRON STORES AND ERYTHROBLAST IRON

Cytology

A Perls' or Prussian blue stain (Figs 1.35 and 1.36) stains haemosiderin in bone marrow macrophages and within erythroblasts and so allows assessment of the amount of iron in reticuloendothelial stores and also the availability of iron to developing erythroblasts.

Assessment of storage iron requires that an adequate number of fragments are obtained since iron is distributed irregularly within the bone marrow macrophages. If only one or two fragments are available it is not possible to quantify iron or to be certain that a negative iron stain does indicate a lack of storage iron. A bone marrow smear or squash will contain both intracellular and extracellular iron, the latter being derived from crushed macrophages. It is usual to base assessment of iron stores mainly on intracellular iron since iron stains are prone to artefactual deposits and it can be difficult to distinguish between extracellular iron and artefact. Iron stores may be assessed as normal, decreased or increased or may be graded as 1+ to 6+ as shown in Table 1.3, grades of 1 to 3+ being considered normal. Alternatively, iron stores may be graded as 1+ to 4+.[33,34]

Examination of a Perls' stain of a bone marrow film allows adequate assessment of erythroblast iron as long as a thinly spread area of the film is examined with optimal illumination. A proportion of normal erythroblasts have a few (one to five) fine iron-containing granules randomly distributed in the cytoplasm. Such erythroblasts are designated sideroblasts. In haematologically normal subjects with adequate iron stores 20−50 per cent of bone marrow erythroblasts are sideroblasts.[35−37] Examination of an iron stain allows detection not only of an increased or decreased proportion of sideroblasts but also of abnormal sideroblasts. The latter include those in which siderotic granules are merely increased in size and number and those in which granules are also distributed abnormally within the cytoplasm, being sited in a ring around the nucleus rather than randomly (ring sideroblasts).

Table 1.2 Mean values and 95 per cent ranges for bone marrow cells in sternal aspirates of healthy adult caucasians

	20–29 years[25] (Males and females, n = 28)	20–30 years[26]		17–45 years[27] (42 males, 8 females, n = 50)	[28] (Males, n = 12)
		(Males, n = 52)	(Females, n = 40)		
Volume aspirated	≤ 0.5 ml	0.2 ml		3 ml	—
M : E ratio	3.34	—	—	6.9	2.3 (1.1–3.5)[§]
Myeloblasts	1.21 (0.75–1.67)	1.32 (0.2–2.5)	1.2 (0.1–2.3)	1.3 (0–3)	0.9 (0.1–1.7)
Promyelocytes	2.49 (0.99–3.99)	1.35 (0–2.9)	1.65 (0.5–2.8)	—[‡]	3.3 (1.9–4.7)
Myelocytes	17.36 (11.54–23.18)	15 (7.5–22.5)	16.6 (11.4–21.8)	8.9 (3–15)	12.7 (8.5–16.9)
Metamyelocytes	16.92 (11.4–22.44)	15.7 (9.2–22)	15.8 (11.0–20.6)	8.8 (4–15)	15.9 (7.1–24.7)
Band cells	8.7 (3.58–13.82)	10.5 (3–17.9)	8.3 (4–12.4)	23.9 (12.5–33.5)	12.4 (9.4–15.4)
Neutrophils	13.42 (4.32–22.52)	20.9 (9.9–31.8)	21.7 (11.3–32)	18.5 (9–31.5)	7.4 (3.8–11)
Eosinophils	2.93 (0.28–5.69)[*]	2.8 (0.1–5.6)[*]	3 (0–7.2)[*]	1.9 (0–5.5)	3.1 (1.1–5.2)[*]
Basophils	0.28 (0–0.69)[*]	0.14 (0–0.38)	0.16 (0–0.46)	0.2 (0–1)	< 0.1 (0–0.2)[‖]
Monocytes	1.04 (0.36–1.72)	2.3 (0.5–4)	1.61 (0.2–3)	2.4 (0–6)	0.3 (0–0.6)
Erythroblasts	19.26 (9.12–29.4)[†]	12.9 (4.1–21.7)	11.5 (5.1–17.9)	9.5 (2.5–17.5)	25.6 (15–36.2)
Lymphocytes	14.6 (6.66–22.54)	16.8 (7.2–26.3)	18.1 (10.5–25.7)	16.2 (7.5–26.5)	16.2 (8.6–23.8)
Plasma cells	0.46 (0–0.96)	0.39 (0–1.1)	0.42 (0–0.9)	0.3 (0–1.5)	1.3 (0–3.5)

* Including eosinophil and basophil myelocytes and metamyelocytes.
† Approximate (sum of ranges for different categories of erythroblast).
‡ Promyelocytes were categorized either with myeloblasts or with myelocytes.
§ Neutrophils plus precursors: erythroblasts.
‖ Including basophil precursors and mast cells.

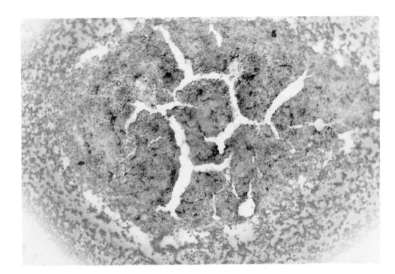

Fig. 1.35 Aspirate of normal BM: bluish-black iron in macrophages in a fragment. Perls' stain × 377.

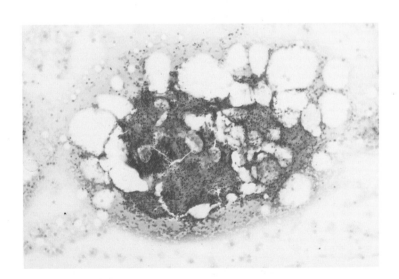

Fig. 1.36 Aspirate of normal BM: a fragment with no stainable iron. Perls' stain × 377.

Table 1.3 Grading of bone marrow storage iron[31,32]

0	No stainable iron
1+	Small iron particles just visible in reticulum cells using an oil objective
2+	Small, sparse iron particles in reticulum cells, visible at lower power
3+	Numerous small particles in reticulum cells
4+	Larger particles with a tendency to aggregate into clumps
5+	Dense, large clumps
6+	Very large clumps and extracellular iron

Histology

Because of the irregular distribution of iron within bone marrow macrophages a biopsy may show the presence of iron when none has been detected in an aspirate. An iron stain (Fig. 1.37) can be successfully carried out on both plastic-embedded and paraffin-embedded biopsies. However plastic-embedded specimens give more reliable results. Decalcification of a paraffin-embedded specimen will lead to some leaching out of iron and may

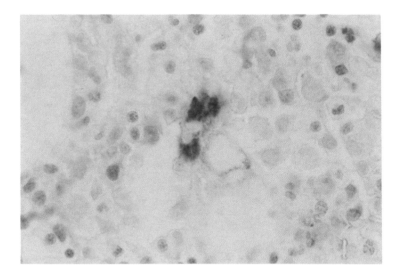

Fig. 1.37 Section of normal BM: macrophage containing iron. Plastic-embedded, Perls' stain × 940.

lessen the amount of iron detected or lead to a failure to detect iron when it is present in an aspirate. Plastic-embedded biopsies are also superior for the detection of ring sideroblasts or other abnormal sideroblasts, although these can sometimes be detected in paraffin-embedded specimens. However no technique for processing and staining a biopsy specimen allows assessment of whether siderotic granules are normal or decreased; this requires an iron stain of an aspirate.

There are conflicting reports on the comparability of iron stains on aspirates and biopsies, not all of which are readily explicable by the factors mentioned above. Lundin et al.[33] found that in eight per cent of cases iron was detectable in a biopsy and not in an aspirate and in another eight per cent the reverse was true; by assessing other factors they were not able to establish that one or other method was more valid. Fong et al.[34] found that in eight per cent of patients iron was present in an aspirate but was not detectable in a biopsy; however this was not due to the process of decalcification since it was noted in sections of marrow fragments as well as in trephine biopsies. Conflicting findings were reported by Krause et al.[38] who found that iron was always detectable in a biopsy when it was present in an aspirate but two-thirds of patients with absent iron in an aspirate had detectable iron on a biopsy. It is clear that minor variations in technique may be crit-

ical. Our own observations are that when specimens are decalcified using manual techniques for processing there may be a failure to detect iron in a trephine biopsy when it is clearly present in an aspirate. Iron stains on aspirates and biopsies should be regarded as complementary.

ASSESSMENT OF BONE MARROW RETICULIN

Histological sections, either particle sections or trephine biopsy specimens, can be stained for reticulin using a silver-impregnation technique and also for collagen using a trichrome stain. Reticulin and collagen deposition can be quantified as shown in Table 1.4[39] and illustrated in Figs 1.38–1.42. The majority of haematologically normal subjects have a reticulin grade of 0 or 1

Table 1.4 Quantification of bone marrow reticulin and collagen[39]

0	No reticulin fibres demonstrable
1	Occasional fine individual fibres and foci of a fine fibre network
2	Fine fibre network throughout most of the section; no coarse fibres
3	Diffuse fibre network with scattered thick coarse fibres but no mature collagen
4	Diffuse often coarse fibre network with areas of collagenization.

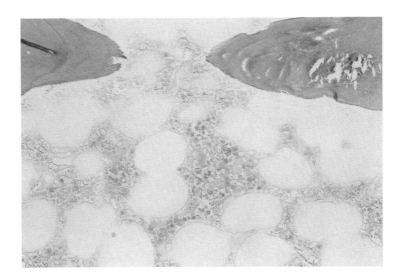

Fig. 1.38 Section of normal BM: reticulin grade 0, showing no stainable fibres. Plastic-embedded, Gomori's reticulin stain × 188.

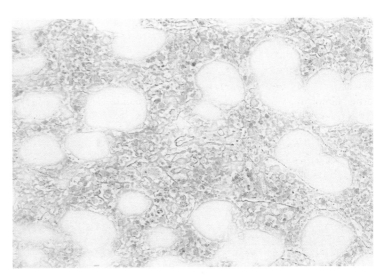

Fig. 1.39 Section of normal BM: reticulin grade 1, showing scattered fine fibres. Plastic-embedded, Gomori's reticulin stain × 188.

but occasional subjects have a grade of 2. There is a tendency for more reticulin to be detected in iliac crest biopsies than in sections of particles aspirated from the sternum. Reticulin is concentrated around blood vessels and close to bone trabeculae and these areas should be disregarded in assessing reticulin deposition.

The term myelofibrosis is used to indicate deposition of collagen in the marrow and sometimes also to indicate increased reticulin deposition. To avoid any ambiguity it is preferable to either grade reticulin/collagen deposition as shown in Table 1.4 or to use the term 'reticulin

fibrosis' for grade 3 fibrosis and 'myelofibrosis' for grade 4. The term myelosclerosis has also been used in various senses; it is best regarded as a synonym for myelofibrosis.

STAINING TECHNIQUES

CYTOCHEMISTRY

Bone marrow films and squashes are routinely stained with a Romanowsky stain such as May Grünwald–Giemsa (MGG) or Wright's stain. An iron stain is also indicated in the great majority

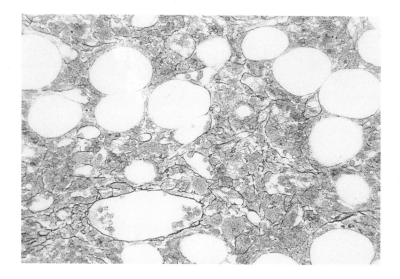

Fig. 1.40 Section of normal BM: reticulin grade 2, showing a fine fibre network but no coarse fibres. Paraffin-embedded, Gomori's reticulin stain × 195.

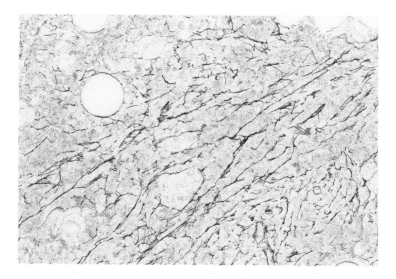

Fig. 1.41 Section of abnormal BM: reticulin grade 3, showing thick coarse fibres. Paraffin-embedded, Gordon–Sweet stain × 188.

of cases. Other cytochemical stains[40] are used selectively. Stains useful in the identification of cells of the granulocytic and monocytic series are very important in the diagnosis and classification of the acute leukaemias. Cytochemical stains identifying cells of granulocyte lineage include myeloperoxidase (MPO), Sudan black B (SBB) and chloroacetate esterase. Those identifying cells of the monocyte lineage include α-naphthyl acetate esterase and other esterase activities collectively referred to as non-specific esterase. Toluidine blue staining is useful in confirming the identity of cells of basophil lineage. Most myeloid and many lymphoid cells show acid phosphatase activity; the demonstration of tartrate-resistant acid phosphatase (TRAP) activity has a place in confirming the diagnosis of hairy cell leukaemia. The periodic acid-Schiff (PAS) stain is positive with a variety of carbohydrates including glycogen; it is of value in the investigation of the acute leukaemias and the myelodysplasias. Oil red O stains lipid droplets including those present in the cytoplasm in some cases of acute leukaemia, particularly cases of L3 subtype (see page 131). Specialized stains for

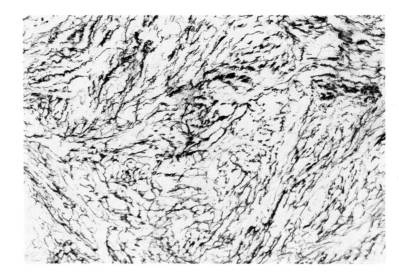

Fig. 1.42 Section of abnormal BM: reticulin grade 4, showing a coarse fibre network; collagen was present. Paraffin-embedded, Gordon–Sweet stain × 188.

micro-organisms can also be applied to bone marrow films (see chapter 2).

IMMUNOCYTOCHEMISTRY

Immunocytochemical stains can be applied to cytospin preparations of washed bone marrow cells. The majority of such stains (with the exception of those for the identification of immunoglobulin or κ and λ light chains) can also be applied to bone marrow films. Techniques which are applicable include direct immuno-fluorescence (in which an antibody is directly labelled with a fluorescent chemical) and indirect techniques (including indirect immunofluor-escence, immunoperoxidase and alkaline phosphatase or alkaline phosphatase–anti-alkaline phosphatase techniques). In indirect techniques the reaction of the primary antibody with the target cell is identified by use of one or more further antibodies which are themselves labelled with a fluorescent chemical, or by attaching to peroxidase or alkaline phosphatase. When such techniques are applied to fixed cells in smears they permit the detection of both membrane and cytoplasmic antigens. Application of similar tech-niques to living cells in suspension permit the detection only of surface membrane antigens. Polyclonal and monoclonal antibodies for the detection of a very large number of membrane and cytoplasmic antigens in haemopoietic cells

are available. Those of most use in diagnosis are discussed by Bain.[41] It is also possible to identify cellular antigens by using a lectin rather than a primary antibody. Monoclonal antibodies capable of detecting carcinoma cells or other non-haemopoietic malignant cells can be applied to bone marrow films when metastatic disease is suspected (see chapter 9).

HISTOCHEMISTRY

Decalcified, paraffin-embedded tissue sections are routinely stained with haematoxylin and eosin (H&E), with Giemsa (a Romanowsky stain), with a stain for reticulin and with a stain for iron such as Perls' stain. A PAS stain can also be employed; it is useful for demonstrating megakaryocytes, neutrophils and certain micro-organisms (see Table 2.1). Other specialized stains for micro-organisms are used in selected cases (see Table 2.1).

The processes employed in decalcifying and paraffin-embedding trephine biopsies render them unsuitable for most enzyme histochemistry as irreversible denaturation of proteins results from the decalcification, dehydration, heating and embedding procedures. Acid phosphatase activity is sometimes retained and when hairy cell leukaemia is suspected a stain for TRAP activity can be useful.

Plastic-embedded specimens can be stained by

all routine stains including H&E, Giemsa, PAS, trichrome, reticulin and iron stains. In addition, a variety of modifications of histochemical techniques have made possible the detection of various enzymes in plastic-embedded specimens.[42,43] Chloroacetate esterase activity is well preserved and excellent results can be achieved with a Leder stain. Acid phosphatase, peroxidase and non-specific esterase (α-naphthyl acetate or α-naphthyl butyrate esterase) activity can also be demonstrated. An alkaline phosphatase stain is positive with osteoblasts, bone marrow stromal cells and endothelial cells.[44] SBB staining is not possible in histological sections.

IMMUNOHISTOCHEMISTRY

Immunohistochemistry using a full range of antibodies can be carried out on frozen sections of bone marrow biopsies[45,46] but technical problems are considerable and this is generally not a suitable technique for a diagnostic laboratory.

Immunohistochemistry can be carried out successfully on decalcified paraffin-embedded sections as long as the antibodies used identify antigens or epitopes which are resistant to the processes employed in embedding.[43,47-50] Both monoclonal and polyclonal antibodies are applicable.

Immunohistochemistry is generally unsatisfactory on plastic-embedded specimens because of strong background staining and difficulty in detecting weak reactions. Some success can be achieved with antibodies to strongly expressed antigens such as the leucocyte common antigen.

The antibodies which have been found most useful in identifying cells or various lineages in decalcified, paraffin-embedded trephine biopsies are summarized in Table 1.5. Those of most value in relation to individual lineages will be discussed.

Granulopoiesis

Early granulocytic cells are stained by CD68 antibodies (KP-1). More mature cells of granulocyte lineage are detected with CD15 antibodies (for example Leu M1); staining is of the membrane and to some extent cytoplasmic. Maturing granulocytes are well shown by the use of anti-

elastase (NP57) or anti-lactoferrin, both of which stain cytoplasmic constituents. Myeloblasts may stain with antibodies to the leucocyte common antigen but staining is weaker than in lymphoid cells. Cases of acute myeloid leukaemia with very little cytoplasmic maturation, FAB M1 category (see page 71), may not give a positive reaction with any antibodies which are specific for myeloid cells but cases of FAB categories M2–M5 are reliably identified by one or more of the above antibodies.[50]

Monocytopoiesis

Monocytes and macrophages can be stained with antibodies to α1 anti-trypsin, α1 anti-chymotrypsin and lysozyme but none of these activities are specific. CD15 monoclonal antibodies and Mac 387 stain both monocytes and granulocytes; CD14 antibodies are more specific for monocytes. CD11c also identifies monocytes. KP-1 (CD68) has been found useful, although immature granulocytic cells, mast cells and occasional lymphoid cells are also positive.[50,51]

Erythropoiesis

Erythropoietic cells can be identified by anti-glycophorin antibodies or by the lectin derived from the common gorse, *Ulex europaeus*.[48] Anti-glycophorin antibodies are specific for the erythroid lineage while *U. europaeus* also stains megakaryocytes. Both stain erythroblasts and mature erythrocytes. In one study of trephine biopsies only the *U. europaeus* lectin was found to identify proerythroblasts[48] although in bone marrow aspirates these early erythroid cells are successfully identified by anti-glycophorin antibodies.

Megakaryocytes

Polyclonal antibodies to factor VIII-related antigen (more correctly von Willebrand antigen) and monoclonal anti-CD61 (anti-platelet glycoprotein IIIa) have been found useful in identifying megakaryocytes and their precursors. We have also found the *U. europaeus* lectin[48] very reliable. Although this lectin stains both erythroid and megakaryocyte lineages the pattern of staining

Table 1.5 Antibodies and lectins useful in decalcified paraffin-embedded trephine biopsies[47-50]

Category	Antibody	Polyclonal/monoclonal	Specificity
—	Anti-glycophorin	P	Erythroid cells
—	U. europaeus lectin	lectin	Erythroid cells, megakaryocytes, endothelial cells, some carcinoma cells
—	Anti-factor VIII-related antigen	P	Megakaryocytes, endothelial cells
CD61	Y2/51, anti-platelet glycoprotein IIIa	M	Megakaryocytes[47]
CD15	Leu M1	M	Promyelocytes to polymorphs, monocytes, Reed–Sternberg cells and mononuclear Hodgkin's cells
CD14	Leu M3	M	Monocytes
—	Anti-elastase (NP57)	M	Some promyelocytes, myelocytes to polymorphs, monocytes
CD11c	Leu M5	M	Monocytes and hairy cells
CD45	PD7/26, 2B11 anti-leucocyte common antigen (LCA)	M	T and B lymphocytes, myeloblasts (weak), mast cells
—	MB2	M	B lymphocytes, endothelial cells, some non-haemopoietic malignant cells
CD3	pT3, anti-CD3	P	T lymphocytes
CD45RO	UCHL1	M	T lymphocytes
CD20	L26	M	B lymphocytes
CD30	Ber H2	M	Reed–Sternberg and mononuclear Hodgkin's cells, some high-grade non-Hodgkin's lymphomas, late erythroblasts (weak), metamyelocytes and polymorphs (weak), some carcinoma cells[48]
CD68	KP-1	M	Monocytes and macrophages, mast cells, myeloblasts, some hairy cells and CLL cells[50]

differs; in megakaryocytes there is granular staining, either in the paranuclear region or throughout the cytoplasm whereas erythroid cells show staining of the membrane. Anti-platelet glycoprotein IIIa (CD61) gives strong homogeneous staining of mature megakaryocytes[47] but also identifies smaller cells, not morphologically identifiable as megakaryocytes, which are probably megakaryocyte precursors.[16] Immunohistochemical staining is particularly valuable in identifying micromegakaryocytes and megakaryoblasts and in distinguishing between megakaryocytes and malignant cells when large abnormal cells are embedded in a dense fibrous stroma.

Mast cells

Mast cells are positive for CD45 and CD68.[51]

Lymphoid cells

The most consistent staining of lymphoid cells is with CD45 monoclonal antibodies detecting the leucocyte common antigen; however some high-grade lymphomas have a weak or negative re-action. Some myeloid precursors also stain for leucocyte common antigen but the reaction is much weaker. CD45RO (monoclonal antibody UCHL1) has been found useful in identifying T lymphocytes in paraffin-embedded tissue; occasional granulocytic precursors and rare B lymphocytes also stain. Unfortunately it has the disadvantage that in decalcified material it commonly stains all nuclei. We have found poly-clonal anti-CD3 to be reliable and useful in detecting T lymphocytes. B cells are well identi-fied with L26 (CD20). The antibody MB2 (no CD number yet assigned) also identifies B lympho-cytes but in our experience L26 is superior. Although T-lineage lymphoblasts can be identi-fied there is as yet no reliable immunohisto-chemical method of identifying B-lineage lympho-blasts in trephine biopsies. Plasma cells are negative for most lymphoid markers including leucocyte common antigen; they are best identi-fied with anti-ϰ and anti-λ antibodies which also demonstrate whether or not an infiltrate is mono-clonal. Reed−Sternberg cells and mononuclear Hodgkin's cells in most histological categories of Hodgkin's disease (see page 182) give negative reactions with CD45 and positive reactions with CD15 and BERH2 (CD30) (the latter is also positive with some high-grade non-Hodgkin's lymphomas known as Ki-1-positive lymphomas, Ki-1 being another antibody of the CD30 cluster). Hairy cells give positive reactions with CD11c (Leu M5). A range of other antibodies suitable for use in decalcified paraffin-embedded sections are available but many of them are less specific or less consistently positive than those described; a number of antibodies are available which stain both T and B lymphocytes but it is more useful, when possible, to use an antibody which will distinguish between these lineages. The anti-

bodies we have found most useful in investigating abnormal cells suspected of being lymphoid are CD45, CD45RO, CD3, CD20 (L26) and anti-ϰ and anti-λ.

INTERPRETATION OF BONE MARROW ASPIRATES AND TREPHINE BIOPSIES

Examination of a bone marrow aspirate in isola-tion permits cytomorphological features to be ascertained but does not permit full interpretation of the findings. The haematologist must also know the age and sex of the patient, the full blood count and relevant clinical details, and must have examined a peripheral blood film. Similarly, examination of a trephine biopsy section in iso-lation permits detection of histomorphological abnormalities but not a full assessment of a case. The pathologist should beware of either over-interpreting biopsy findings or failing to offer an adequate interpretation because of lack of con-sideration of clinical and haematological features and aspirate findings. It is desirable that trephine biopsies are either reported by a haematopatho-logist able also to interpret bone marrow aspirates or that the histopathologist and haematologist work closely together and examine aspirate films and biopsy sections together. Reports should distinguish between factual statements and opinions. It is useful if a description of relevant features is followed by a summary which may include explanation or interpretation so that the significance of morphological features is apparent to clinical staff reading a report.

Examination of bone marrow aspirate films

A minimum of two or three films should always be examined. If there is a likelihood of infiltration of the marrow and the first films do not show any abnormality it is important to stain and examine a larger number.

Bone marrow films should first be examined under low power (× 10 objective) in order to assess cellularity and megakaryocyte numbers and to scan the entire film for any abnormal infiltrate. The film should then be examined with a × 40 or × 50 objective which will allow appreciation of most morphological features. At this stage all cell lineages should be specifically and systematically examined from the point of view of both numbers and morphology — the erythroid series, granulocytic lineages including eosinophils and basophils, megakaryocytes, lymphocytes and plasma cells. Consideration should be given as to whether there is an increased number of mast cells, macrophages, osteoblasts or osteoclasts and whether any non-haemopoietic cells are present. Only when a thorough assessment of several films has been carried out with a × 40 or × 50 objective should the film be examined under high power (× 100) with oil immersion in order to assess fine cytological detail. A differential count of cells in the trails behind several fragments is best carried out under high power, but only with a prior assessment of whether there is any increase of minority populations, for example blasts cells or plasma cells, which is confined to one film or to the cell trail behind one fragment. Films stained for iron would be similarly examined under low power to assess storage iron, with a × 40 or × 50 objective to detect abnormally prominent siderotic granulation and with a × 10 objective to assess whether siderotic granulation is reduced, normal or increased.

Films of squashed bone fragments should be similarly examined in a systematic manner.

Examination of trephine biopsy sections

The interpretation of trephine biopsy sections is often viewed as one of the more difficult areas of surgical pathology. This is probably because the organized structure of haemopoietic tissue is not as readily apparent as that of many other tissues. However, as the preceding part of this chapter illustrates, the bone marrow is actually highly organized, with the various elements maturing in different micro-anatomical sites. Failure to recognize this and failure to identify individual categories of cell may lead to the lack of a systematic analysis, with diagnoses being made by a process of 'pattern recognition'. Conversely, the haematologist, although experienced in cytology, may be unfamiliar with the interpretation of tissue sections, where architectural features are often of prime importance.

A systematic approach, which is essential for accurate diagnosis, requires a working knowledge of the normal micro-anatomy and the pathological changes that may occur, coupled with a methodical examination of the various component parts. Initially, the whole section should be examined at low power, preferably using a × 4 objective. This allows a general impression of the biopsy to be gained, including overall cellularity and megakaryocyte number and distribution. Abnormalities of the bone are often apparent at this magnification, and it should also be noted if the biopsy specimen is too small, or is composed largely of cortical bone and subcortical marrow, or shows crushing artefact and distortion of the architecture. Focal lesions such as granulomas, or infiltrates of metastatic tumour or lymphoma are often better appreciated on low power examination. Following this, the bone, haemopoietic elements and marrow stromal elements should be studied using medium power (× 10 or × 20 objective) and a high dry objective (× 40); examination under oil immersion (× 100 objective) is not necessary as a routine, but is often useful for study of fine cytological detail. The bone should be examined for trabecular thickness, number of osteoblasts and osteoclasts, and presence and number of Howship's lacunae; undecalcified plastic sections should be assessed for the quantity of osteoid (see chapter 10). With a little experience, visual estimations of the marrow cellularity, of the relative amounts of granulocytic and erythroid elements, and of any deviations from normal can easily be made. The next step is to examine the various haemopoietic elements for the following features:

Erythroid series. The presence and appearance of erythroblastic islands, the morphology and degree of maturation of the erythroblasts, and evidence of dyserythropoiesis.

Granulocytic series. The morphology and relative proportions of immature and mature granulocytic precursors, and the position of the immature precursors (promyelocytes and myeloblasts).

Megakaryocytes. The number, morphological features, localization and presence or absence of clusters, with special attention being paid to cell size and nuclear morphology.

Lymphoid series. The number, localization, and morphology of plasma cells and the presence, position and morphology of lymphoid aggregates.

Macrophages. Marrow macrophages may be increased in number, and show evidence of haemophagocytosis, phagocytosis of micro-organisms (usually fungi or protozoa) or lysosomal storage diseases, such as Gaucher's disease.

It is often easy to neglect to examine the stromal elements, yet these are disturbed in a variety of conditions. The important changes include: gelatinous change; fibrosis; ectasia of sinusoids; oedema; and, less commonly, amyloidosis and vasculitis.

Routine stains for reticulin and iron should be examined in every case. Choice of further special stains is dependent on the clinical and histological findings.

Obviously, in many cases, as when there is heavy infiltration by leukaemic cells or metastatic carcinoma, the above scheme is modified.

The report should include: an estimate of the cellularity (usually it is adequate to state whether cellularity is normal, increased or reduced); a statement of whether the erythroid, granulocytic or megakaryocytic elements are normal and if they are abnormal, a description of the abnormalities; a description of any other abnormalities; an assessment of the reticulin pattern and of the iron stores. Finally, the findings should be interpreted in the light of clinical, blood film and marrow aspirate data.

REFERENCES

1 Hashimoto M (1962) Pathology of bone marrow. *Acta Haematol (Basel)*, **27**, 193–216.
2 de Bruyn PPH (1981) Structural substrates of bone marrow function. *Semin Hematol*, **18**, 179–193.
3 Wickramasinghe SN. *Human Bone Marrow.* Blackwell Scientific Publications, Oxford, 1975.
4 Bennike T, Gormsen H and Moller B (1956) Comparative studies of bone marrow punctures of the sternum, the iliac crest, and the spinous process. *Acta Med Scand*, **155**, 377–396.
5 Kerndrup G, Pallesen G, Melsen F and Mosekilde L

(1980) Histomorphometric determination of bone marrow cellularity in iliac crest biopsies. *Scand J Haematol*, **24**, 110–114.
6 Al-Adhadh AN and Cavill I (1983) Assessment of cellularity in bone marrow fragments. *J Clin Pathol*, **36**, 176–179.
7 Frisch B, Lewis SM, Burkhardt R and Bartl R. *Biopsy Pathology of Bone and Marrow.* Chapman and Hall, London, 1985.
8 Hartsock RJ, Smith EB and Petty CS (1965) Normal variations with ageing of the amount of hematopoietic tissue in bone marrow from the anterior iliac crest; a study made from 177 cases of sudden death examined by necropsy. *Am J Clin Pathol*, **43**, 326–331.
9 Meunier P, Aaron J, Edouard C, Vignon G (1971) Osteoporosis and the replacement of cell populations of the marrow by adipose tissue. *Clin Orthopaed*, **80**, 147–154.
10 Courpron P, Meunier P, Edouard C, Bernard J, Bringuier J-P, Vignon G (1973) Données histologiques quantitatives sur le vieillissement osseux humain. *Rev Rhum*, **40**, 469–482.
11 Bryon PA, Gentilhomme O and Fiere D (1979) Étude histologique quantitative du volume et de l'hétérogénéité des adipocytes dans les insuffisance myéloïdes globales. *Pathol Biol*, **27**, 209–213.
12 Bessis M (1958) L'îlot érythroblastique, unité fonctionelle de la moelle osseuse. *Rev Hematol*, **13**, 8–11.
13 Mohandas N and Prenant M (1978) Three-dimensional model of bone marrow. *Blood*, **51**, 633–643.
14 Queisser U, Queisser W and Spiertz B (1971) Polyploidization of megakaryocytes in normal humans and patients with idiopathic thrombocytopenia and with pernicious anaemia. *Br J Haematol*, **20**, 489–501.
15 Tavassoli M and Aoki M (1989) Localization of megakaryocytes in the bone marrow. *Blood Cells*, **15**, 3–14.
16 Thiele J and Fischer R (1991) Megakaryocytopoiesis in human disorders: diagnostic features of bone marrow biopsies. An overview. *Virchows Archiv (A)*, **418**, 87–97.
17 Johnstone JM (1954) The appearance and significance of tissue mast cells in the human bone marrow. *J Clin Pathol*, **7**, 275–280.
18 Rosse C, Kraemer MJ, Dillon TL, McFarland R and Smith NJ (1977) Bone marrow cell populations of normal infants: the predominance of lymphocytes. *J Lab Clin Med*, **89**, 1225–1240.
19 Thaler J, Greil R, Dietze O and Huber H (1989) Immunohistology for quantification of normal bone marrow lymphocyte subsets. *Br J Haematol*, **73**, 576–577.

20 Steiner ML and Pearson HA (1966) Bone plasmacytic values in children. *J Pediatr*, **68**, 562–568.

21 Dresch C, Faille A, Poieriero O and Kadouche J (1974) The cellular composition of normal human bone marrow according to the volume of the sample. *J Clin Pathol*, **27**, 106–108.

22 Glaser K, Limarzi L and Poncher HG (1950) Cellular composition of the bone marrow in normal infants and children. *Pediatrics*, **6**, 789–824.

23 Gairdner D, Marks J and Roscoe JD (1952) Blood formation in infancy. Part I. The normal bone marrow. *Arch Dis Child*, **27**, 128–133.

24 Diwany M (1940) Sternal marrow puncture in children. *Arch Dis Child*, **15**, 159–170.

25 Jacobsen KM (1941) Untersuchungen über das Knochenmarkspunktat bei normalen Individuen verschiedener Altersklassen. *Acta Med Scand*, **106**, 417–446.

26 Segerdahl E (1935) Über sternalpunktionen. *Acta Med Scand*, **64**, suppl, 1–105.

27 Vaughan SL and Brockmyr F (1947) Normal bone marrow as obtained by sternal puncture. *Blood*, **1** (special issue), 54–59.

28 Wintrobe MM, Lee RG, Boggs DR, Bithell TC, Athens JW and Foerster J. *Clinical Hematology*, 7th edition. Lea and Febiger, Philadelphia, 1974.

29 Dancy JT, Deubelbeiss KA, Harker LA and Finch CA (1976) Neutrophil kinetics in man. *J Clin Invest*, **58**, 705–715.

30 Wilkins BS and O'Brien CJ (1988) Techniques for obtaining differential cell counts from bone marrow trephine biopsy specimens. *J Clin Pathol*, **41**, 558–561.

31 Rath CE and Finch CA (1948) Sternal marrow hemosiderin; a method for determining available iron stores in man. *J Lab Clin Med*, **33**, 81–86.

32 Gale E, Torrance J and Bothwell T (1963) The quantitative estimation of total iron stores in human bone marrow. *J Clin Invest*, **42**, 1076–1082.

33 Lundin P, Persson E and Weinfeld A (1964) Comparison of hemosiderin estimation in bone marrow sections and bone marrow smears. *Acta Med Scand*, **175**, 383–390.

34 Fong TP, Okafor LA, Thomas W and Westerman MP (1977) Stainable iron in aspirated and needle-biopsy specimens. *Am J Hematol*, **2**, 47–51.

35 Douglas AS and Dacie JV (1953) The incidence and significance of iron-containing granules in human erythrocytes and their precursors. *J Clin Pathol*, **6**, 307–313.

36 Bainton DF and Finch CA (1964) The diagnosis of iron deficiency anemia. *Am J Med*, **37**, 62–70.

37 Hansen HA and Weinfeld A (1965) Hemosiderin estimations and sideroblast counts in the differential diagnosis of iron deficiency and other anemias. *Acta Med Scand*, **165**, 333–356.

38 Krause JR, Brubaker D and Kaplan S (1979) Comparisons of stainable iron in aspirated and needle biopsy specimens of bone marrow. *Am J Clin Pathol*, **72**, 68–70.

39 Bauermeister DE (1971) Quantification of bone marrow reticulin—a normal range. *Am J Clin Pathol*, **56**, 24–31.

40 Hayhoe FGJ and Quaglino D. *Haematological Cytochemistry*, 2nd edition. Churchill Livingstone, Edinburgh, 1988.

41 Bain BJ. *Leukaemia Diagnosis: a Guide to the FAB Classification*. Gower Medical Publishing, London, 1990.

42 Beckstead JH, Halvarsen PS, Ries CA and Bainton D (1981) Enzyme histochemistry and immunohisto-chemistry on biopsy specimens of pathologic human bone marrow. *Blood*, **57**, 1088–1098.

43 Beckstead JH (1986) The bone marrow biopsy: a diagnostic strategy. *Arch Pathol Lab Med*, **110**, 175–179.

44 Dilly SA and Jagger CJ (1990) Bone marrow stromal cell changes in haematological malignancies. *J Clin Pathol*, **43**, 942–946.

45 Nash JRG, Smith SR and Mackie MJ (1989) An immunocytochemical study of lymphocyte and macrophage populations in the bone marrow of patients with non-Hodgkin's lymphoma. *J Pathol*, **154**, 141–149.

46 Chilosi M, Pizzolo G, Fiore-Danti L, Boffil M and Janossy G (1983) Routine immunofluorescent and histochemical analysis of bone marrow involvement of leukaemia: the use of cryostat sections. *Br J Cancer*, **48**, 763–775.

47 Gatter KC, Cordell JL, Turley H, Heryet A, Kieffer N, Anstee DJ and Mason DY (1988) The immuno-histological detection of platelets, megakaryocytes and thrombi in routinely processed specimens. *Histopathology*, **13**, 257–267.

48 van der Valk P, Mullink H, Huijgens PC, Tadema TM, Vos W and Meijer CJLM (1989) Value of a panel of monoclonal antibodies on routinely processed bone marrow biopsies. *Am J Surg Pathol*, **13**, 97–106.

49 Davey FR, Elghetany MT and Kurec AS (1990) Immunophenotyping of hematologic neoplasms in paraffin-embedded tissue sections. *Am J Clin Pathol*, **93**, suppl 1, 17–26.

50 Kurec AS, Cruz VE, Barrett D, Mason DY and Davey FR (1990) Immunophenotyping of acute leukemias using paraffin-embedded tissue sections. *Am J Clin Pathol*, **93**, 502–509.

51 Horny H-P, Schaumeberg-Lever G, Bolz S, Geertz ML and Kaiserling E (1990) Use of monoclonal antibody KP1 for identifying normal and neoplastic human mast cells. *J Clin Pathol*, **43**, 719–722.

2: Infection and Reactive Changes

INFECTION

The response of the bone marrow to infection is very variable, depending on the nature and chronicity of the infection, the age of the subject and the presence of any associated diseases. The response differs, depending on whether the infection is bacterial, viral, rickettsial or fungal.

Peripheral blood

In adults the usual haematological response to a bacterial infection is neutrophil leucocytosis with a left shift (an increase of band forms and possibly the appearance of neutrophil precursors in the peripheral blood) (Fig. 2.1). The neutrophils usually show toxic granulation and may show Döhle bodies and cytoplasmic vacuolation. Rarely neutrophils contain phagocytosed bacteria. The presence of bacteria, either extracellularly or within neutrophils, is usually seen only in overwhelming infections, particularly when there is associated hyposplenism. In relapsing fever, however, the characteristic spiral borrelia appears episodically in the bloodstream and are seen lying free between red cells. When there is very severe bacterial infection and in neonates, alcoholics and patients with reduced bone marrow reserve, neutrophilia does not occur, but there is a left shift with the above 'toxic' changes in neutrophils. Certain bacterial infections, specifically typhoid, paratyphoid and tularaemia, are characterized by neutropenia rather than neutrophilia. In severe infection, particularly if there is shock or hypoxia, nucleated red blood cells may appear in the blood, the presence of both granulocyte precursors and nucleated red cells being referred to as leuco-erythroblastosis. The lymphocyte count is reduced but a few atypical lymphocytes including plasmacytoid lymphocytes may be present; plasma cells are sometimes seen. Monocytosis occurs in some chronic infections (Fig. 2.2). The

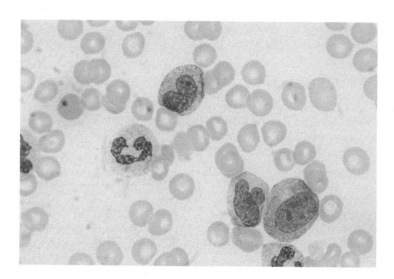

Fig. 2.1 PB, bacterial infection, left shift and toxic granulation. MGG × 940.

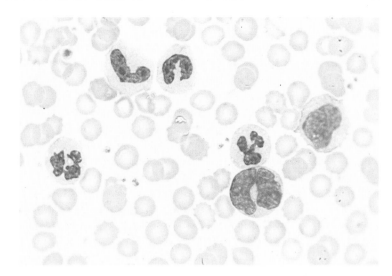

Fig. 2.2 PB, bacterial infection, monocytosis and neutrophilia. MGG × 940.

eosinophil count is reduced during acute infection but eosinophilia can occur during recovery. Children may respond to bacterial infection with lymphocytosis rather than neutrophilia, and certain bacterial infections, particularly whooping cough and sometimes brucellosis, are characterized by lymphocytosis. In bacterial infection the platelet count is often reduced but sometimes increased and if the infection persists anaemia develops and rouleaux formation is increased. The anaemia develops the characteristics of the anaemia of chronic disease with the cells produced being hypochromic and microcytic. Certain bacterial infections can be complicated by haemolytic anaemia. Infection by *Escherichia coli* or shigella can be followed by a microangiopathic haemolytic anaemia as part of a haemolytic uraemic syndrome. Sepsis due to *Clostridium welchii* can be complicated by acute haemolysis with spherocytic red cells. Mycoplasma infection is commonly associated with the production of cold auto-antibodies so that red cell agglutinates are present in blood films made at room temperature and haemolytic anaemia sometimes occurs.

Viral infections usually provoke lymphocytosis. Often the cells which are produced are morphologically fairly normal but sometimes they have atypical features. Infectious mononucleosis consequent on infection by the EB virus is characterized by the production of large numbers of atypical lymphocytes, often referred to as atypical mononuclear cells (Fig. 2.3). These are pleomorphic, usually large, and often have abundant basophilic cytoplasm and nuclei with a diffuse chromatin pattern and nucleoli. The presence of large numbers of atypical mononuclear cells in not specific for infection by the EB virus; it may also be seen in infection by other viruses (cytomegalovirus, human immunodeficiency virus (during the primary infection), hepatitis A, adenovirus) and in toxoplasmosis as well as in hypersensitivity reactions to drugs. Smaller numbers of similar atypical lymphocytes are seen in a wider variety of infective (and non-infective) conditions. Viral infections which may be associated with marked lymphocytosis without many atypical features include those due to Coxsackie virus, various adenoviruses and the human immunodeficiency virus (HIV); other haematological abnormalities produced by HIV are discussed below (see page 57). Viral infections, particularly those due to herpes viruses, may be associated with a haemophagocytic syndrome (see page 55) with the peripheral blood showing consequent pancytopenia. In a few individuals viral hepatitis, particularly non-A non-B hepatitis, is followed in a period of a few weeks or months by pancytopenia consequent on aplastic anaemia. In certain subjects who are unable to mount a normal immune response to EBV, infection by this virus may also be followed by chronic pancytopenia due to bone marrow aplasia. Parvovirus

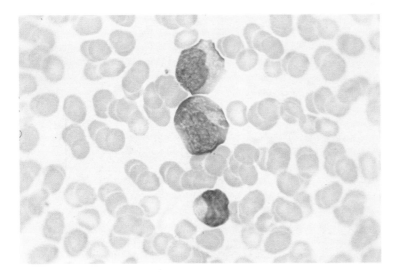

Fig. 2.3 PB, infectious mononucleosis, atypical lymphocytes. MGG × 940.

commonly causes transient pure red cell aplasia but unless red cell survival is reduced this may go unnoticed; less often it is a cause of neutropenia or thrombocytopenia. Viral infections may be complicated by cytopenias consequent on either damage to cells by immune complexes or auto-antibody production. Rubella and less often other viral infections may be followed by transient thrombocytopenia consequent on damage to platelets by immune complexes. Infectious mononucleosis may be complicated by either auto-immune thrombocytopenia or auto-immune haemolytic anaemia due to a cold antibody with anti-i specificity; in these cases there are red cell agglutinates and occasional spherocytes. Rarely viral infections, particularly measles, are followed by acute haemolysis due to an autoantibody with anti-P specificity (paroxysmal cold haemoglobinuria); in these cases the blood film usually shows only occasional spherocytes and subsequently polychromasia.

Rickettsial infections cause varied haematological effects which may include neutrophilia, neutropenia, lymphocytosis and thrombocytopenia which is sometimes severe.

Fungal infections have no specific haematological features. Some fungal diseases, for example actinomycosis and coccidioidomycosis, are associated with neutrophilia. Occasionally in systemic fungal infections, such as candidiasis or histoplasmosis, fungi are seen in the peripheral blood.

Occasionally severe infections are associated with a haematological picture which simulates leukaemia, designated a leukaemoid reaction. This is most often seen in association with very severe bacterial infection, particularly when there is coexisting megaloblastic anaemia. The bone marrow response to miliary tuberculosis can also simulate leukaemia. In a leukaemoid reaction anaemia and thrombocytopenia are common. The white cell count is sometimes low with neutropenia and sometimes high; the blood film may show granulocyte precursors or be leucoerythroblastic. Specific features suggestive of infection are also present.

Bone marrow cytology

In severe bacterial infection the bone marrow features reflect those of the peripheral blood. There is granulocytic hyperplasia with associated toxic changes. In overwhelming infection the marrow sometimes shows an increase of granulocyte precursors but with few maturing cells. Erythropoiesis is depressed and erythroblasts show reduced siderotic granulation. When there is thrombocytosis, megakaryocytes may be increased. Macrophages are increased and in a minority of patients with severe infection prominent

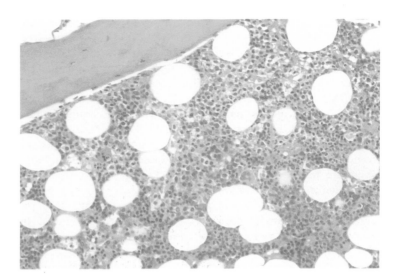

Fig. 2.4 BM trephine biopsy, bacterial infection with leukaemoid reaction: there is increased cellularity and granulocytic hyperplasia with left shift; note emperipolesis of a mature neutrophil by a megakaryocyte. Paraffin-embedded, H&E × 195.

haemophagocytosis occurs (see page 55). When infection is chronic an increase of iron stores is apparent. In tuberculosis the bone marrow aspirate shows only non-specific features such as increased iron stores and an increase in macrophages, often with haemophagocytosis; mycobacteria may be detected and specific staining and cultures should always be performed when this diagnosis is suspected. In typhoid fever also, bone marrow culture can be useful since in only two-thirds of patients with a positive bone marrow culture is there also a positive culture of the peripheral blood.[1] In Whipple's disease the causative organisms may be seen within bone marrow macrophages.[2] Bacteria visible within macrophages have also been reported in bacterial endocarditis.

In viral infection the bone marrow shows an increase of lymphocytes, either typical or atypical. In some infections, particularly by herpes viruses, haemophagocytosis is prominent (see page 55). When haemolytic anaemia occurs erythroid hyperplasia will be apparent whilst in pure red cell aplasia there are prominent, very large proerythroblasts with a striking lack of more mature cells. When there is thrombocytopenia due to increased platelet destruction megakaryocytes are present in normal or increased numbers.

Fungi are rarely seen in the bone marrow aspirate. The exception is in severely immuno-compromised patients such as those with HIV infection or following bone marrow transplantation when aspergillus, histoplasma and cryptococcus may be seen. Organisms may be within macrophages or free.

Bone marrow histology

In immunocompetent individuals severe viral, bacterial or fungal infection is usually accompanied by an increase in marrow cellularity due to granulocytic hyperplasia. There is often left shift of the granulocytic series — that is, an increase in the numbers of immature precursors (myelocytes and promyelocytes) in relation to mature polymorphonuclear neutrophils (Fig. 2.4). However, the normal topographical arrangement of granulopoiesis is retained, with the more immature cells (mainly promyelocytes) found predominantly in the paratrabecular region.[3] Megakaryocytes are often increased in number;[4] they are morphologically normal, but there may be an increase in 'bare' megakaryocyte nuclei. Erythropoiesis is often reduced although morphologically normal. Plasmacytosis of the bone marrow is a common response to a wide variety of infections, as well as to many other inflammatory and neoplastic conditions[5] (see page 53). Very rarely, there may be up to 50 per cent plasma cells in the marrow in benign conditions. The differential diagnosis of increased numbers of plasma cells in the marrow is discussed on page 53. In infections the plasma cells are distributed through the marrow in an interstitial manner, often with focal pericapillary accentuation. This may be accompanied by plasma cell satellitosis, in which a central macrophage is surrounded by three or more plasma cells. The plasma cells have mature nuclear and cytoplasmic characteristics, although there are often occasional binucleate forms and cells containing Russell bodies. Benign lymphoid aggregates are seen more frequently (see page 52). Macrophages may be increased and commonly contain ingested granulocytes. A wide variety of infectious agents may cause a secondary haemophagocytic syndrome (see page 55). Stromal changes include an increase in the number of sinusoids, focal reticulin fibrosis, and rarely, in very severe chronic infections, gelatinous change (see page 63). A decrease in marrow cellularity and loss of fat spaces usually accompany gelatinous change.[6]

All the above changes are non-specific and may be seen in many other conditions, including carcinoma, Hodgkin's disease, non-Hodgkin's lymphoma and auto-immune disorders such as systemic lupus erythematosus. In addition to these reactive changes there may be features that are more specific for certain types of infection. Many infective conditions result in bone marrow granulomas (see page 46). Atypical lymphoid cells, morphologically identical to those in the peripheral blood, can be seen in the marrow in EBV and CMV infection; in CMV infection eosinophilic intranuclear inclusions are occasionally seen in endothelial cells and in cells, probably macrophages, within granulomas or interspersed among haemopoietic cells.[7] In systemic fungal infections, particularly in immunocompromised patients such as those with AIDS (see page 57), organisms can sometimes be identified in the marrow. The histological features of the important fungi that can be seen in histological sections of the bone marrow are summarized in Table 2.1. Cases of disseminated infection caused by unusual fungi not previously recognized as pathogenic are also being recognized in patients with AIDS.[8]

Immunocompromised patients are more prone to infections that involve the bone marrow; moreover such infections are more likely to be overlooked because of the lack of a tissue response to

Table 2.1 Differential diagnosis of fungal and protozoal pathogens

Species	Tissue forms	Special stains
Fungi		
Candida albicans	Non-branching pseudohyphae and small (2–4 μm) budding yeast forms	PAS* and GMS
Cryptococcus neoformans	Yeast forms (5–10 μm), thick capsule, narrow-based unequal buds (Fig. 2.13)	PAS*, GMS and mucicarmine
Histoplasma capsulatum	Small (2–5 μm) yeast forms (Fig. 2.11)	PAS* and GMS
Protozoa		
Toxoplasma gondii	Tachyzoites (ovoid 3 × 6 μm, tiny nucleus, 'single dot' appearance) (Fig. 2.6); occasionally cysts with numerous small bradyzooites	Giemsa
Leishmania donovani	Small (3 μm) intracellular amastigote, nucleus and paranuclear kinetoplast gives 'double dot' appearance (Fig. 2.5)	Giemsa

PAS, Periodic acid-Schiff.
GMS, Grocott's methenamine silver stain.
* Pretreatment with diastase to remove glycogen considerably reduces positive staining of neutrophils and megakaryocytes and facilitates the detection of micro-organisms.

the infective agent. Because of this it is essential to use special stains that detect mycobacteria, fungi and protozoa as a routine on biopsies from these patients.

The other marrow findings in HIV infection are discussed on page 57.

PARASITIC DISEASES

Peripheral blood

Parasitic infections in which there is infiltration of tissues often provoke eosinophilia. The presence of parasites within the bowel may lead to blood loss with consequent iron deficiency anaemia. In malaria and babesiosis parasites are seen within red cells and in leishmaniasis phagocytosed parasites are occasionally detectable within peripheral blood monocytes. Other parasites detectable free in the peripheral blood are trypanosomes and microfilariae.

Bone marrow cytology

A bone marrow aspirate is very useful in the diagnosis of leishmaniasis (Fig. 2.5). Trypanosomes are sometimes detected in the bone marrow, but less often than leishmania. Malaria parasites are sometimes also detected in red cells in a bone marrow aspirate. Other parasites are rarely detected in the bone marrow, except in

severely immunosuppressed patients in whom pneumocystis[9] and toxoplasma have sometimes been found. Features useful in identifying various protozoan parasites are shown in Table 2.1. An increase of bone marrow eosinophils and their precursors is often apparent when there is tissue infiltration by parasites.

Bone marrow histology

In visceral leishmaniasis there may be granuloma formation. In more severe cases there is a diffuse increase of macrophages. The organisms are often seen within macrophages; their small size (3 μm) sometimes leads to their being confused with the fungus *Histoplasma capsulatum*. However leishmania fail to stain with PAS or silver stains and a Giemsa stain will demonstrate a small paranuclear basophilic body, known as the kinetoplast giving the organism a characteristic 'double dot' appearance.

Granulomas are also seen in toxoplasmosis; rarely, in immunosuppressed individuals, organisms are seen in the marrow (Fig. 2.6). These usually take the form of tachyzoites, which are 3–6 μm in diameter and have a tiny single nucleus. Occasionally cysts containing numerous bradyzoites are present. These are of a similar size to tachyzoites and also have a single nucleus; the lack of a kinetoplast helps to distinguish them from leishmania.

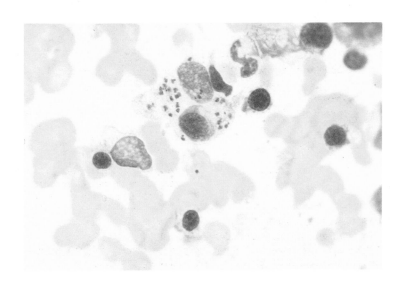

Fig. 2.5 BM aspirate, leishmaniasis, showing a macrophage containing numerous organisms which in addition to a nucleus have a small paranuclear kinetoplast giving them a characteristic 'double-dot' appearance. MGG × 940.

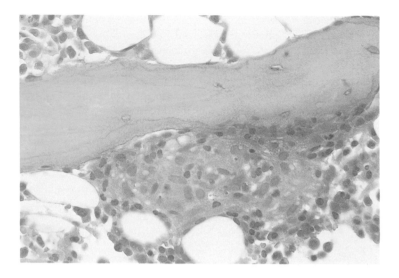

Fig. 2.6 BM trephine biopsy, toxoplasmosis showing a small granuloma in a paratrabecular position containing several small organisms with a single nucleus consistent with the tachyzoites of *Toxoplasma gondii*; fungal stains were negative and the patient had raised serum IgM antibodies to *Toxoplasma*. Plastic-embedded, H&E × 390.

Extra-pulmonary infection with *Pneumocystis carinii* is rare; it is invariably secondary to pulmonary disease, and appears to be more common in those patients who have received aerosolized pentamidine therapy. Approximately a third of patients with extra-pulmonary infection have marrow involvement.[10] There are areas of 'frothy' exudate which is pink on an H&E stain; Grocott's methenamine silver stain demonstrates the cysts which are 4–6 μm in diameter and often have a crumpled or cup-shaped appearance.

BONE MARROW GRANULOMAS

A granuloma is a compact aggregate of modified macrophages. These cells, known as epithelioid cells, have large amounts of pale pink cytoplasm and ovoid or elongated nuclei with a dispersed chromatin pattern. Often several epithelioid cells fuse to form a giant cell. Two types of giant cells are recognized in granulomas: Langhans' type, which has numerous nuclei arranged around the periphery of the cell, and foreign body type with nuclei scattered throughout the cell. Other cell types including lymphocytes, plasma cells, neutrophils, eosinophils and fibroblasts may be found within granulomas, but these are not a constant feature.

A wide range of aetiological agents are associated with marrow granulomas (Table 2.2). It should be noted that patients with immuno-deficiency, such as AIDS, may fail to produce granulomas in response to infection with organisms that stimulate granuloma formation in normal individuals; this is probably consequent on the important role of T cells in facilitating formation of some types of granuloma.

Peripheral blood

There are no specific peripheral blood findings associated with the presence of bone marrow granulomas. The blood film may show features associated with the primary disease or, if bone marrow disease is extensive, there may be anaemia or pancytopenia with a leucoerythroblastic blood film. Lymphopenia is also common.[11]

Bone marrow cytology

There are no specific features in the bone marrow aspirate in patients with bone marrow granulomas. Occasionally it is possible to recognize epithelioid cells.

Bone marrow histology

Lipid granulomas. Lipid granulomas were previously reported to be the most common type of granuloma seen in the marrow, being present in up to nine per cent of biopsies.[21] In our experience they are considerably less common than this.

Table 2.2 Bone marrow granulomas[11-13]

Infection	Tuberculosis
	Atypical mycobacterial infection
	Disseminated bacillus Calmette−Guerin (BCG) infection[14]
	Brucellosis
	Leprosy
	Syphilis
	Typhoid fever
	Legionnaire's disease
	Tularaemia[11]
	Q fever
	Rocky Mountain spotted fever[11]
	Leishmaniasis
	Toxoplasmosis
	Histoplasmosis
	Cryptococcosis
	Saccharomyces[11]
	Blastomycosis
	Coccidioidomycosis[15]
	Paracoccidioidomycosis
	herpes viruses (infectious mononucleosis, CMV, *herpes zoster*)
	Hantaan virus (Korean haemorrhagic fever)[16]
	Cat scratch disease[16]
Sarcoidosis	
Malignant disease	Hodgkin's disease
	Multiple myeloma
	Non-Hodgkin's lymphoma
	Mycosis fungoides[11]
	Acute lymphoblastic leukaemia[11,13,16]
	Myelodysplastic syndrome[13]
Drug hypersensitivity	Phenytoin
	Procainamide
	Phenylbutazone[11] and oxyphenbutazone
	Chlorpropamide
	Sulphasalazine[17]
	Ibuprofen[11]
	Indomethacin[11]
	Allopurinol
Associated with eosinophilic interstitial nephritis	
Reaction to foreign substances	Anthracosis and silicosis[13,16,18]
	Talc[19]
	Berylliosis[20]

They are of no clinical importance and must be distinguished from epithelioid granulomas which they can sometimes resemble. Similar lesions may be seen in the liver, spleen and lymph nodes and these have been reported to be associated with the ingestion of mineral oil.[22] In the marrow they are usually located close to sinusoids or lymphoid nodules and measure from 0.2 to 0.8 mm in diameter. They contain fat vacuoles which vary in size but are usually smaller than the vacuoles in marrow fat cells; these are found both within macrophages and extra-cellularly. Lipid granulomas usually have plasma cells, eosinophils and lymphocytes within them, and

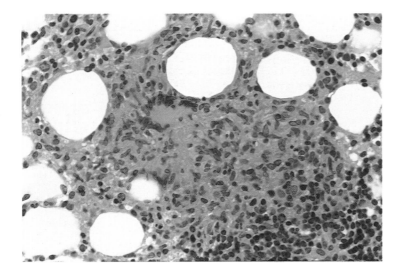

Fig. 2.7 BM trephine biopsy, miliary tuberculosis, showing an epithelioid granuloma containing a Langhans' giant cell and with numerous lymphocytes at its periphery. Paraffin-embedded, H&E × 390.

approximately five per cent contain giant cells. Occasionally the fat vacuoles may be small and easily overlooked giving the granulomas a sarcoid-like appearance.

Other granulomas. Unless a specific organism can be demonstrated within a granuloma, there are usually no histological features that allow a definitive diagnosis to be made.[23] Because of this, it is important for the pathologist to be aware of all the relevant clinical details, in order to be able to suggest an appropriate differential diagnosis. All biopsies with granulomas should have special stains for acid-fast bacilli and fungi performed. Ideally, in those cases in which marrow granulomas with an infective aetiology are possible, for example in patients with a pyrexia of unknown origin, part of the marrow aspirate should be cultured for mycobacteria and fungi.

Granulomas are found on marrow biopsy in 15−40 per cent of patients with miliary tuberculosis (Fig. 2.7). Tuberculous granulomas usually contain Langhans' type giant cells and caseation is present in approximately half the cases with marrow involvement.[23] Acid-fast bacilli cannot be demonstrated in most cases, and when seen

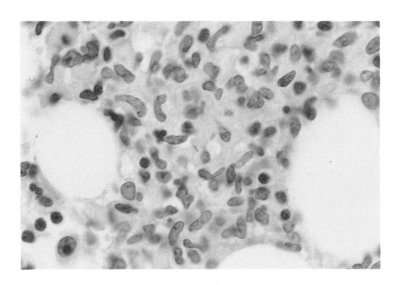

Fig. 2.8 BM trephine biopsy, miliary tuberculosis, showing a granuloma containing an acid-fast bacillus. Paraffin-embedded, Ziehl−Neelson stain × 970.

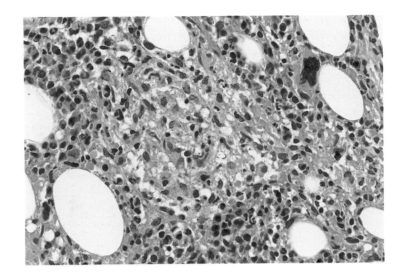

Fig. 2.9 BM trephine biopsy from a patient with AIDS and disseminated *M. avium intracellulare* infection showing a poorly formed granuloma made up of epithelioid macrophages many of which have vacuolated cytoplasm. Paraffin-embedded, H&E × 390.

they are usually scanty (Fig. 2.8). Approximately 50 per cent of patients with disseminated *Mycobacterium avium intracellulare* infection have marrow granulomas (Fig. 2.9), ranging from small ill-defined lymphohistiocytic aggregates to larger, more solid lymphohistiocytic lesions and small well-formed epithelioid granulomas.[24] Giant cells are only present in a minority of lesions and necrosis is not usually seen. Atypical mycobacteria may be demonstrated by special stains, sometimes in large numbers; they tend to be longer, more curved and more coarsely beaded than tubercle bacilli (Fig. 2.10). They are PAS-

positive, whereas *M. tuberculosis* is PAS-negative. Marrow granulomas containing foamy macrophages are occasionally seen in patients with leprosy; a Fite stain will demonstrate the acid fast bacilli of *M. leprae*.[25] Foamy macrophages may also be a feature of granulomas due to typhoid. Small poorly formed epithelioid granulomas are found in the bone marrow in most cases of brucellosis. Distinctive 'doughnut type' granulomas may be seen in the marrow in Q fever,[26] although they do not appear to be specific for this disease.[7] This type of granuloma often has a central empty space, surrounded

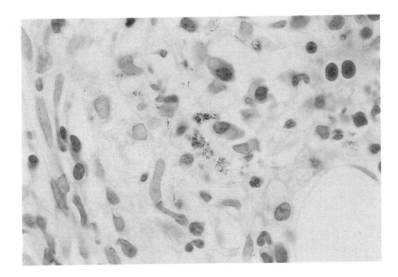

Fig. 2.10 BM trephine biopsy, *M. avium intracellulare* infection (same case as Fig. 2.9), showing large numbers of acid-fast bacilli; note the coarse beading of the organisms. Paraffin-embedded, Ziehl−Neelson stain × 970.

by neutrophils, lymphocytes, histiocytes and concentrically arranged, laminated fibrinoid material; more haphazardly arranged lesions without a central space also occur, as do small areas of fibrinoid necrosis.[26]

Disseminated infection by the fungus *H. capsulatum* usually involves the bone marrow; in normal hosts there are numerous granulomas, often with Langhans' giant cells and necrosis. Discrete granulomas are only present in a minority of immunodeficient hosts; more commonly such patients have ill-defined lymphohistiocytic aggregates or sheets of macrophages infiltrating

between haemopoietic cells[27] (Fig. 2.11). Tiny yeast forms, $2-5\,\mu m$ in diameter, some of which show unequal budding, are present within macrophages. The organisms may be seen on an H&E stain, but are best visualized using Gomori's methenamine silver (GMS) stain. *Cryptococcus neoformans* may cause granulomas. The organisms seen in tissue sections are yeasts ($5-10\,\mu m$ in diameter) with a wide capsular halo, and narrow-based unequal budding (Figs 2.12 and 2.13); with a mucicarmine stain the capsule of the yeast is red. Infection with the protozoans *Leishmania donovani* (Fig. 2.5) and *T. gondii*

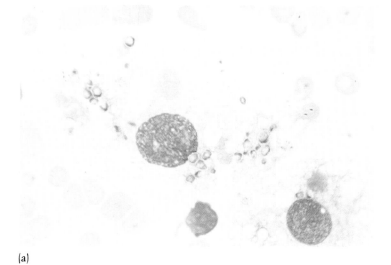

(a)

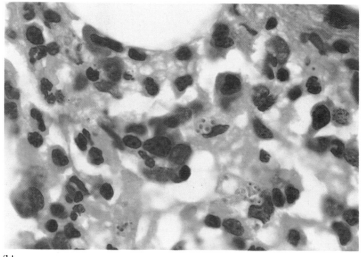

(b)

Fig. 2.11 (a) BM aspirate, histoplasmosis, showing numerous organisms within a macrophage. MGG × 940. (b) BM trephine biopsy, *H. capsulatum* infection in a patient with AIDS showing numerous organisms present within macrophages; the yeast forms have a clear unstained capsule surrounding them. Paraffin-embedded, H&E × 970.

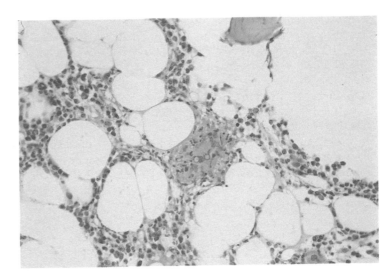

Fig. 2.12 BM trephine biopsy, *C. neoformans*, showing a small epithelioid granuloma containing large yeast forms with broad-based unequal budding. Paraffin-embedded, PAS × 195.

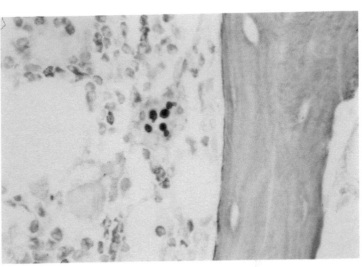

Fig. 2.13 BM trephine biopsy, *C. neoformans* (same case as Fig. 2.12), showing budding yeast forms. Paraffin-embedded, GMS × 390.

(Fig. 2.6) may involve the marrow and provoke granuloma formation (see page 45).

Up to 60 per cent of patients with infectious mononucleosis have small epithelioid granulomas on marrow biopsy; Langhans' giant cells and necrosis are not seen. Marrow granulomas are seen less commonly in other viral infections.

Granulomas may be seen in Hodgkin's disease,[28] non-Hodgkin's lymphoma (Fig. 2.14) and multiple myeloma (Fig. 2.15) in association with neoplastic infiltration of the marrow. In both Hodgkin's disease and non-Hodgkin's lymphoma granulomas also occur in the absence of marrow involvement; these are usually small, well-formed epithelioid granulomas, although larger poorly formed lymphohistiocytic lesions have also been reported.[29] Since patients with lymphoma have an increased susceptibility to many of the infections associated with marrow granulomas, these should always be excluded before attributing the granulomas to the underlying neoplastic disease.

The bone marrow is commonly involved in sarcoidosis; granulomas were seen in nine out of 21 patients in a biopsy series.[23] Often patients with marrow granulomas have evidence

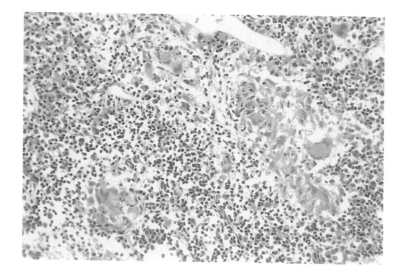

Fig. 2.14 BM trephine biopsy showing a reactive granuloma in a patient with diffuse bone marrow involvement by low-grade non-Hodgkin's lymphoma (ML-centroblastic-centrocytic). Paraffin-embedded, H&E × 195.

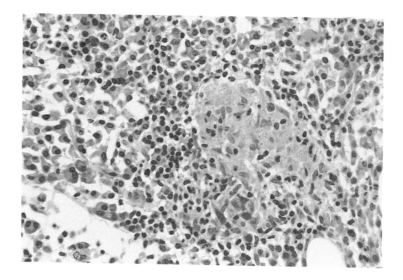

Fig. 2.15 BM trephine biopsy, multiple myeloma showing large numbers of plasma cells and an epithelioid granuloma (centre); no evidence of an infective cause for the granuloma was found in this patient. Paraffin-embedded, H&E × 390.

of multisystem involvement, such as hepato-splenomegaly, although in some chest radiography may be normal.[30] Typically there are numerous, well-formed epithelioid granulomas which, in approximately a third of cases, contain Langhans' giant cells (Fig. 2.16); necrosis is seen very rarely.

The granulomas associated with drug hypersensitivity are poorly circumscribed lympho-histiocytic lesions often containing eosinophils. Rarely they are accompanied by a systemic vasculitis which may involve the vessels in the marrow.

BENIGN LYMPHOID AGGREGATES

Benign lymphoid aggregates are commonly present in the bone marrow, their incidence increasing with age. An increased frequency has been reported in association with infection, inflammation, haemolysis, myeloproliferative disorders and auto-immune diseases such as rheumatoid arthritis and thyrotoxicosis. Patients with low-grade lymphoma have also been found to have an increased incidence of bone marrow lymphoid aggregates assessed histologically as benign.[31]

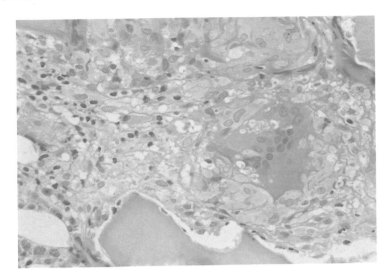

Fig. 2.16 BM trephine biopsy, sarcoidosis, showing a granuloma with a giant cell containing asteroid bodies. Plastic-embedded, H&E × 390.

Peripheral blood

There are no specific peripheral blood features associated with the presence of benign lymphoid aggregates in the bone marrow.

Bone marrow cytology

The bone marrow aspirate is usually normal but may show an increase in normal, mature lymphocytes.

Bone marrow histology

Benign lymphoid aggregates are usually few in number, not paratrabecular in position, well circumscribed and composed of small mature lymphocytes interspersed with some plasma cells and macrophages and sometimes occasional eosinophils, mast cells and immunoblasts[31–33] (see Fig. 1.31). They may be associated with small blood vessels. The lymphocytes show more pleomorphism than those in neoplastic lymphoid aggregates. Occasionally germinal centres are seen.[34] Reticulin fibres are increased within lymphoid nodules. Bone marrow biopsies showing benign lymphoid aggregates have an increased incidence of lipid granulomas and plasmacytosis. When lymphoid nodules are relatively large or numerous, immunohistochemical demonstration of a normal κ : λ ratio may be necessary to confirm their reactive nature.[33]

PLASMACYTOSIS

A reactive increase of polyclonal plasma cells is common and is associated with a variety of conditions including infections, chronic inflammatory diseases, haemopoietic and non-haemopoietic malignant disease, cirrhosis, diabetes mellitus, iron deficiency, megaloblastic anaemia and haemolytic anaemia.[5,35] A reactive increase in plasma cells needs to be distinguished from bone marrow infiltration by neoplastic plasma cells such as occurs in multiple myeloma and in many cases of immunocyte-derived amyloidosis, systemic light-chain disease, and monoclonal gammopathy of undetermined significance (see chapter 6).

Peripheral blood

Patients with reactive bone marrow plasmacytosis commonly show non-specific abnormalities in the peripheral blood consequent on the underlying disease. There is often anaemia which may have the features of the anaemia of chronic disease (either a normocytic, normochromic anaemia or, if the inflammatory process is severe, a microcytic, hypochromic anaemia). Rouleaux formation is commonly increased as a consequence of an increased concentration of polyclonal immunoglobulins and other reactive changes in plasma proteins. Occasionally patients with reactive plasmacytosis have plasma cells in the peripheral blood, usually in small numbers.

Bone marrow cytology

In reactive plasmacytosis the bone marrow shows an increased number of plasma cells, not usually exceeding 10–20 per cent of nucleated cells, but in rare cases up to 50 per cent. The plasma cells are predominately mature (see Fig. 1.32) although occasional cells may have nucleoli, a diffuse chromatin pattern or some degree of nucleo-cytoplasmic asynchrony. Small numbers of bi- or trinucleated forms can be present. The plasma cells may contain cytoplasmic vacuoles or inclusions, or intranuclear inclusions. Large homogeneous hyaline inclusions, often single, 2–3 μm in diameter and displacing the nucleus are designated Russell bodies; on an MGG stain they often dissolve leaving a single large vacuole. Cells containing multiple vacuoles or inclusions are referred to as Mott cells, grape cells or morular cells. Cells may contain cytoplasmic crystals. Cells may have a pyknotic nucleus and voluminous pale-staining cytoplasm, consequent on greatly dilated endoplasmic reticulum; such cells are designated thesaurocytes indicating they are storing the products they have synthesized. Cells which synthesize carbohydrate may have flaming pink cytoplasm ('flaming cells'). All these inclusions and unusual tinctorial qualities are consequent on increased immunoglobulin synthesis within the rough endoplasmic reticulum. Nuclear inclusions are consequent on invagination from the cytoplasm. Cells of these various types are characteristic of conditions with immune stimulation but neoplastic plasma cells sometimes show similar features.

Bone marrow histology

A trephine biopsy section in reactive plasmacytosis shows an interstitial infiltrate of plasma cells, particularly adjacent to capillaries (see Fig. 1.33). Plasma cells are sometimes clustered around macrophages. A minority of cases have small clusters of plasma cells but large homogeneous nodules, which are a feature of multiple myeloma, are not seen. The variety of inclusions described above may also be apparent on histological sections (Fig. 2.17) and some degree of cellular immaturity may be noted. Russell bodies stain pink on an H&E stain and show variable PAS staining. In reactive plasmacytosis immunocytochemistry shows that κ- and λ-expressing plasma cells are present in a ratio of approximately 2:1. About half the plasma cells express γ heavy chain, about a third α and the remainder μ.[36]

Plasmacytosis may be associated with other reactive changes such as granulocytic hyperplasia and the presence of benign lymphoid aggregates and increased numbers of macrophages. The

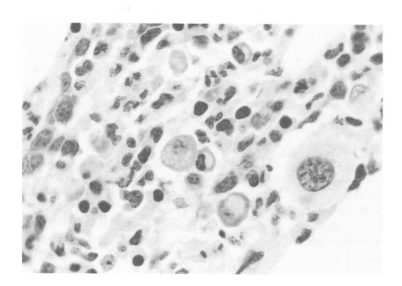

Fig. 2.17 BM trephine biopsy, myelodysplastic syndrome, showing prominent plasma cells including one with multiple cytoplasmic vacuoles (Mott cell). Plastic-embedded, H&E × 940.

macrophages may have enhanced haemophago-cytic activity and an increased iron content.

MAST CELLS

Small numbers of mast cells are present in normal bone marrow. Increased numbers are present in systemic mastocytosis, when the infiltrating cells are neoplastic, and as a reactive change in association with a variety of pathological processes. Increased numbers have been noted in infection, inflammation, renal failure, lymphoproliferative disorders and reactive lymphocytosis, aplastic anaemia, paroxysmal nocturnal haemoglobinuria, myeloproliferative disorders and the myelodysplastic syndromes.[37-39] Mast cells accumulate in areas of connective tissue proliferation, for example in fracture callus and in zones of osteitis fibrosa in patients with renal failure.

Peripheral blood

There are no specific peripheral blood features associated with a reactive increase of bone marrow mast cells.

Bone marrow cytology

The cytological features of bone marrow mast cells have been described on page 19. Lymphocytosis and plasmacytosis may coexist with an increase in mast cells.

Bone marrow histology

The characteristics of mast cells in histological sections have been described on page 20 and the features of systemic mastocytosis will be described on page 119. In histological sections mast cells may be confused with fibroblasts or macrophages, consequent on their elongated shape, oval nuclei and the failure of their granules to stain with H&E. The lesions associated with drug hypersensitivity previously designated 'eosinophilic fibrohistiocytic lesions'[40] are now known to represent proliferation of eosinophils and mast cells.

When mast cells are increased there may be an associated increase in plasma cells and lymphocytes.

HAEMOPHAGOCYTIC SYNDROMES

Haemophagocytic syndromes result from increased proliferation of macrophage or histiocyte precursors associated with haemophagocytosis which, when marked, leads to various cytopenias. Common clinical features are hepatomegaly, splenomegaly and fever. The proliferating macrophages may be part of a malignant clone (malignant histiocytosis) (see page 98) or may be reactive (Table 2.3). Reactive haemophagocytic syndromes are commonly caused by bacterial or viral infection, occurring either in previously healthy subjects or as a terminal complication in patients with a defective immune response. Haemophagocytic syndromes are relatively common when viral or mycobacterial infections occur in patients with AIDS or with haemopoietic or other malignancy. Haemophagocytosis may also be prominent in patients with lymphoma, particularly T-cell lymphoma, when there is no evidence of infection; it is likely that in these cases there is increased proliferation of macrophage precursors and enhanced phagocytic activity in response to lymphokines secreted by the lymphoma cells. The cause of familial haemophagocytic lymphohistiocytosis remains unknown; since the cytological and histological features cannot be distinguished from those of infection-induced haemophagocytosis the diagnosis must rest on clinical differences.[52]

Malignant histiocytosis (see page 98) may be regarded as the tissue equivalent of acute monocytic leukaemia (AML of M5b type); with disease progression there is increasing bone marrow infiltration by malignant cells and increasing numbers of malignant cells appear in the peripheral blood. Phagocytosis is minor in comparison with that seen in reactive conditions.

Peripheral blood

The haemophagocytic syndromes are characterized by pancytopenia. Phagocytic macrophages are rarely present in the peripheral blood, although in malignant histiocytosis there may be small numbers of monoblasts. The blood film may also show the features of the primary condition, for example atypical lymphocytes in patients with EBV infection.

Table 2.3 Conditions associated with a haemophagocytic syndrome[12,41−52]

Malignant histiocytosis	
Reactive haemophagocytic syndromes	Induced by viral infection
	herpes viruses
	EB virus (including fatal infectious mononucleosis in
	X-linked lymphoproliferative syndrome)
	herpes simplex
	herpes zoster
	cytomegalovirus
	other viruses
	adenovirus
	measles (vaccine virus)
	influenza A[41]
	para-influenza
	vaccinia
	rubella (congenital)
	parvovirus B19[42]
	Kyasanur forest disease
	Induced by bacterial infection
	Salmonella typhi
	brucellosis
	staphylococcal,[43] streptococcal and *E. Coli*[44] infection
	legionnaires' disease (*Legionella pneumophila*)
	Mycobacterium tuberculosis
	atypical mycobacterial infection
	Induced by rickettsiae
	Rocky Mountain spotted fever
	Q fever[45]
	dengue[46]
	Induced by protozoan and other parasites
	toxoplasmosis
	leishmaniasis
	babesiosis[47]
	Induced by fungi
	histoplasmosis
	candidiasis[44]
	Associated with certain lymphomas particularly T-cell
	lymphomas[48−50]
	Kawasaki's disease
	Anticonvulsant lymphadenopathy
	Sarcoidosis[50]
	As a terminal complication in patients with various
	immunodeficiencies and malignant conditions (ALL, CLL, HD,
	NHL, hairy cell leukaemia, AML, carcinoma, Chediak−Higashi
	syndrome)−probably as a complication of infection
	In graft-versus-host disease[51]
Familial haemophagocytic lymphohistiocytosis[52]	

Bone marrow cytology

In the secondary haemophagocytic syndromes there are increased numbers of macrophages and haemophagocytosis is usually prominent with many macrophages having ingested numerous cells of various haemopoietic lineages (Fig. 2.18). The macrophages are mainly mature and lack

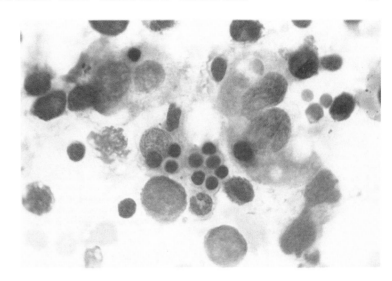

Fig. 2.18 BM aspirate, reactive haemophagocytosis in a patient with AIDS and miliary tuberculosis. MGG × 940.

atypical features. The bone marrow aspirate may also show other abnormalities due to the primary disease. For example, in viral infections there is usually an increase of lymphocytes which may be immature or atypical and in bacterial infection there is granulocytic hyperplasia with toxic changes in the neutrophil lineage. In familial haemophagocytic lymphohistiocytosis the bone marrow findings are identical to those of infection-induced haemophagocytosis. Repeated bone marrow examination may be needed to establish the diagnosis since abnormalities are detected at presentation in less than a third of patients.[52] When haemophagocytosis is secondary to a T-cell lymphoma the marrow may show closely intermingled lymphoma cells and macrophages but cases have also been reported in which the bone marrow shows only haemophagocytosis with the lymphomatous infiltrate being confined to other tissues.[49]

In malignant histiocytosis the bone marrow infiltrate may be initially very scanty. The abnormal population includes a much larger proportion of monoblasts and promonocytes while mature histiocytes are relatively less common. Phagocytic activity is not prominent.

Bone marrow histology

The marrow in secondary haemophagocytic syndromes usually shows hypoplasia of erythroid and myeloid lines; megakaryocyte numbers are either normal or increased. The degree of macrophage infiltration is variable (Fig. 2.19); in some cases it is inconspicuous, while in others there is diffuse replacement of the marrow by mature macrophages with a low nucleo-cytoplasmic ratio, dispersed chromatin, inconspicuous nucleoli and abundant cytoplasm which is often vacuolated. Haemophagocytosis is often less apparent than in marrow smears.[44,53] Features of the underlying disease may be present. Atypical lymphoid cells are seen in some cases of EBV infection. Granulomas may be present in tuberculosis[54] and a variety of other infections associated with a haemophagocytic syndrome (page 46).

In malignant histiocytosis the marrow biopsy is often normal in the early stages of the disease. Later infiltration may occur, initially focal then diffuse.

HIV INFECTION AND THE ACQUIRED IMMUNE DEFICIENCY SYNDROME (AIDS)

In infection by the human immunodeficiency virus the main indications for examination of the bone marrow are pyrexia of unknown origin and various cytopenias. It may also be required as part of a staging procedure in patients with lymphoma. A biopsy is very often useful, particularly in patients with a hypocellular aspirate. Part of any

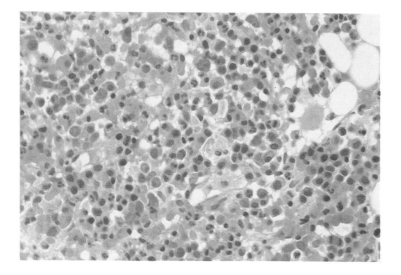

Fig. 2.19 BM trephine biopsy, AIDS, showing increased cellularity, dyserythropoiesis and numerous macrophages, some of which contain erythrocytes and apoptotic normoblasts (haemophagocytosis). Paraffin-embedded, H&E × 390.

aspirate from a febrile patient should be submitted for microbiological culture. In addition to routine stains, all biopsied tissues should be stained for acid-fast bacilli and fungi.

Peripheral blood

The earliest haematological manifestations of the human immunodeficiency virus occur at the time of primary infection when atypical lymphocytes appear in the peripheral blood, often in association with a febrile illness which clinically can resemble infectious mononucleosis. Acute infection by HIV also occasionally causes transient pancytopenia. Patients with established infection may have lymphocytosis or isolated thrombocytopenia consequent on peripheral destruction of platelets. Late in the course of the disease pancytopenia, including marked lymphopenia, is usual. Red cells may show anisocytosis and poikilocytosis. The reticulocyte count is reduced. Because of the frequency of opportunistic infections the peripheral blood may also show non-specific reactive changes such as increased rouleaux formation, left shift and toxic changes in neutrophils and the presence of immature monocytes and reactive lymphocytes. The haematological effects of the primary viral infection and secondary infections may be compounded by the effects of therapy; patients taking zidovudine

are usually markedly macrocytic and may have marked dysplastic changes in blood cells.

Bone marrow cytology

Early in the course of infection the bone marrow is of normal cellularity or, during the course of infection, shows granulocytic hyperplasia. When there is immune thrombocytopenia megakaryocyte numbers are normal or increased. Common non-specific changes are infiltration by lymphocytes and plasma cells and an increase of macrophages or eosinophils. Erythropoiesis may show mild dysplastic features such as nuclear irregularity and fragmentation. In patients taking zidovudine, erythropoiesis is megaloblastic and dyserythropoiesis is more marked; dysplastic changes such as nuclear fragmentation are also noted in the granulocytic series. With disease progression the bone marrow becomes progressively more hypocellular and aspiration becomes difficult due to increased reticulin deposition. Cachectic patients may show gelatinous transformation. Bone marrow necrosis is sometimes seen. In patients with advanced disease the bone marrow aspirate may provide evidence of miliary tuberculosis, atypical mycobacterial infection or disseminated fungal or parasitic infection. Because of the deficient host response, mycobacterial infection may be associated with the pres-

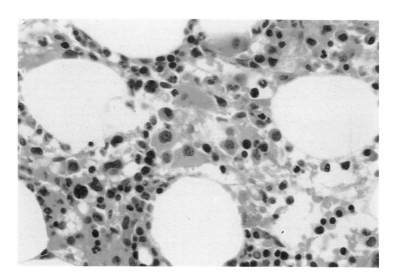

Fig. 2.20 BM trephine biopsy, AIDS showing clustering of megakaryocytes, H&E × 390.

ence of numerous bacteria within macrophages which may be foamy or may morphologically resemble Gaucher's cells. Haemophagocytic syndromes (see page 55) secondary to tuberculosis or other infections are relatively common in patients with AIDS (Fig. 2.18). Spread to the bone marrow is common when lymphoma, either Burkitt's or non-Burkitt's, complicates AIDS.

Bone marrow histology

A wide variety of non-specific reactive changes are commonly seen in HIV infection.[55–57] The cellularity is increased in approximately 40 per cent of cases, and decreased in 20–40 per cent; hypocellularity is more common in patients on zidovudine therapy. Frequently the haemopoietic marrow has an oedematous appearance with the cells being separated by clear spaces. Focal gelatinous transformation (see page 63) is seen in up to 20 per cent of cases. Dyserythropoiesis is common (Fig. 2.19); the erythroblastic islands are often large and poorly organized, and megaloblastic change may be present, particularly in patients taking zidovudine. Granulocytic hyperplasia with left shift is seen in some patients, usually in response to infection. Megakaryocytes are usually present in normal or increased numbers, bare nuclei are a frequent finding, and occasionally dysplastic forms are seen. Clustering

of megakaryocytes may occur (Fig. 2.20). Plasma cells are increased in 50–60 per cent of biopsies and lymphoid aggregates are seen in approximately one-third. The lymphoid aggregates are often large and poorly circumscribed. They consist largely of small lymphocytes, with variable numbers of plasma cells, macrophages, and eosinophils (Figs 2.21 and 2.22); sometimes there is proliferation of small vessels within the lesion. In some cases with a mixed infiltrate of lymphocytes and inflammatory cells the lesions may resemble a peripheral T lymphoma.[7] Increased reticulin is seen in the majority of cases (Fig. 2.23). Rarely, the combination of marked marrow hypercellularity, severe reticulin fibrosis and increased numbers and clustering of megakaryocytes may closely resemble the appearance of a myeloproliferative disorder.

In all cases a careful search should be made for evidence of opportunistic infections, in particular tuberculosis and atypical mycobacterial infection (see page 48), fungal infection (see Table 2.1), and protozoal diseases (leishmaniasis, toxoplasmosis and infection by *P. carinii* (see page 46). Approximately 15 per cent of biopsies contain granulomas; the commonest cause is atypical mycobacterial infection; other causes include tuberculosis, histoplasmosis, cryptococcal infection, and leishmaniasis (see page 46). Atypical mycobacteria can be cultured from the marrow in

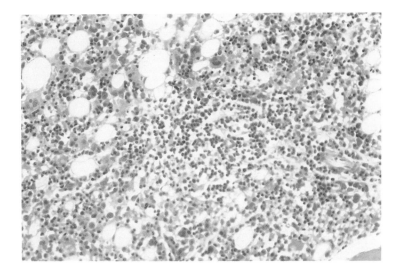

Fig. 2.21 BM trephine biopsy, AIDS showing increased cellularity and a polymorphous lymphoid aggregate (centre). Paraffin-embedded, H&E × 195.

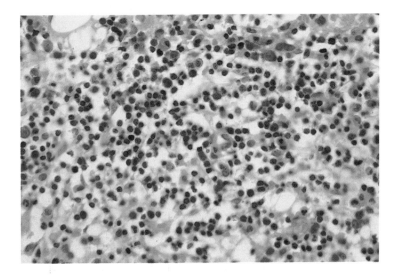

Fig. 2.22 BM trephine biopsy, AIDS showing a polymorphous lymphoid aggregate, composed of lymphocytes and small numbers of macrophages, eosinophils and plasma cells. Paraffin-embedded, H&E × 390.

up to 20 per cent of cases of AIDS. Granulomas are present in approximately 50 per cent of culture-positive cases and acid-fast bacilli can be seen on special stains in 60 per cent. Atypical mycobacteria may be seen in biopsies in the absence of granulomas, usually within macrophages scattered throughout the marrow; occasionally cells which morphologically resemble Gaucher cells (see page 234) are seen. Focal areas of epithelioid angiomatosis have been observed in the marrow of an HIV-positive patient with bacillary angiomatosis, an infective condition consequent on infection with a Rickettsia-like organism; it is likely that a Warthin–Starry stain would demonstrate the causative organisms although it was not applied to the marrow in this case.[58]

Marrow involvement is common in non-Hodgkin's lymphoma associated with AIDS. These are almost always high-grade lymphomas, either Burkitt's lymphoma or large cell lymphoma of B lineage. Infiltration is diffuse (see Fig. 5.38). Metastatic Kaposi's sarcoma occurs but is rare.[59]

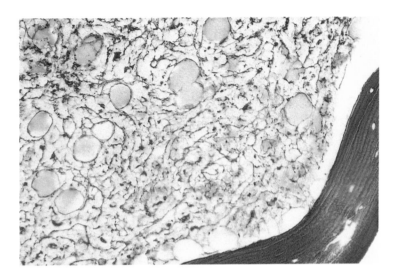

Fig. 2.23 BM trephine biopsy, AIDS, showing reticulin fibrosis (grade 3). Paraffin-embedded, Gordon–Sweet stain × 195.

BONE MARROW NECROSIS

Bone marrow necrosis indicates the death of bone marrow stromal cells and haemopoietic cells. There may be associated death of bone cells and of bone. Bone marrow necrosis results from impairment of the blood supply, often in association with a hypercellular marrow. Causes are multiple (Table 2.4). Necrosis is followed either by haemopoietic regeneration with small fibrotic scars or occasionally by extensive fibrosis. Bone marrow necrosis commonly occurs at multiple sites. Clinical features include bone pain and fever.

Peripheral blood

If bone marrow necrosis is extensive, pancytopenia occurs. The blood film shows leucoerythroblastic features. Recovery is associated with a rise in the reticulocyte count and recovery of haemoglobin, platelets and white cells.

Bone marrow cytology

A bone marrow aspirate is often macroscopically abnormal. It is sometimes opaque and whitish and sometimes reddish-purple. The stained film shows amorphous pink-staining material in which the faint outlines of necrotic cells can be seen (Fig. 2.24). Necrotic nuclei appear as darker-staining smudges. Some intact cells may also be present.

Bone marrow necrosis is more often noted in bone marrow trephine sections than in aspirates. This may be partly because a larger volume is sampled and partly because necrotic cells mixed with intact cells in an aspirate are often dismissed as an artefact.

Bone marrow histology

The appearances depend to some extent on the condition underlying the necrosis. In cases in which the necrosis is secondary to infiltration by leukaemia or lymphoma (Fig. 2.25) low-power examination may reveal hypercellularity and loss of fat cells. In the early stages there is nuclear pyknosis and the cells have granular cytoplasm with indistinct margins. Later there is nuclear karyorrhexis and complete loss of cell outlines. Finally, all that remains is amorphous eosinophilic debris. Marrow necrosis is often accompanied by necrosis of the adjacent bone. In some patients the necrosis is very extensive and biopsy of several different sites may be necessary before a diagnostic sample is obtained. Necrotic marrow eventually repopulates with haemopoietic cells; the only signs of previous necrosis are small areas of fibrous scarring around bony trabeculae that have lost osteocytes.[63] Occasionally there is extensive fibrosis (Fig. 2.26).

Table 2.4 Causes of bone marrow necrosis[12,60–62]

Relatively common associations	Sickle cell anaemia and haemoglobin S/C disease (particularly during pregnancy) Acute myeloid leukaemia Acute lymphoblastic leukaemia Metastatic carcinoma Caisson disease

Less common associations	Chronic granulocytic leukaemia
	Lymphoma
	Chronic lymphocytic leukaemia
	Multiple myeloma
	Malignant histiocytosis
	Myelofibrosis
	Other haemoglobinopathies (S/D, S/β thalassaemia and sickle cell trait)
	Megaloblastic anaemia plus infection
	Acute haemolytic anaemia
	Embolism of the bone marrow, e.g. by vegetations from cardiac valves or tumour embolism[60]
	Disseminated intravascular coagulation
	Hyperparathyroidism
	Systemic lupus erythematosus[61]
	Infections
	  Typhoid fever
	  Gram-positive infections, e.g. streptococcus, staphylococcus
	  Gram-negative infections, e.g. *E. coli*
	  Diphtheria
	  Miliary tuberculosis
	  Cytomegalovirus[62]
	  Q fever
	  Mucormycosis
	  Histoplasmosis

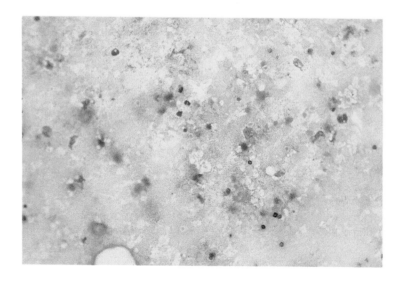

Fig. 2.24 BM aspirate, bone marrow necrosis, showing amorphous debris containing karyorrhectic nuclei. MGG × 940.

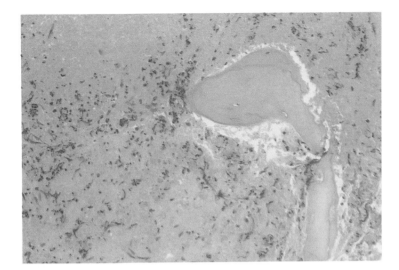

Fig. 2.25 BM trephine biopsy, necrosis in a marrow infiltrated by high-grade lymphoma. Note the necrosis of both the lymphoma cells infiltrating the marrow and of osteocytes within the bone trabecula. Paraffin-embedded, H&E × 195.

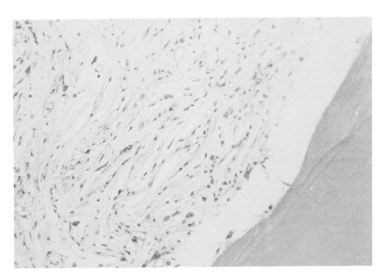

Fig. 2.26 BM trephine biopsy. Repair following marrow necrosis, showing collagen fibrosis. Paraffin-embedded, H&E × 188.

GELATINOUS TRANSFORMATION

Gelatinous transformation, also known as serous degeneration or serous atrophy, is a condition in which there is loss of fat cells and haemopoietic cells from the bone marrow with these cells being replaced by an increased amount of in ground substance. Common causes include anorexia nervosa and cachexia due to chronic debilitating illnesses such as carcinoma and tuberculosis or other chronic infection. The condition has also been observed in AIDS and in association with renal failure, coeliac disease[64] and severe hypo-thyroidism.[65] It occurs at sites exposed to high-dose X-irradiation. Gelatinous transformation can also develop rapidly and is seen in acute severe illnesses with multiple organ failure[6] and in severe acute infections.

Peripheral blood

The peripheral blood shows variable cytopenia, often pancytopenia. In patients with anorexia nervosa acanthocytes are seen but their presence has not been noted in other patients with gelatinous transformation.

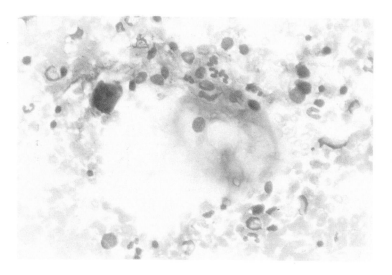

Fig. 2.27 BM aspirate, gelatinous transformation, showing amorphous purplish-pink material. MGG × 377.

Bone marrow cytology

The aspirate may not spread normally on film preparation. It contains amorphous material, sometimes fibrillar or finely granular, which is composed of acid muco-polysaccharide with a high content of hyaluronic acid. On Romanowsky stains it is pink or pinkish-purple (Fig. 2.27). This abnormal ground substance is weakly positive on a periodic acid-Schiff stain, the reaction being diastase resistant. Positive staining also occurs with alcian blue; this reaction is stronger at pH 2.5 than pH 1.[6] A toluidine blue stain is weakly positive.

Bone marrow histology

The changes are usually focal; less commonly the whole of a biopsy section is affected. There is atrophy of fat cells, which are both reduced in number and of variable size, and in the affected areas there is a mild to marked hypoplasia of haemopoietic cells. Both fat and haemopoietic cells are replaced by amorphous material which on an H&E stain has a light blue to pale pink colour and a finely granular appearance (Fig. 2.28). Its other staining characteristics are identical to those seen on marrow smears (see above).

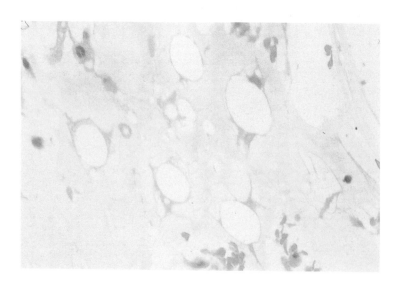

Fig. 2.28 BM trephine biopsy, gelatinous transformation, showing replacement of haemopoietic marrow and fat cells by amorphous pink material. H&E × 390.

BONE MARROW FIBROSIS

Bone marrow fibrosis indicates an increase of reticulin or of reticulin and collagen in the bone marrow. Such fibrosis may be focal or generalized. Reticulin and collagen deposition are graded 0 to ++++ as shown in Table 1.4. Some patients with grade ++++ fibrosis also have osteosclerosis. Increased reticulin formation and even collagen deposition can revert to normal if the causative condition is amenable to treatment.

An increase in bone marrow reticulin is common and is a useful non-specific indication that the marrow is abnormal. It is also of some use in differential diagnosis; for example, it may be increased in hypoplastic acute myeloid leukaemia but is not increased in aplastic anaemia.

Collagen deposition is uncommon and of greater diagnostic significance than an increase in reticulin. It is therefore useful to distinguish between these two degrees of abnormality, either by grading the fibrosis or by using the terms 'reticulin fibrosis' for a grade +++ abnormality and 'fibrosis' or 'myelofibrosis' for a grade ++++ abnormality. Causes of bone marrow fibrosis are shown in Table 2.5.

Table 2.5 Causes of grade 4 bone marrow fibrosis[12,66]

Generalized myelofibrosis	Malignant disease
	Primary (idiopathic) myelofibrosis* (myelofibrosis with myeloid metaplasia)
	Myelofibrosis secondary to essential thrombocythaemia or polycythaemia rubra vera*
	Chronic granulocytic leukaemia*
	Transitional myeloproliferative syndrome
	Acute megakaryoblastic leukaemia*
	Other acute myeloid leukaemias
	Acute lymphoblastic leukaemia[67]
	Systemic mastocytosis*
	The myelodysplastic syndromes (particularly secondary MDS)
	Paroxysmal nocturnal haemoglobinuria
	Hodgkin's disease
	Non-Hodgkin's lymphoma
	Multiple myeloma
	Waldenström's macroglobulinaemia
	Secondary carcinoma*
	Bone diseases
	Marble bone disease — osteopetrosis
	Primary and secondary hyperparathyroidism
	Nutritional and renal rickets (vitamin D deficiency)
	Osteomalacia
	Miscellaneous
	Tuberculosis
	Other granulomatous diseases
	Grey platelet syndrome
	Systemic lupus erythematosus
	Systemic sclerosis
	Prior thorium dioxide administration
Focal or localized	Osteomyelitis
	Paget's disease
	Following bone marrow necrosis
	Following irradiation of the bone marrow
	Adult T-cell leukaemia/lymphoma
	Healing fracture
	Site of previous trephine biopsy

* Osteosclerosis may also occur.

Peripheral blood

Bone marrow fibrosis is commonly associated with a leucoerythroblastic anaemia; red cells show anisocytosis and poikilocytosis with tear drop poikilocytes often being prominent. When fibrosis is extensive there may also be thrombocytopenia and leucopenia. The blood may also show abnormalities related to the primary disease which has caused the fibrosis. When bone marrow fibrosis has developed acutely, as in acute megakaryoblastic leukaemia, there may be little anisocytosis and poikilocytosis and the blood film is not necessarily leucoerythroblastic.

Bone marrow cytology

Bone marrow fibrosis often leads to failure to aspirate marrow or to aspiration of peripheral blood or a diluted marrow specimen. Otherwise the aspirate may show carcinoma cells or the specific features of the primary disease which has led to the fibrosis. If there is associated osteosclerosis the aspirate may contain increased numbers of osteoblasts and osteoclasts.

Bone marrow histology

The appearances of primary myelofibrosis (myelofibrosis with myeloid metaplasia) are described on page 114. In secondary fibrosis findings range from a mild increase of fibroblasts and the presence of scattered collagen fibres to a dense fibrosis which obliterates normal haemopoietic tissue. An increase of reticulin can be suspected on an H&E stain by the distortion and angularity of fat cells and by the 'streaming' of haemopoietic cells held between parallel reticulin fibres. Fibrosis may also be suspected when vascular channels, which normally are collapsed, are held open. Increased reticulin deposition is confirmed by a silver impregnation technique such as the Gomori stain. Collagen fibres are detected as eosinophilic fibres which may be in bundles. The oval nuclei of fibroblasts are apparent in relation to the collagen fibres. It is important not to confuse either endothelial cells of collapsed capillaries or mast cells with fibroblasts. The presence of collagen is confirmed by a trichrome stain. The distribution of reticulin and collagen within the marrow depends on the causative condition. In hyperparathyroidism fibrosis is paratrabecular. When associated with a myeloproliferative disorder or with the grey platelet syndrome fibrosis may be spatially related to megakaryocytes.

REFERENCES

1 Farooqui BJ, Khurshid M, Ashfaq MK and Khan MA (1991) Comparative yield of salmonella typhi from blood and bone marrow cultures in patients with fever of unknown origin. *J Clin Pathol*, **44**, 258–259.

2 Rausing A (1973) Bone marrow biopsy in the diagnosis of Whipple's disease. *Acta Med Scand*, **193**, 5–8.

3 Schmid C, Frisch B, Beham A, Jager K and Kettner G (1990) Comparison of bone marrow histology in early chronic granulocytic leukaemia and in leukaemoid reaction. *Eur J Haematol*, **44**, 154–158.

4 Thiele J, Holgado S, Choritz H and Georgii A (1983) Density distribution and size of megakaryocytes in inflammatory reaction of the bone marrow (myelitis) and chronic myeloproliferative disorders. *Scand J Haematol*, **31**, 329–341.

5 Hyun BH, Kwa D, Gabaldon H and Ashton JK (1976) Reactive plasmacytic lesions of the bone marrow. *Am J Clin Pathol*, **65**, 921–928.

6 Amos RJ, Deane M, Ferguson C, Jeffries G, Hinds CJ and Amess JAL (1990) Observations on the haemopoietic response to critical illness. *J Clin Pathol*, **43**, 850–856.

7 Brunning RD. Bone marrow. In: *Ackerman's Surgical Pathology*, 7th edition, volume 2, Rosai J (ed). C.V. Mosby, St Louis, 1989.

8 Piehl MR, Kaplan RL and Haber MH (1988) Disseminated penicilliosis in a patient with acquired immunodeficiency syndrome. *Arch Pathol Lab Med*, **112**, 1262–1264.

9 Grimes MM, La Pook JD, Bar MH, Wasserman HS and Dwork A (1987) Disseminated *Pneumocystis carinii* infection in a patient with acquired immunodeficiency syndrome. *Hum Pathol*, **18**, 307–308.

10 Telsak EE, Cote RJ, Gold JMW, Campbell SW and Armstrong D (1990) Extrapulmonary *Pneumocystis carinii* infections. *Reviews of Infectious Diseases*, **12**, 380–386.

11 Bodem CR, Hamory BH, Taylor HM and Kleopfer L (1983) Granulomatous bone marrow disease. A review of the literature and clinicopathological analysis of 58 cases. *Medicine (Baltimore)*, **62**, 372–383.

12 Bain BJ and Wickramasinghe SNW. Pathology of the bone marrow: general considerations. In: *Systemic Pathology, Blood and Bone Marrow,*

Wickramasinghe SNW (ed), Symmers W St C (series ed). Churchill Livingstone, Edinburgh, 1986.

13 Vilalta-Castel E, Váldes-Sanchez MD, Guerra-Vales JM, et al. (1988) Significance of granulomas in bone marrow: a study of 40 cases. Eur J Haematol, 41, 12–14.

14 Epstein HD and Kruskall MS (1988) Spurious leukopenia due to in vitro granulocyte aggregation. Am J Clin Pathol, 89, 652–655.

15 Ampel NM, Ryan KJ, Carry PJ, Wieden MA and Schifman RB (1986) Fungemia due to Coccidioides immitis. An analysis of 16 episodes in 15 patients and a review of the literature. Medicine (Baltimore), 65, 312–321.

16 Hyun BH. Colour Atlas of Clinical Hematology. Igaka-Shoin Med US, New York, 1986.

17 Poland GA and Love KR (1986) Marked atypical lymphocytosis, hepatitis, and skin rash in sulfasalazine drug allergy. Am J Med, 81, 707–708.

18 Pelstring RJ, Kim K, Lower EE and Swerdlow SH (1988) Marrow granulomas in coal workers' pneumoconiosis. Am J Clin Pathol, 89, 553–556.

19 Lewis JH, Sundeen JT, Simon GL, et al. (1985) Disseminated talc granulomatosis: acquired immunodeficiency syndrome and fatal cytomegalovirus infection. Arch Pathol Lab Med, 109, 147–150.

20 Davis S and Trubowitz S. Pathologic reactions involving the bone marrow. In: The Human Bone Marrow: Anatomy, Physiology and Pathophysiology, volume 2, Trubowitz S and Davis S (eds). CRC Press, Boca Raton, 1982.

21 Rywlin AM and Ortega R (1971) Lipid granulomas of the bone marrow. Am J Clin Pathol, 57, 457–462.

22 Hudson P and Robertson GM (1966) Demonstration of mineral oil in splenic lipid granulomas. Lab Invest, 15, 1134–1135.

23 Pease GL (1956) Granulomatous lesions in bone marrow. Blood, 11, 720–734.

24 Farhi DC, Mason UG and Horsburgh CR (1984) The bone marrow in disseminated Mycobacterium avium intracellulare infection. Am J Clin Pathol, 83, 463–468.

25 Lawrence C and Schreiber AJ (1979) Leprosy's footprints in bone marrow histiocytes. N Eng J Med, 300, 834–835.

26 Okun DB, Sun NCJ and Tanaka KR (1979) Bone marrow granulomas in Q-fever. Am J Clin Pathol, 71, 117–121.

27 Kurtin PJ, McKinsey DS, Gupta MR and Driks M (1989) Histoplasmosis in patients with acquired immunodeficiency syndrome. Hematologic and bone marrow manifestations. Am J Clin Pathol, 93, 367–372.

28 Kadin ME, Donaldson SS and Dorfman RF (1970) Isolated granulomas in Hodgkin's Disease. N Eng J Med, 283, 859–861.

29 Yu NC and Rywlin AM (1982) Granulomatous lesions of the bone marrow in non-Hodgkin's lymphoma. Hum Pathol, 13, 905–910.

30 Browne PM, Sharma OP and Salkin D (1978) Bone marrow sarcoidosis. JAMA 240, 2654–2655.

31 Faulkner-Jones BE, Howie AJ, Boughton BJ and Franklin IM (1988) Lymphoid aggregates in bone marrow: study of eventual outcome. J Clin Pathol, 41, 768–775.

32 Rywlin AM, Ortega RS and Dominguez CJ (1974) Lymphoid nodules of bone marrow. Blood, 43, 389–400.

33 Sangster G, Crocker J, Nar P and Leylan MJ (1986) Benign and malignant (B cell) focal lymphoid aggregates in bone marrow trephines shown by means of an immunogold-silver technique. J Clin Pathol, 39, 453–457.

34 Farhi DC (1989) Germinal centres in the bone marrow. Hematol Pathol, 3, 133–136.

35 Klein H and Block M (1953) Bone marrow plasmacytosis. Blood, 8, 1034–1041.

36 Crocker J and Curran RC (1981) Quantitative study of the immunoglobulin-containing cells in trephine samples of bone marrow. J Clin Pathol, 34, 1080–1082.

37 Peart KM and Ellis HA (1972) Quantitative observations on iliac crest bone marrow mast cells in chronic renal failure. J Clin Pathol, 28, 947–955.

38 Yoo D, Lessin LS and Jensen WN (1978) Bone marrow mast cells in lymphoproliferative disorders. Ann Intern Med, 88, 753–757.

39 Prokimer M and Polliack A (1980) Increased bone marrow mast cells in preleukemic syndromes, acute leukaemia, and lymphoproliferative disorders. Am J Clin Pathol, 75, 34–38.

40 Rywlin AM, Hoffman EP and Ortega RS (1972) Eosinophilic fibrohistiocytic lesions of bone marrow: a new morphologic finding probably related to drug hypersensitivity. Blood, 40, 464–472.

41 Potter MN, Foot ABM and Oakhill A (1991) Influenza A and virus-associated haemophagocytic syndrome: cluster of three cases in children with acute leukaemia. J Clin Pathol, 44, 297–299.

42 Komp DM, Buckley PJ, McNamara J and van Hoff J (1989) Soluble interleukin-2 receptors in hemophagocytic histiocytosis. Pediatr Hematol Oncol, 6, 253–264.

43 Manoharan A and Catovsky D. Histiocytic medullary reticulosis revisited. In: Haematology and Blood Transfusion, volume 27, Disorders of the Monocyte Macrophage System, Schmalzl F, Huhn D and Schaefer HE (eds). Springer-Verlag, Berlin, 1981.

44 Risdall RJ, Brunning RD, Hernandez JI and Gordon DH (1984) Bacteria associated hemophagocytic syndrome. Cancer, 54, 2968–2972.

45 Estrov Z, Bruck R, Shtalrid M, Berrebi A and Resnitzky P (1983) Histiocytic hemophagocytosis in Q-fever. *Arch Pathol Lab Med*, **108**, 7.

46 Nelson ER, Bierman HR and Chulajata R (1966) Hematologic phagocytosis in postmortem bone marrow of dengue hemorrhagic fever. *Am J Med Sci*, **252**, 68–74.

47 Auerbach M, Haubenstock A and Soloman G (1980) Systemic babebiosis. Another cause of the hemophagocytic syndrome. *Am J Med*, **80**, 301–303.

48 Jaffe ES, Costa J and Fauci AS (1981) Erythrophagocytic Tγ lymphoma. *New Engl J Med*, **305**, 103–104.

49 Chan E, Pi D, Chan GT, Todd D and Ho FC (1989) Peripheral T-cell lymphoma presenting as hemophagocytic syndrome. *Hematol Oncol*, **7**, 275–285.

50 Sonneveld P, van Lom K, Kappers-Klunne M, Prins MER and Abels J (1990) Clinico-pathological diagnosis and treatment of malignant histiocytosis. *Br J Haematol*, **75**, 511–516.

51 Janka GE (1989) Familial hemophagocytic lymphohistiocytosis: diagnostic problems and differential diagnosis. *Pediatr Hematol Oncol*, **6**, 219–226.

52 Aricó M, Caselli D and Burgio GR (1989) Familial hemophagocytic lymphohistiocytosis: clinical features. *Pediatr Hematol Oncol*, **6**, 247–251.

53 Risdall RJ, McKenna RW, Nesbitt ME, *et al.* (1979) Virus-associated hemophagocytic syndrome: a benign histiocytic proliferation distinct from malignant histiocytosis. *Cancer*, **44**, 993–1002.

54 Campo E, Condom E, Miro M-J, Cid M-C and Romagosa V (1986) Tuberculosis associated haemophagocytic syndrome. *Cancer*, **58**, 2640–2645.

55 Osborne BM, Guarda LA and Butler JJ (1984) Bone marrow biopsies in the acquired immunodeficiency syndrome. *Hum Pathol*, **15**, 1048–1053.

56 Scheider DR and Picker LJ (1985) Myelodysplasia in the acquired immunodeficiency syndrome. *Am J Clin Pathol*, **84**, 144–152.

57 Castella A, Croxson TS, Mildvan D, Witt DH and Zalusky R (1985) The bone marrow in AIDS. *Am J Clin Pathol*, **84**, 425–432.

58 Relman DA, Loutit JS, Schmidt TM, Falkow S and Tompkins LS (1990) The agent of bacillary angiomatosis—an approach to the identification of uncultured pathogens. *New Engl J Med*, **323**, 1573–1580.

59 Karcher DS and Frost AR (1991) The bone marrow in human immunodeficiency virus (HIV)-related disease: morphology and clinical correlation. *Am J Clin Pathol*, **95**, 63–71.

60 Laso F-J, González-Diaz M, Paz J-I and De Castro S (1983) Bone marrow necrosis associated with tumor emboli and disseminated intravascular coagulation. *Arch Intern Med*, **143**, 2220.

61 Upchurch KS (1988) Case records of the Massachusetts General Hospital. Case 38–1988. *New Engl J Med*, **319**, 768–781.

62 Rustgi VK, Sacher RA, O'Brien P and Garagusi VF (1983) Fatal disseminated cytomegalovirus infection in an apparently normal adult. *Arch Intern Med*, **143**, 372–373.

63 Kiraly JF and Wheby MS (1976) Bone marrow necrosis. *Am J Med*, **60**, 361–368.

64 Clarke BE, Brown DJ and Xipell JM (1983) Gelatinous transformation of the bone marrow. *Pathology*, **15**, 85–88.

65 Savage RA and Sipple C (1987) Marrow myxedema: gelatinous transformation of marrow ground substance in a patient with severe hypothyroidism. *Arch Pathol Lab Med*, **111**, 375–377.

66 McCarthy DM (1985) Fibrosis of the bone marrow: content and causes. *Br J Haematol*, **59**, 1–7.

67 Hann IM, Evans DIK, Marsden HB, Jones PM and Palmer MK (1978) Bone marrow fibrosis in acute lymphoblastic leukaemia of childhood. *J Clin Pathol*, **31**, 313–315.

3: Acute Myeloid Leukaemia, the Myelodysplastic Syndromes and Malignant Histiocytosis

Acute myeloid leukaemia (AML) is a disease resulting from the neoplastic proliferation of a clone of myeloid cells characterized by uncoupling of proliferation and maturation. The leukaemic clone may be derived from a pluripotent stem cell (capable of giving rise to both myeloid and lymphoid lineages), from a multipotent stem cell (capable of giving rise to more than one myeloid lineage) or from a committed precursor cell (for example, one capable of giving rise only to granulocyte and monocyte lineages). Normal haemopoietic marrow is largely replaced by immature myeloid cells, mainly blast cells, which show a limited ability to differentiate into mature cells of the different myeloid lineages. Pancytopenia is common, as a result both of the replacement of normal bone marrow and of the defective capacity for maturation of the leukaemic clone.

The myelodysplastic syndromes (MDS) resemble acute myeloid leukaemia in that normal polyclonal haemopoietic bone marrow is largely replaced by a neoplastic clone, usually derived from a multipotent stem cell. The neoplastic clone is characterized by defective maturation so that haemopoiesis is usually both morphologically dysplastic and functionally ineffective. In the great majority of patients with MDS the bone marrow is hypercellular but there is increased intramedullary death of haemopoietic precursors leading to defective production of mature cells of one or more haemopoietic lineages; this process, which leads to anaemia, cytopenia or both, is what is meant by ineffective haemopoiesis. In the MDS, as in AML, there is imbalance between proliferation and maturation but the degree of abnormality is less than in AML so that the proportion of blast cells is lower. The neoplastic clone in MDS shows a tendency to clonal evolu-

tion; emergence of a subclone with more 'malignant' characteristics may be manifest clinically as transformation to acute leukaemia. The myelodysplastic syndromes may therefore be regarded as preleukaemic conditions.

Acute myeloid leukaemia

AML is a heterogeneous disease. In different patients the leukaemic clone shows differing patterns of differentiation and maturation.[1,2] An international co-operative group, the FAB (French–American–British) group have devised a classification of acute myeloid leukaemia which is now widely accepted. It is based on differentiation shown (for example: granulocytic, monocytic, erythroid, megakaryocytic) and the extent of maturation (for example: myeloblast, promyelocyte, granulocyte). Both differentiation and maturation are assessed on the basis of the predominant cell types in peripheral blood and bone marrow. The FAB classification is summarized in Table 3.1.

Acute myeloid leukaemia occurs at all ages but becomes increasingly common with advancing age. The incidence rises from one to 10/100 000/ year between the ages of 20 and 70. The incidence is somewhat higher in men than in women.

The different categories of AML have many clinical features in common but some differences. Some degree of hepatomegaly and splenomegaly are common in AML, particularly in those categories with a prominent monocytic component (M5 and, to a lesser extent, M4 AML.) Lymphadenopathy and infiltration of the skin, the gums and the tonsils are also more common in AML with a prominent monocytic component. As a consequence of pancytopenia patients commonly exhibit pallor and bruises and show susceptibility

Table 3.1 The FAB classification of acute myeloid leukaemia[1,2]

Criteria for diagnosis of AML	FAB category	Criteria for classification as specific FAB subtype of AML		Equivalent name
	M1	• Blasts ≥ 90% of bone marrow NEC (non-erythroid cells) • ≥ 3% of blasts MPO- or SBB-positive • Maturing monocytic component in bone marrow ≤ 10% • Maturing granulocytic component in bone marrow ≤ 10%		Acute myeloblastic leukaemia without maturation
	M2	• Blasts 30–89% of BM NEC • BM maturing granulocytic component ≥ 10% NEC • BM monocytic component ≤ 20% of NEC and other criteria of M4 not met		Acute myeloblastic leukaemia with maturation
	M3	• Characteristic morphology		Acute promyelocytic leukaemia
Blasts ≥ 30% of bone marrow cells*	M3v	• Characteristic morphology		Variant form of acute promyelocytic leukaemia
≥ 3% of blasts SBB or MPO positive†	M4	• Blasts ≥ 30% of BM NEC • Granulocytic component ≥ 20% of BM NEC • Monocytic component ≥ 20% of BM NEC and *either* PB monocytes ≥ 5 × 10⁹/l *or* BM like M2 but PB monocytes ≥ 5 × 10⁹/l and cytochemical proof of monocytic differentiation		Acute myelomonocytic leukaemia
	M5a	• Blasts ≥ 30% of NEC • BM monocytic component ≥ 80% of NEC	• Monoblasts ≥ 80% of BM monocytic component	Acute monoblastic leukaemia
	M5b		• Monoblasts < 80% of BM monocytic component	Acute monocytic leukaemia
	M6	• Erythroid cells ≥ 50% of BM cells • BM blasts ≥ 30% of NEC		Acute erythroleukaemia
	M7	• Blasts shown to be predominantly megakaryoblasts		Acute megakaryoblastic leukaemia
	M0	• < 3% of blasts MPO or SBB positive • Lymphoid markers negative • Immunological or ultrastructural evidence of myeloid differentiation		Acute myeloid leukaemia with minimal evidence of myeloid differentiation

* Except in some M3 and some M6.
† Except in M0 and some M5a.

to infection. A more marked bleeding tendency is usual in acute promyelocytic leukaemia (M3 AML), in which disseminated intravascular coagulation (DIC) is a frequent feature.

The different categories of AML have certain haematological features in common although the morphological features of the predominant leukaemic cells differ. Normocytic normochromic anaemia, neutropenia and thrombocytopenia are common. The total white cell count is usually elevated as a consequence of the presence of circulating leukaemic cells but some patients have a normal or low total count with few circulating leukaemic cells. A normal or low count is most often observed in M3 and M7 AML. M7 AML commonly presents with the features of acute myelofibrosis, that is with pancytopenia, few circulating immature cells and a bone marrow which, as a consequence of bone marrow fibrosis, cannot be aspirated. (However, not all cases of acute myelofibrosis are examples of M7 AML.)

The blood film and bone marrow aspirate features are of prime importance in the diagnosis of AML. The bone marrow biopsy is of secondary importance except in those cases in which an adequate aspirate cannot be obtained. Assignment to a FAB category is most readily performed on the basis of the blood and aspirate findings and is not always straightforward on tissue sections. It may also be impossible on tissue sections to distinguish M1 and M0 AML from ALL unless immunohistochemistry is employed.

ACUTE MYELOBLASTIC LEUKAEMIA
(M1 AND M2 AML)

The term acute myeloblastic leukaemia indicates leukaemia in which lineage commitment (differentiation) is to one of the granulocyte lineages, usually the neutrophil lineage. Cases can be divided between the FAB categories M1 and M2, depending on whether leukaemic cells are predominantly myeloblasts or whether, alternatively, further maturation to promyelocytes and later cells is occurring (see Table 3.1).

Peripheral blood

Anaemia, thrombocytopenia and a high white cell count are usual. Neutropenia is common in M1 AML but cases of M2 AML may have a normal or high neutrophil count. The majority of cases have considerable numbers of circulating myeloblasts. These are large cells, usually about twice the diameter of an erythrocyte. They have a high nucleo-cytoplasmic ratio. The nucleus has a diffuse chromatin pattern and one or more nucleoli. The cytoplasm is weakly or moderately basophilic and may contain scanty azurophilic granules. In some cases, particularly but not exclusively M2, the blasts contain Auer rods; these are cytoplasmic crystals formed by fusion of primary granules with which they share staining characteristics. In M2 the peripheral blood may also contain morphologically abnormal promyelocytes and other maturing cells. Occasional patients with M2 AML have eosinophilia or basophilia.

Various subtypes of AML, characterized by specific chromosomal abnormalities, are included within the FAB M1 and M2 categories.[3] Of these the commonest is M2 AML associated with t(8;21); peripheral blood features in this condition include the presence of large blasts with basophilic cytoplasm and often a single long thin Auer rod, and the presence of morphologically abnormal maturing cells. A much less common subtype is that associated with t(6;9) in which blasts are of basophil lineage; the peripheral blood basophil count is commonly elevated and blasts often contain Auer rods.

Bone marrow cytology

The bone marrow is markedly hypercellular. Numbers of megakaryocytes and developing erythroid cells are usually reduced. In M1 AML the bone marrow is almost totally replaced by myeloblasts, some of which may contain scanty granules or Auer rods (Fig. 3.1). In M2 AML myeloblasts are relatively less numerous and there are considerable numbers of maturing cells (Fig. 3.2). Many of these are morphologically abnormal and often difficult to categorize; abnormalities include hypogranularity, bizarre nuclear shapes and the presence of Auer rods, not only in blasts but sometimes also in promyelocytes, myelocytes and neutrophils. In some cases of M2 AML the maturing granulocytic component includes or is comprised of basophils or

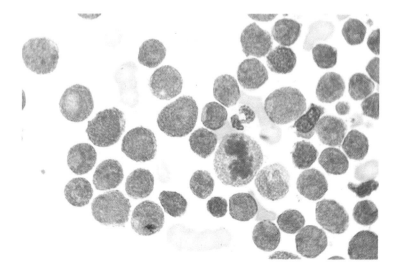

Fig. 3.1 BM aspirate, M1 AML. Note that some of the blasts resemble lymphoblasts in that they are small and round with a high nucleo-cytoplasmic ratio and no granules. The presence of an agranular neutrophil and occasional blasts with granules suggests the correct diagnosis. MGG × 940.

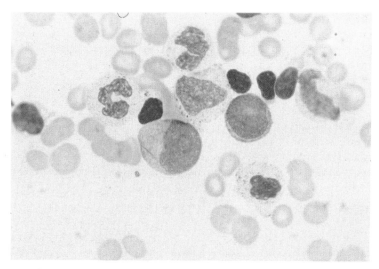

Fig. 3.2 BM aspirate, M2 AML, showing two myeloblasts, one of which contains a long slender Auer rod, and abnormal maturing cells. MGG × 940.

eosinophils. In both M1 and M2 AML the erythrocytes and megakaryocytes may show dysplastic features.

In M2 AML associated with t(8;21) the bone marrow, in addition to maturing cells of neutrophil lineage, commonly shows increased eosinophils; these are usually cytologically normal. Erythroid cells and megakaryocytes do not show dysplastic features. In M2 AML associated with t(6;9) the bone marrow commonly shows not only blasts of basophil lineage but also increased numbers of mature basophils; there is often associated myelodysplasia. In M2 AML associated

with 12p- blasts are also of basophil lineage but there is very little maturation so that they may appear undifferentiated by light microscopy.

The myeloid nature of M2 AML is evident from the features of differentiation observable in MGG stained films but in M1 AML cytochemical staining[4] is often necessary to confirm the diagnosis. Either a myeloperoxidase (MPO) or a Sudan black B (SBB) stain must be positive in at least three per cent of blasts to satisfy the FAB criteria of AML;[1] usually both stains are positive. These stains are also very useful in identifying Auer rods and reveal their presence in some cases in

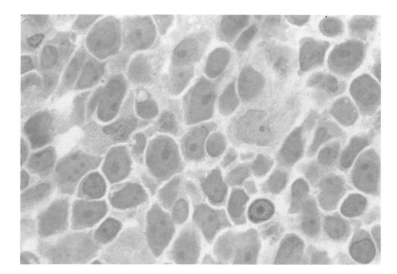

Fig. 3.3 Section of BM trephine biopsy, M1 AML. There is a relatively uniform population of small blasts with a high nucleo-cytoplasmic ratio and prominent nucleoli. Plastic-embedded, H&E ×970.

which they are not identifiable in the MGG stain. A naphthol AS-D chloroacetate esterase stain is also positive in myeloblasts in the majority of cases of M1 and M2 AML. Metachromatic staining with toluidine blue or SBB is useful in the diagnosis of cases with basophil differentiation but with little maturation, for example cases of M2Baso AML associated with 12p-.

Bone marrow histology

The marrow is markedly hypercellular (greater than 95 per cent cells) in most cases. Often the cellularity seen in the biopsy sections is greater than that estimated from aspirated fragments in films.[5] The morphology of the neoplastic cells in tissue sections is different from that seen in smears of aspirates. In tissue sections myeloblasts have large round to oval nuclei, delicate chromatin, one or more small well-defined nucleoli and scant basophilic cytoplasm (Fig. 3.3). In a half to two-thirds of all cases there is a dense homogeneous infiltrate of blasts, whereas in the remainder there is a mixture of blasts, more mature haemopoietic cells and inflammatory cells such as plasma cells, lymphocytes and mast cells.[5,6] Evidence of maturation is often apparent in M2 AML. Leder's chloroacetate esterase stain is usually positive in M2 AML, but is often negative in M1 AML. Dysplastic changes are commonly detected in megakaryocytes and erythroid

precursors (see page 90). In M2 AML associated with t(8;21) there is often a prominent infiltrate of eosinophils scattered amongst the blasts. Reticulin fibrosis is present in up to a third of cases,[7] but collagen fibrosis is rare. Areas of bone marrow necrosis are sometimes present. Following chemotherapy the marrow is hypoplastic and often shows necrosis, stromal oedema and gelatinous change. Residual leukaemic cells are often more apparent in tissue sections than in aspirate smears. However, they can be difficult to distinguish from foci of immature regenerating granulocytic or erythroid precursors.

ACUTE (HYPERGRANULAR) PROMYELOCYTIC LEUKAMIA (M3 AML)

The majority of cases of acute promyelocytic leukaemia have hypergranular promyelocytes and are therefore designated acute hypergranular promyelocytic leukaemia or M3 AML. The minority of cases have abnormal promyelocytes which are either microgranular or hypogranular when examined by light microscopy; such cases are referred to as the variant form of acute promyelocytic leukaemia or M3 variant.

Peripheral blood

In M3 AML the peripheral blood white cell count is not usually greatly elevated and the number

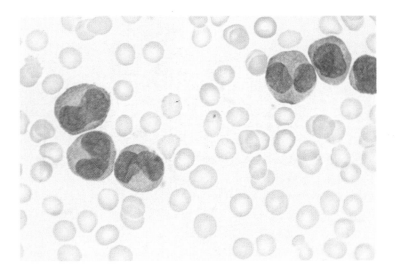

Fig. 3.4 PB film, M3 variant AML, showing hypogranular promyelocytes with characteristic deeply lobulated nuclei. Several cells have very fine granules. MGG × 940.

of circulating leukaemic cells tends to be low. There is usually anaemia. The platelet count may be disproportionately low as a consequence of complicating disseminated intravascular coagulation. The abnormal promyelocytes are large cells, usually two to three times the diameter of an erythrocyte. Their cytoplasm is packed with granules which stain bright pink or reddish-purple. Some cells contain bundles of Auer rods ('faggot cells') or giant granules. No Golgi zone is apparent. The nucleus is usually round or oval but the cytoplasmic granulation is so marked that the nuclear outline is difficult to discern.

In M3 variant AML the white cell count is usually elevated. Again there is usually anaemia and marked thrombocytopenia. Abnormal promyelocytes are characteristically more frequent in the peripheral blood in M3 variant than in M3 AML. The promyelocytes may appear completely agranular or may have fine dust-like reddish granules (Fig. 3.4). Some cells contain bundles of Auer rods or other crystalline inclusions. The nucleus is usually deeply lobed; often there are two large lobes joined by a narrow bridge. The cytoplasm is usually weakly or moderately basophilic but some cases have promyelocytes with more marked basophilia and with cytoplasmic protrusions or blebs. A careful search in cases of M3 variant AML often discloses a minor population of more typical hypergranular promyelocytes occasionally with multiple Auer rods.

Bone marrow cytology

The bone marrow is often difficult to aspirate since the hypercoagulable state leads to clotting of the specimen, even during aspiration. However, the bone marrow aspirate is important in diagnosis since in M3 AML there may be only infrequent leukaemic cells in the peripheral blood and in M3 variant AML the bone marrow often contains a higher proportion of typical hypergranular cells than does the peripheral blood.

The bone marrow aspirate is intensely hypercellular. The number of blasts is relatively low since the predominant cell is an abnormal promyelocyte (Fig. 3.5); in the majority of cases there are fewer than 30 per cent of blasts in the marrow. In M3 AML the predominant cell is a hypergranular promyelocyte while in M3 variant the predominant cell is a hypogranular promyelocyte with a variable admixture of hypergranular forms. There is a marked reduction in the number of normal maturing granulocytes. Erythroid cells and megakaryocytes are also considerably reduced in number but are cytologically normal.

Bone marrow histology

There is marked hypercellularity and a homogeneous infiltrate of abnormal promyelocytes (Fig. 3.6). These have a characteristic appearance; they have prominent large granules that fill the

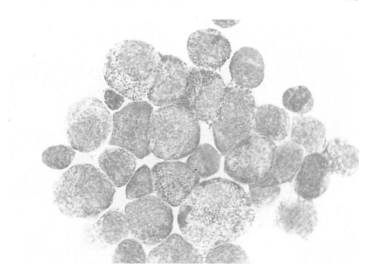

Fig. 3.5 BM aspirate, M3 AML, showing heavily granulated promyelocytes, one of which contains a giant granule. MGG × 940.

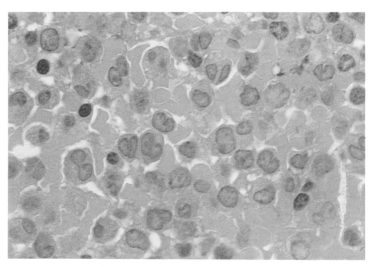

Fig. 3.6 Section of BM trephine biopsy, M3 AML, showing abnormal promyelocytes with irregular, often bi-lobulated, nuclei containing prominent nucleoli and prominent cytoplasmic granules. Plastic-embedded, H&E × 970.

cytoplasm and often obscure the nucleus. The nucleus may be oval or bi-lobed and has a single prominent nucleolus. In M3 variant the granules are much smaller and may be inconspicuous; the nuclei are often bi-lobed.

ACUTE MYELOMONOCYTIC LEUKAEMIA (M4 AML)

Acute myelomonocytic leukaemia, M4 AML, shows evidence of both significant granulocytic differentiation and significant monocytic differentiation (Fig. 3.7). The granulocytic differen-

tiation is usually neutrophilic but in some variants it is eosinophilic (M4Eo) or basophilic (M4Baso).

Peripheral blood

There is usually anaemia and thrombocytopenia with an elevated white cell count and circulating leukaemic cells of both granulocytic and monocytic lineages. Myeloblasts and monoblasts show the usual cytological features of these lineages (see below). Maturation of leukaemic cells is usual so that the leukaemic cell population commonly

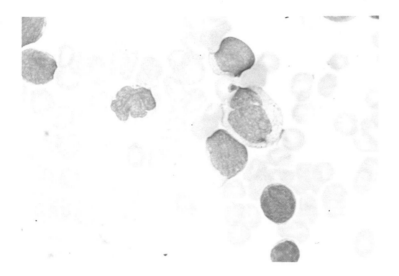

Fig. 3.7 BM aspirate, M4 AML, showing four myeloblasts, one monoblast and a monocyte. MGG × 940.

includes both monocytes and neutrophils. However, some cases of M4 AML have no evidence in the peripheral blood of the significant monocytic component which is present in the bone marrow.

There are several subtypes within the M4 AML category. In acute myelomonocytic leukaemia with eosinophilia (M4Eo), which is usually associated with inversion of chromosome 16, inv(16), the peripheral blood may show a few eosinophils; they are usually cytologically normal. Similarly, peripheral blood basophilia is a feature of some cases of acute myelomonocytic leukaemia with basophilic differentiation (M4Baso), a subtype which may be associated with t(6;9).

Bone marrow cytology

The bone marrow is hypercellular and shows a variable mixture of cells of granulocytic and monocytic lineages (Fig. 3.7). In the majority of cases maturation of leukaemic cells is occurring and mature monocytes as well as maturing cells of granulocytic lineage can be readily recognized. However there are a minority of cases in which, despite a peripheral blood monocytosis, the bone marrow cannot be distinguished morphologically from that of M2 AML; the significant monocytic component can be confirmed either by cytochemistry (see below) or by assays of serum or urinary lysozyme. The explanation of such cases is probably twofold. First, leukaemic monocytes

may be infrequent in the bone marrow because of early migration to the peripheral blood. Secondly, promonocytes can be difficult to distinguish morphologically from promyelocytes.

Megakaryocytes and erythroid precursors are usually reduced. Dysplastic features are sometimes present in these lineages.

In myelomonocytic leukaemia with eosinophilia (M4Eo) the bone marrow usually shows a mixture of cells of monocyte and eosinophil lineages but cells of neutrophil lineage are relatively infrequent (Fig. 3.8). Some basophils may also be present. The cells of eosinophil lineage are a mixture of myelocytes and mature eosinophils. In the great majority of cases the eosinophil myelocytes are morphologically abnormal with prominent basophilic granules mixed with eosinophilic granules. The mature eosinophils may show cytological abnormalities such as nuclear hyper- or hypolobulation or the presence of occasional basophilic granules. Some cells of granulocyte lineage, mainly but not entirely immature cells, show Auer rods. There is usually maturation in the monocyte lineage so that mature monocytes are present. Megakaryocytes and erythroid cells do not show dysplastic features. In M4Baso associated with t(6;9) the bone marrow commonly but not invariably shows an increase of mature basophils and sometimes an increase of eosinophils. There are associated myelodysplastic features.

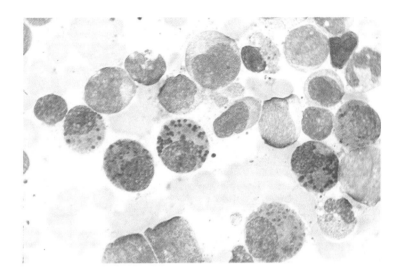

Fig. 3.8 BM aspirate, M4 AML with eosinophilia (M4 Eo), showing characteristic eosinophil myelocytes, eosinophils, a monocyte and blasts. MGG × 940.

Cytochemistry is important to confirm the monocytic component of M4 AML. The cytochemical reactions are those expected of cells of neutrophil and monocyte lineages. In addition, in M4Eo, there may be aberrant cytochemical reactions, eosinophils which are normally negative for chloroacetate esterase activity being positive. In addition SBB and MPO stains may show Auer rods in occasional eosinophils and their precursors as well as in neutrophil precursors. A toluidine blue stain is useful in confirming basophil differentiation in M4Baso.

Bone marrow histology

The marrow is markedly hypercellular and there is an infiltrate composed of variable numbers of myeloblasts, monoblasts and maturing cells of both lineages (Fig. 3.9). Monoblasts have large irregular nuclei with delicate chromatin and prominent nucleoli; cytoplasm is abundant and may be vacuolated. The distribution of monoblasts is not uniform; they are often seen in small clusters, particularly in the paratrabecular areas.[5] Dysplastic changes are often seen in other

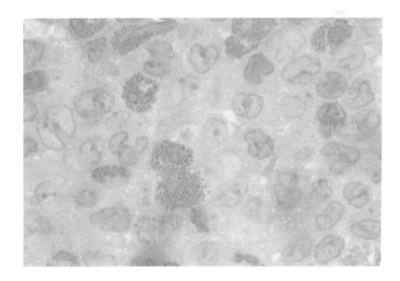

Fig. 3.9 Section of BM trephine biopsy, M4 Eo AML, showing monoblasts, myeloblasts, eosinophil myelocytes and eosinophils. Plastic-embedded, H&E × 970.

haemopoietic lineages and reticulin fibrosis may be present. Eosinophils are increased in M4Eo (Fig. 3.9).

ACUTE MONOCYTIC/MONOBLASTIC LEUKAEMIA (M5 AML)

AML showing predominantly or entirely monocytic differentiation is categorized as acute monocytic or acute monoblastic leukaemia, the former showing maturation of leukaemic cells to mature monocytes and the latter showing little maturation. The FAB group have assigned to these categories (designated M5) those cases of AML in which there is monocytic differentiation and in which less than 20 per cent of bone marrow non-erythroid cells are granulocytes or their precursors. Cases are further divided into acute monoblastic leukaemia (M5a) and acute monocytic leukaemia (M5b) on the basis of whether or not the leukaemic clone is showing maturation (see Table 3.1).

Peripheral blood

The peripheral blood usually shows anaemia, thrombocytopenia and leucocytosis with circulating leukaemic cells which are variously monoblasts, promonocytes or monocytes. Monoblasts are larger than myeloblasts, usually with a diameter about three times that of an erythrocyte.

Their shape varies from round to oval or irregular. The cytoplasm is voluminous and varies from weakly to strongly basophilic; it may contain very infrequent granules. The nucleus ranges from round to lobulated and is usually nucleolated; nucleoli vary from being large, single and prominent to being smaller and multiple. Promonocytes are large cells with moderately basophilic cytoplasm which contains moderately numerous azurophilic granules. Monocytes in M5 AML resemble normal monocytes in having lobulated nuclei and weakly basophilic, sometimes vacuolated cytoplasm. They may show cytological abnormalities such as nuclei of bizarre shape. In M5b AML the peripheral blood shows monocytes and a variable number of promonocytes and monoblasts. In some cases of M5a AML the peripheral blood contains large numbers of monocytes and promonocytes, even though the predominant cell in the bone marrow is a monoblast; in other cases the peripheral blood leukaemic cells, like those in the marrow, are almost exclusively monoblasts.

Bone marrow cytology

The bone marrow is hypercellular and numbers of megakaryocytes and erythroid precursors are reduced. In M5a AML (Fig. 3.10) the great majority of cells are monoblasts. All cases in which at least 80 per cent of bone marrow non-erythroid

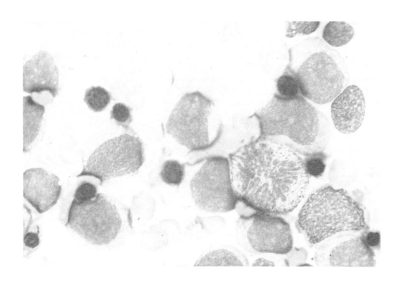

Fig. 3.10 BM aspirate, M5a AML, showing large blasts with moderately abundant cytoplasm. MGG × 940.

cells are monoblasts are classified as M5a, regardless of whether there are maturing cells in the peripheral blood. In M5b AML the marrow contains a mixture of monoblasts, promonocytes and monocytes (Fig. 3.11).

Cytochemical stains[4] are useful in confirming the nature of M5 AML, particularly in those cases of M5a with negligible maturation. Monoblasts are often negative for MPO and SBB, although positive results are obtained in promonocytes. The most useful stains are those for 'non-specific' esterases such as α-naphthyl acetate esterase or α-naphthyl butyrate esterase. An alternative is the demonstration of strong, fluoride-sensitive positivity for naphthol-AS-acetate esterase, another 'non-specific' esterase. Monocyte differentiation can also be demonstrated by using a suspension of the bacterium *Micrococcus lysodeikticus* to show lysozyme activity. However, this test is less used since the availability of monoclonal antibodies has provided another means of confirming monocyte differentiation. Positive reactions with monoclonal antibodies such as those of the CD11b and CD14 clusters provide useful confirmation of the diagnosis of M5 AML in cases with negative reactions for non-specific esterases.

Subtypes of M5 AML include those associated with deletions and translocations involving a chromosome 11q23 breakpoint; the association of this karyotypic abnormality is most strongly with M5a but otherwise there are no specific cytological features. The subtype associated with t(8;16) is also most often M5a but is distinguished by the frequent occurrence of haemophagocytosis by the leukaemic cells (and clinically by a relatively high incidence of coagulation abnormalities).

Bone marrow histology

The marrow is intensely hypercellular. In M5a AML there is an homogeneous infiltrate of monoblasts, whereas in M5b (Fig. 3.12) there is a variable proportion of more mature cells of monocyte lineage. The monoblasts are similar to those seen in M4 AML. The more mature monocytoid cells are smaller than monoblasts and have irregular, often convoluted or lobulated nuclei with delicate chromatin, but without nucleoli. Cytochemical stains to confirm the monocyte lineage are not generally applicable to tissue sections.

ACUTE ERYTHROLEUKAEMIA (M6 AML)

Acute erythroleukaemia describes an acute myeloid leukaemia in which erythroid cells represent a major part of the leukaemic population. The FAB group has recommended that cases be assigned to this category (M6) when at least 50 per cent of bone marrow cells are erythroid and at least 30 per cent of the remaining

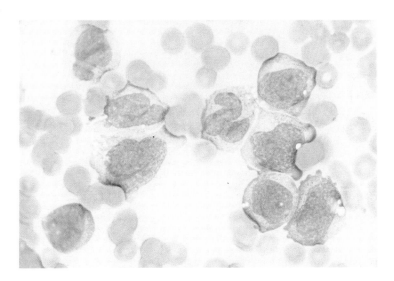

Fig. 3.11 BM aspirate, M5b AML, showing monoblasts, promonocytes and a monocyte. MGG × 940.

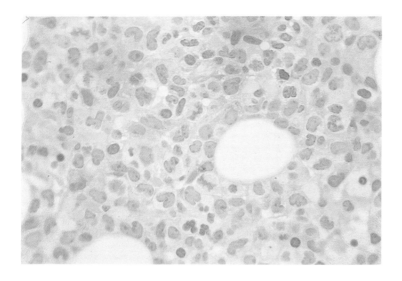

Fig. 3.12 BM trephine biopsy, M5b AML, showing replacement of haemopoietic marrow and fat spaces by a mixture of monoblasts, promonocytes and monocytes. Plastic-embedded, H&E × 390.

non-erythroid cells are blasts (see Table 3.1). Others have considered that a case can also reasonably be classified as erythroleukaemia if there are between 30 and 50 per cent of erythroid cells in the bone marrow but these show prominent cytological abnormalities.[8] There is a problem in assigning to an FAB category cases with almost exclusively erythroid cells including many very primitive erythroid cells. Such cases may have fewer than 30 per cent of non-erythroid cells being blasts and may thus fail to meet the FAB criteria for M6 AML; nevertheless this seems to be the category where they fit most naturally.

It appears likely that a very high proportion of cases of M6 AML represent transformation of underlying MDS.

Peripheral blood

The peripheral blood almost always shows anaemia, neutropenia and thrombocytopenia and usually some circulating blasts.

Bone marrow cytology

The bone marrow is hypercellular and shows both erythroid hyperplasia and a significant population of blasts (Fig. 3.13). The morphology of erythroid cells varies between cases. In some patients erythroid cells show striking cytological abnormalities which may include nuclear lobulation, karyorrhexis, multinuclearity, gigantism

or megaloblastic or sideroblastic erythropoiesis. In other patients cytological abnormalities are quite minor. The associated blasts are usually myeloblasts, which may contain Auer rods, or a mixed population including monoblasts or megakaryoblasts. Maturing granulocytes often show dysplastic features such as hypogranularity and nuclear hypolobulation. Megakaryocytes are also commonly dysplastic with features such as nuclear hypolobulation or the presence of micromegakaryocytes.

Cytochemical stains may show various abnormalities. SBB, MPO and chloroacetate esterase can be employed to confirm the nature of myeloblasts and the former two stains to demonstrate Auer rods. An α-naphthyl acetate esterase stain can be used to identify monoblasts. Erythroblasts may be positive with a periodic acid-Schiff (PAS) stain; such positivity is not shown by normal erythroid precursors but it is not confined to neoplastic erythroblasts. Erythroblasts in M6 AML may also show focal staining for α-naphthyl acetate esterase and acid phosphatase. An iron stain may show the presence of ring sideroblasts.

Bone marrow histology

There is marked hypercellularity of the marrow with intense erythroid hyperplasia (Fig. 3.14). The erythroid precursors are usually markedly abnormal and may have a bizarre appearance. They often show nuclear lobulation or fragmen-

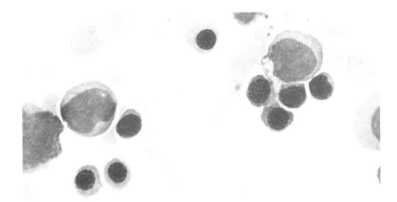

Fig. 3.13 BM aspirate, M6 AML, showing two myeloblasts and numerous erythroblasts. MGG × 940.

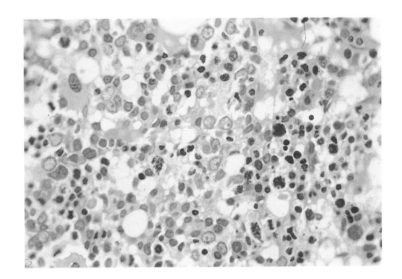

Fig. 3.14 Section of BM trephine biopsy, M6 AML, showing a disorganized marrow containing large numbers of dysplastic erythroblasts and numerous myeloblasts. Paraffin-embedded, H&E × 390.

tation, marked variation in size or megaloblastic change. They are arranged in sheets without the formation of normal erythroblastic islands. Megakaryocytic dysplasia is often seen. Non-erythroid blasts (myeloblasts or monoblasts) may be relatively inconspicuous, although by definition they must make up more than 30 per cent of the non-erythroid cells in the marrow.

ACUTE MEGAKARYOBLASTIC LEUKAEMIA (M7 AML)

Acute megakaryoblastic leukaemia has blasts constituting at least 30 per cent of bone marrow cells, with megakaryoblasts being the predominant form. There may be an admixture with other lineages, for example with myeloblasts. The diagnosis is often difficult because of the paucity of leukaemic cells in the peripheral blood and the difficulty in obtaining a bone marrow aspirate. The trephine biopsy is then of critical importance in making the diagnosis.

Peripheral blood

Commonly the peripheral blood shows only pancytopenia with very infrequent or no circulating leukaemic blasts. Such patients usually lack organomegaly and have a fibrotic marrow; this condition has been described as 'acute myelofibrosis'. Other patients have features more typical of acute leukaemia, with hepatomegaly, splenomegaly and significant numbers of circulating blasts. Megakaryoblasts are similar in size to myeloblasts. They have a high nucleo-cytoplasmic ratio and agranular, moderately basophilic cytoplasm. In some cases there are distinctive features which suggest their nature, such as formation of peripheral cytoplasmic blebs or an association with circulating micromega-karyocytes, but in other cases there are no features to suggest lineage.

Bone marrow cytology

Aspiration may be impossible or a poor aspirate containing scanty blasts may be obtained (Fig. 3.15). In addition to megakaryoblasts, the aspirate may contain some micromegakaryocytes or other markedly dysplastic megakaryocytes. There may be an admixture with myeloblasts. Erythroid precursors sometimes show dysplastic features.

Cytochemistry is often not very useful. SBB, MPO and chloroacetate esterase stains are negative, except in any associated myeloblasts. PAS, acid phosphatase and α-naphthyl acetate esterase stains may be positive in cells showing cyto-plasmic maturation but not in more immature cells of megakaryocyte lineage. The PAS stain sometimes shows a distinctive pattern with positivity being confined to cytoplasmic blebs. The differential staining pattern with α-naphthyl acetate esterase (positive) and α-naphthyl butyrate esterase (negative) can be useful in distinguishing megakaryoblasts from monoblasts since the latter cells give positive reactions with both these non-specific esterases. Immunocytochemistry with monoclonal antibodies directed at platelet glyco-proteins is now the most practicable way to confirm the diagnosis.

Bone marrow histology[9,10]

The marrow histology is very variable. In those cases that present clinically as acute myelofib-rosis the marrow is largely replaced by fibrous tissue containing blasts and dysplastic mega-karyocytes (Fig. 3.16). In other cases the marrow is very hypercellular with an infiltrate of blasts; in some cases the blasts are relatively small and monomorphic, while in others they are large and pleomorphic. Cases with a hypercellular marrow usually show increased reticulin and scattered collagen fibres. Dyserythropoiesis is common. Immunocytochemical staining for factor VIII-related antigen or for platelet GP IIIa is useful in the identification of megakaryoblasts.

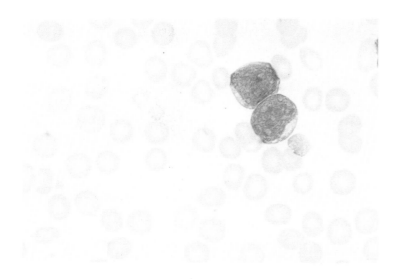

Fig. 3.15 BM aspirate of a patient with Down's syndrome and M7 AML showing two megakaryocytes and two giant platelets. MGG × 940.

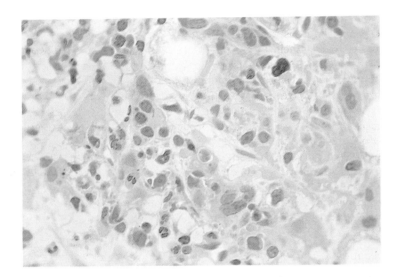

Fig. 3.16 Section of BM trephine biopsy, M7 AML. There is collagen fibrosis and an infiltrate of dysplastic megakaryocytes and small blasts. Plastic-embedded, H&E × 390.

ACUTE MYELOID LEUKAEMIA WITH MINIMAL EVIDENCE OF MYELOID DIFFERENTIATION (M0 AML)

The availability of ultrastructural cytochemistry and of monoclonal antibodies detecting antigens specific for myeloid cells has revealed cases of acute leukaemia which are negative for markers of lymphoid lineages but have insufficient evidence of myeloid differentiation to meet the original FAB criteria for AML. Such cases have fewer than three per cent SBB or MPO-positive blasts; blasts are also negative for α-naphthyl acetate esterase and lysozyme activity. When such cases can be demonstrated to have peroxidase activity at ultrastructural level or to be positive for myeloid antigens such as CD13, CD14 and CD33 they should be classified as acute myeloid leukaemia. The FAB group have suggested the designation AML M0.[11]

Peripheral blood

The peripheral blood usually shows anaemia, neutropenia, thrombocytopenia and the presence of circulating blasts (Fig. 3.17). The blasts are

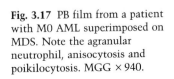

Fig. 3.17 PB film from a patient with M0 AML superimposed on MDS. Note the agranular neutrophil, anisocytosis and poikilocytosis. MGG × 940.

agranular and have cytological features similar to those of the blasts of AML M1, ALL L2 or, more rarely, ALL L1 (see page 130). They tend to be large blasts with prominent nucleoli and abundant, often basophilic cytoplasm but there are no constant features permitting the diagnosis on cytomorphology alone.

Bone marrow cytology

The bone marrow features do not differ from those of AML M1 except that the blasts have scanty if any granules, have no Auer rods and are negative with all the cytochemical stains which are usually used to identify cells of various myeloid lineages. Immunocytochemistry for the above antigens will confirm the diagnosis.

Bone marrow histology

The trephine biopsy appearances do not differ from those of M1 AML. It is also often not possible to distinguish M0 AML from ALL, although the presence of dysplastic features suggests a diagnosis of AML. The diagnosis of AML cannot be confirmed by the Leder stain which is uniformly negative in M0 AML. Immunological markers, however, can permit the distinction. Lymphoblasts usually stain positively for CD45 and may stain with the B cell marker L26, whereas myeloblasts stain negatively for L26 and are often CD45 negative.

HYPOPLASTIC AML

A minority of cases of AML have a bone marrow which is hypocellular rather than hypercellular. Hypoplastic AML is variously defined, for example as AML with bone marrow cellularity less than 50 per cent[12] or less than 40 per cent.[13] Blasts constitute at least 30 per cent of nucleated cells. Cases of hypoplastic AML may belong to various FAB categories, but not M3. They may arise apparently *de novo* or be preceded by a hypoplastic variant of myelodysplasia. Clinical and haematological features differ from those of typical cases of AML with a hypercellular bone marrow. Hepatomegaly and splenomegaly are not commonly present. The median age is higher

than that of AML in general.[12] The prognostic significance of hypoplastic AML is not yet clear. In one series patients who were treated had a low remission rate and treated patients, overall, did not survive longer than those who received no specific treatment.[12] However, in another series, treated patients had a high remission rate and improved survival.[13]

Hypoplastic AML needs to be distinguished from aplastic anaemia and from myelodysplastic syndromes with hypoplasia. Both bone marrow aspirates and trephine biopsies are generally useful in making the distinction from aplastic anaemia whereas a trephine biopsy is usually the most useful procedure for making the distinction from hypoplastic myelodysplasia since it shows the foci of blasts.

Peripheral blood

In contrast to cases of typical AML, pancytopenia is usual and peripheral blood blasts are often absent or infrequent. Blasts may contain Auer rods.

Bone marrow cytology

The bone marrow aspirate is often hypocellular and may therefore not be optimal for diagnosis. Blasts are increased and commonly show granulocytic rather than monocytic differentiation. There may be associated dysplastic features.

Bone marrow histology

Because a poor aspirate is often obtained, trephine biopsy is usually important in diagnosis. The marrow shows irregular hypoplasia (Fig. 3.18) with small foci of blasts separated by fat cells (Fig. 3.19). The blasts make up more than 30 per cent of the nucleated cells in the marrow. There are often dysplastic changes in the other haemopoietic lineages. Reticulin may be increased.

The myelodysplastic syndromes

As discussed at the beginning of this chapter the myelodysplastic syndromes are diseases consequent on clonal disorders of haemopoïesis char-

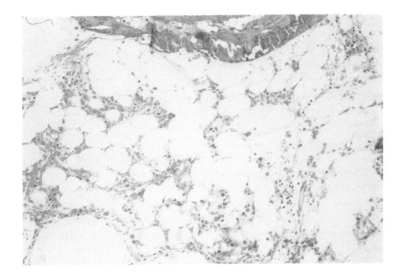

Fig. 3.18 Section of BM trephine biopsy, hypoplastic AML. The marrow is hypocellular with preservation of fat cells. However, normal haemopoietic cells are not seen. Plastic-embedded, H&E × 97.

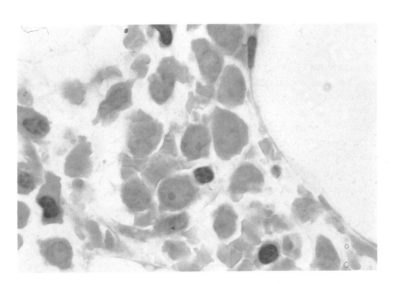

Fig. 3.19 Section of BM trephine biopsy, hypoplastic AML, same case as Fig. 3.18. High-power examination reveals most of the cells present to be myeloblasts. Plastic-embedded, H&E × 970.

acterized by dysplastic, ineffective haemopoiesis. There is thus often a discrepancy between a hypercellular bone marrow and peripheral cytopenia. In any one patient different haemopoietic lineages are not necessarily affected to the same degree and there may be defective production of cells of one lineage while in another lineage normal numbers of cells are produced. There may even be increased production of cells of one or more lineages—for example, neutrophils, monocytes or platelets—despite other features typical of MDS.

The MDS are predominantly diseases of the elderly with an incidence of the order of 70 cases/ 100 000/year.

Clinical features of MDS are consequent on the various cytopenias; there may be haemorrhage, susceptibility to infections, and symptoms of anaemia. Some patients have hepatomegaly and splenomegaly. The MDS show a tendency to evolve into more severe forms of MDS and into acute leukaemia. These conditions may be secondary to exposure of the bone marrow to known mutagens such as alkylating agents or may be apparently primary. There are some differences in laboratory and clinical features between primary and secondary MDS.

Diagnosis of MDS requires consideration of clinical, peripheral blood and bone marrow features. Peripheral blood and bone marrow aspirate findings are most important and in a straightforward case may be all that is required for diagnosis. Bone marrow biopsy in general offers only supplementary information; however, sometimes it is necessary for confirmation of the diagnosis as, for example, when an excess of blasts or an abnormal localization of blasts is detected in a patient who has other features suggestive but not diagnostic of MDS. Bone marrow biopsy is particularly important in patients with secondary MDS in whom a hypocellular bone marrow with increased fibrosis often leads to a non-diagnostic aspirate. In some patients a firm diagnosis cannot be made on cytological and histological features alone, but diagnosis is possible when these are supplemented by cytogenetic analysis or information on clonality. An iron stain should be performed in all patients with suspected myelo-dysplasia; this demonstrates any ring sideroblasts as well as permitting an assessment of iron stores. A MPO or SBB stain should be performed at least in all patients with any increase in blasts; this will facilitate the detection of Auer rods which are of importance both in diagnosis and in classification.

The MDS are a heterogeneous group of disorders with very variable prognoses. They can be divided into various disease categories which have more uniform clinicopathological characteristics. The most widely used categorization is that proposed by the FAB group.[1,2,14] The FAB classification is based on the presence or absence of significant sideroblastic erythropoiesis, on the numbers of monocytes in the peripheral blood and on the number of blasts in the peripheral blood and bone marrow (Table 3.2). The FAB categories are: (i) refractory anaemia (RA) or refractory cytopenia (ii) refractory anaemia with ring sideroblasts (RARS) (iii) refractory anaemia with excess of blasts (RAEB) (iv) chronic myelomonocytic leukaemia (CMML), and (v) refractory anaemia with excess of blasts in transformation (RAEB-t).

Table 3.2 The FAB classification of the myelodysplastic syndromes[1-3,14]

Category	Peripheral blood			Bone marrow
Refractory anaemia (RA) or refractory cytopenia*	Anaemia* Blasts $\leqslant 1\%$ Monocytes $\leqslant 1 \times 10^9/l$		*and*	Blasts $<5\%$, Ringed sideroblasts $\leqslant 15\%$ of erythroblasts
Refractory anaemia with ringed sideroblasts (RARS)	Anaemia Blasts $\leqslant 1\%$ Monocytes $\leqslant 1 \times 10^9/l$		*and*	Blasts $<5\%$, Ringed sideroblasts $>15\%$ of erythroblasts
Refractory anaemia with excess of blasts (RAEB)	Anaemia Blasts $>1\%$ Blasts $<5\%$ Monocytes $\leqslant 1 \times 10^9/l$		*or* *and*	Blasts $\geqslant 5\%$ Blasts $\leqslant 20\%$
Chronic myelomonocytic leukaemia (CMML)	Blasts $<5\%$ Monocytes $>1 \times 10^9/l$ Granulocytes often increased		*and*	Blasts up to 20% Promonocytes often increased
Refractory anaemia with excess of blasts in transformation (RAEB-t)	Blasts $\geqslant 5\%$ *or*	Auer rods in blasts in blood or marrow	*or*	Blasts $>20\%$ *but* $<30\%$

* Or in the case of refractory cytopenia either neutropenia or thrombocytopenia. Reproduced, with permission, from Bain.[3]

Although the myelodysplastic syndromes are heterogeneous they also have many features in common. We will therefore describe these syndromes as a group before discussing specific categories of disease. Some morphological abnormalities are characteristic of the MDS without being specific for them while others shows sufficient specificity to be useful in confirming the diagnosis.

Peripheral blood

Anaemia is seen in the great majority of patients. Red cells are usually normochromic and either normocytic or macrocytic. In patients with sideroblastic erythropoiesis there is commonly a dimorphic blood film with a mixture of a minority population of hypochromic microcytes and a majority population of normochromic cells which are either normocytic or, more commonly, macrocytic; Pappenheimer bodies, the nature of which can be confirmed with an iron stain, may be present. Microcytosis is seen in certain rare variants including acquired haemoglobin H disease. Some patients have occasional circulating erythroblasts which may include dysplastic forms such as megaloblasts and, in patients with sideroblastic erythropoiesis, ring sideroblasts.

Neutropenia is common, particularly in RAEB and RAEB-t, while neutrophilia is common in CMML. Neutrophils often show dysplastic features including reduced granulation and the acquired or pseudo-Pelger–Hüet anomaly. Hypogranular and agranular neutrophils (Fig. 3.20) are consequent on defective formation of secondary granules; agranular neutrophils are highly specific for the MDS.[15] The acquired Pelger–Hüet anomaly refers to hypolobulation of nuclei associated with dense chromatin clumping (Fig. 3.20); nuclei of mature neutrophils may be completely non-lobed, dumb-bell or peanut shaped, or bilobed with the shape resembling a pair of spectacles. This abnormality resembles the inherited Pelger–Hüet anomaly hence the name. The acquired anomaly is highly characteristic of the MDS and almost pathognomonic.[15] Eosinophil and basophil counts are commonly reduced but in a small minority of patients are increased; dysplastic forms with abnormalities of either nuclear shape or cytoplasmic granulation can occur. Monocytosis is an essential feature of CMML but is also sometimes present in other categories of MDS; monocytes may show cytological abnormalities such as increased cytoplasmic basophilia or nuclei of unusual shape. Blast cells may be present in the peripheral blood in all categories of MDS but particularly in RAEB and RAEB-t. They usually have the cytological features of myeloblasts with scanty cytoplasm and few granules. Auer rods are sometimes present. Other granulocyte precursors are quite uncommon in the peripheral blood.

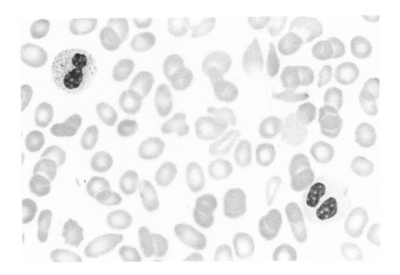

Fig. 3.20 PB film, MDS, showing anisocytosis, poikilocytosis and two pseudo-Pelger–Hüet neutrophils, one of which is also hypogranular. MGG × 940.

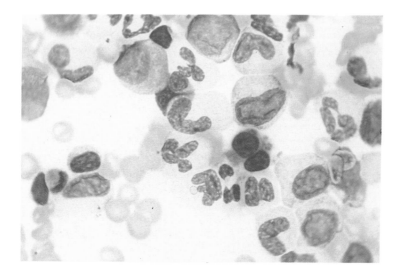

Fig. 3.21 BM aspirate, RA, showing a binucleate micromegakaryocyte which is budding platelets. MGG × 940.

The platelet count is usually either normal or reduced. In a minority of patients it is increased. Dysplastic features which may be noted in platelets include hypogranular and agranular forms ('grey' platelets) and the presence of giant platelets.

Bone marrow cytology

The bone marrow is hypercellular in the majority of patients but is sometimes normocellular and in about 10 per cent of patients is hypocellular. Hypercellularity may be consequent on hyperplasia of erythroid or granulocytic series or both.

Erythropoiesis may be normoblastic, macronormoblastic or megaloblastic. A feature sometimes of use in distinguishing megaloblastic erythropoiesis due to MDS from that consequent on deficiency of vitamin B_{12} or folic acid is the lack of associated white cell changes — giant metamyelocytes and hypersegmented neutrophils — in the former group. In patients with sideroblastic erythropoiesis there are some erythroblasts with poorly haemoglobinized or vacuolated cytoplasm. Other dysplastic features may include: binuclearity and multinuclearity; internuclear bridges; lobulation, irregularity or fragmentation of nuclei; gigantism; increased pyknosis; basophilic stippling.

Granulopoiesis is usually hyperplastic. Defects of granulation may be apparent from the pro-myelocyte stage onwards and defects of nuclear lobulation may also be present.

Megakaryocyte numbers are usually normal or increased but sometimes decreased. One of the features most specific for the MDS is the presence of micromegakaryocytes,[15] cells of about the size of a blast with one or two small round nuclei (Fig. 3.21). Megakaryocytes may also be of normal size but have a large non-lobulated nucleus (Fig. 3.22); this abnormality is less specific for MDS but is characteristic of cases with 5q− as an acquired chromosomal abnormality.[16] Other megakaryocyte abnormalities include bizarre nuclear shapes and the presence of multiple separate nuclei. Poor granulation of megakaryocyte cytoplasm is also common in the MDS and has been found to be highly specific.[17]

The bone marrow aspirate may show non-specific abnormalities such as an increase of macrophages, lymphocytes, plasma cells or mast cells.

The cytochemical stain of most value is an iron stain which should be performed in all cases of suspected MDS, in order to quantify iron stores and detect and enumerate ring sideroblasts and other abnormal sideroblasts. Ring sideroblasts have iron-positive granules in a circle close to the nuclear membrane (Fig. 3.23). Other abnormal sideroblasts have scattered iron-positive granules which are both larger and more numerous than those of normal siderocytes. Ring sideroblasts are

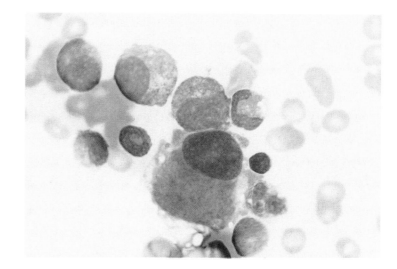

Fig. 3.22 BM aspirate, RA, 5q− syndrome, showing a megakaryocyte of normal size with a hypolobulated nucleus. MGG × 940.

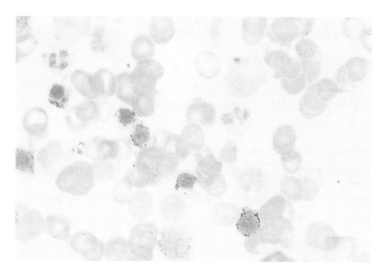

Fig. 3.23 BM aspirate, RARS, showing numerous ring sideroblasts several of which can be seen to have defectively haemoglobinized cytoplasm. Perls' × 940.

highly suggestive of MDS if the other known causes of sideroblastic erythropoiesis (see page 205) can be eliminated. Abnormal sideroblasts other than ring sideroblasts are common both in MDS and in other disorders of erythropoiesis so are not useful in the differential diagnosis of suspected MDS. Other cytochemical stains are of use in identifying abnormal cells of megakaryocyte lineages, in characterizing blasts and in detecting Auer rods. MPO and SBB stains will identify myeloblasts and may also show cells of the neutrophil lineage to have defective primary granules. Non-specific esterase stains are useful for identifying monoblasts, and non-specific esterase and PAS stains for identifying abnormal megakaryocytes.

Bone marrow histology

In the majority of cases the marrow is hypercellular (Fig. 3.24), but a significant minority have a hypocellular marrow.[18,19] There may be considerable variation of the cellularity between adjacent intertrabecular spaces.[20] In addition to the cytological evidence of dysplasia there is derangement of the normal architecture. In

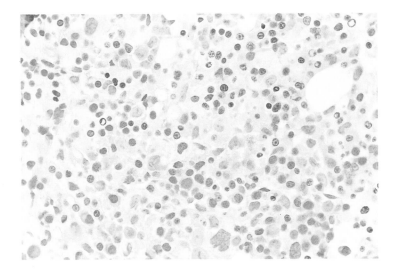

Fig. 3.24 BM trephine biopsy, RA, showing marked hypercellularity with disorganization of haemopoiesis and marked dyserythropoiesis. Note the apoptotic erythroblast with peripheral condensation of its nuclear chromatin. Plastic-embedded, H&E × 390.

histological sections dysplasia is most obvious in the erythroid precursors and megakaryocytes; however, in good plastic-embedded sections features of granulocytic dysplasia such as pseudo-Pelger–Hüet neutrophils may be identified. Disturbance of normal architecture results in groups of granulocytic precursors being found in the intertrabecular spaces (Fig. 3.25) and erythroid precursors and megakaryocytes in the paratrabecular regions. Erythroblastic islands are poorly formed and erythroid precursors may be multinucleated or show megaloblastic change, nuclear

budding or fragmentation, or cytoplasmic vacuolation. Megakaryocytic dysplasia is present in the vast majority of cases and is usually more apparent in histological sections than in marrow smears. They are usually increased in number and clustering is often seen (Fig. 3.26). Typically they have hypolobulated nuclei which are often hyperchromatic; the small dysplastic megakaryocytes are usually referred to as micromegakaryocytes.[19,21] Immunocytochemical staining with anti-Gp IIIa may be used to accentuate the abnormal megakaryocytes.[22] Increased numbers

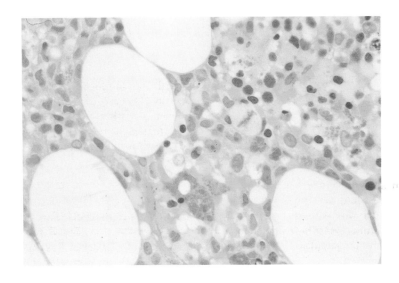

Fig. 3.25 BM trephine biopsy, RAEBt, showing increased numbers of blasts forming a small cluster (centre) (ALIP). Plastic-embedded, H&E × 970.

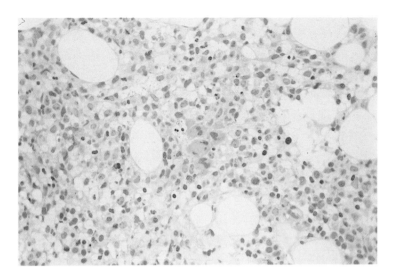

Fig. 3.26 BM trephine biopsy, RAEB, showing a cluster of dysplastic megakaryocytes. Plastic-embedded, H&E × 195.

of apoptotic erythroid (Fig. 3.24) and granulocytic precursors are commonly seen in MDS consequent on ineffective haematopoiesis.[23] Reticulin fibrosis is found in almost half of all cases, being more common in chronic myelomonocytic leukaemia than in other subtypes.[19] However, severe collagen fibrosis is rare in all subtypes.[19] Other non-specific reactions are commonly seen including oedema, ectasia of sinusoids, increased numbers of plasma cells, and increased numbers of lymphoid follicles. Haemosiderin-laden macrophages are a frequent finding, particularly in patients who have received transfusions.

One feature that has been the subject of much debate is the significance of small groups of immature granulocytic precursors (promyelocytes and myeloblasts) in an intertrabecular position (Fig. 3.25). This has been termed abnormal localization of immature precursors (ALIP) and some studies have found it to be an independent predictor of prognosis and to be associated with an increased incidence of leukaemic transformation.[24] Although ALIP is more frequent in the subtypes of myelodysplasia with increased numbers of blasts in the marrow, several recent studies have failed to confirm any independent influence on prognosis.[19,20,25] It should also be noted that it can be difficult to distinguish between small groups of immature erythroid precursors and ALIP, particularly in paraffin-embedded sections.

The FAB categories and other identified subtypes of MDS

REFRACTORY ANAEMIA

Refractory anaemia (RA) is characterized by ineffective erythropoiesis, with or without ineffective granulopoiesis and thrombopoiesis but, as defined by the FAB group, there are insufficient monocytes, blast cells or ring sideroblasts for the case to qualify for inclusion in other categories of MDS (see Table 3.2). Refractory anaemia is usually either an incidental diagnosis in the elderly or is diagnosed because of symptoms of anaemia.

Peripheral blood

Often morphological and numerical abnormalities are confined to the erythroid series, but some patients, particularly those with secondary MDS, manifest anomalies of other lineages. A minority of cases have thrombocytosis.

Bone marrow cytology

The bone marrow is usually hypercellular, consequent on erythroid hyperplasia (Fig. 3.27). A minority of patients show marked erythroid hypoplasia, sometimes with an apparent arrest

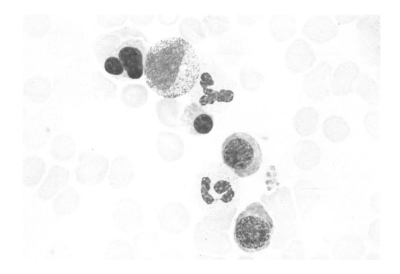

Fig. 3.27 BM aspirate, RA, showing erythroid hyperplasia and hypogranular neutrophils; note a dysplastic binucleated erythroblast. MGG × 940.

of erythropoiesis at the proerythroblast stage. Erythropoiesis usually shows dysplastic features but in some patients erythropoiesis is ineffective although dysplastic features are quite minor. Ring sideroblasts may be present but constitute no more than 15 per cent of erythroblasts.

In RA the granulocyte series and the megakaryocytes may be apparently normal or may be hyperplastic or dysplastic (see Figs 3.21 and 3.22).

Bone marrow histology

There are often no histological features of diagnostic importance in trephine biopsies of patients with refractory anaemia. The marrow is usually hypercellular but hypocellular forms do occur. Erythroid hyperplasia and dyserythropoiesis are usually present and are easily seen in tissue sections (see Fig. 3.24). The granulocytic series may appear relatively normal. Dysplastic megakaryocytes are found in most cases; however they are not universally present and in their absence the diagnosis of myelodysplasia may be easily overlooked if the clinical and cytological features are not taken into account.

REFRACTORY CYTOPENIA

A small proportion of patients with MDS are not anaemic but have refractory neutropenia or thrombocytopenia. The FAB group has re-commended that if such cases lack the features of the other categories of MDS they should be grouped with refractory anaemia and be designated refractory cytopenia.

Patients with refractory neutropenia show abnormalities predominantly of the neutrophil lineage while patients with refractory thrombocytopenia have increased and dysplastic megakaryocytes are often dysplastic platelets.

REFRACTORY ANAEMIA WITH RING SIDEROBLASTS

Refractory anaemia with ring sideroblasts (RARS) is also referred to as primary acquired sideroblastic anaemia. The FAB group criteria for this diagnosis are the presence of more than 15 per cent of ring sideroblasts among bone marrow erythroblasts, with monocytes and blast cells being insufficiently increased to permit assignment to other MDS categories (see Table 3.2). Sideroblastic anaemia is usually either an incidental diagnosis in the elderly or is diagnosed because of symptoms of anaemia.

Peripheral blood

There is anaemia which is sometimes normocytic but more often macrocytic. The film is dimorphic, consequent on the presence of a minor population of hypochromic and microcytic red cells.

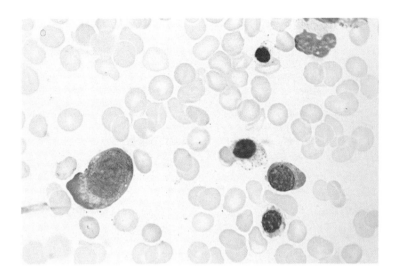

Fig. 3.28 BM aspirate, RARS, showing five erythroblasts, two of which show defectively haemoglobinized, heavily granulated cytoplasm. MGG × 940.

Occasional cells contain Pappenheimer bodies. There may be a small number of circulating erythroblasts, among which may be some ring sideroblasts. Abnormalities of neutrophils and platelets can occur but are uncommon. A significant minority of patients have thrombocytosis.

Bone marrow cytology

The bone marrow is usually hypercellular and shows erythroid hyperplasia. Erythropoiesis is usually normoblastic or macronormoblastic. A proportion of erythroblasts, which correspond to the ring sideroblasts, are micronormoblasts or show defective haemoglobinization or cytoplasmic vacuolation (Fig. 3.28). Other dysplastic features in red cells are uncommon. Abnormalities may occur in other lineages but they are uncommon except when the MDS is secondary.

By definition in RARS an iron stain shows that more than 15 per cent of erythroblasts are ring sideroblasts (see Fig. 3.23); they may be as frequent as 70 or 80 per cent of erythroblasts and may be associated with other abnormal sideroblasts. Iron stores are commonly increased.

Bone marrow histology

Trephine biopsy is not usually very useful in the diagnosis of RARS. Bone marrow histology may be relatively normal with the only abnormality being erythroid hyperplasia with large poorly formed erythroblastic islands. There is often an increase in stainable iron within macrophages. Ring sideroblasts can be seen in plastic-embedded sections of trephine biopsies and paraffin-embedded sections of marrow clot sections (Fig. 3.29); they are often not visible in paraffin-embedded sections of trephine biopsy specimens. The granulocytic series is usually normal. Dysplastic megakaryocytes are present in some cases.

REFRACTORY ANAEMIA WITH EXCESS OF BLASTS

Refractory anaemia with excess of blasts (RAEB) as defined by the FAB group (see Table 3.2) has *either* an increase of peripheral blood blasts to more than one but less than five per cent *or* an increase of bone marrow blasts to at least five per cent but not more than 20 per cent; the monocyte count must be less than $1 \times 10^9/l$ or the case falls into the CMML category (see below). Diagnosis of RAEB usually follows the development of symptoms of anaemia or the occurrence of bruising, bleeding or infection.

Peripheral blood

The peripheral blood shows normocytic or macrocytic anaemia and may also show some hypochromic microcytic cells. In addition there may

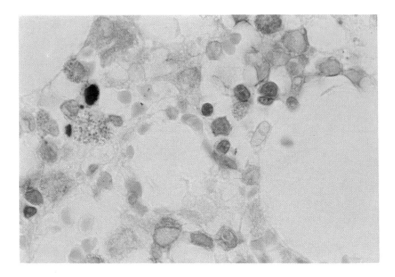

Fig. 3.29 BM clot section, RARS, showing two ring sideroblasts with blue iron-containing granules arranged around the nucleus. Paraffin-embedded, Perls' stain × 970.

be neutropenia, mild monocytosis or thrombocytopenia. Dysplastic features in neutrophils and platelets are commonly present. There may be some circulating blasts, which are usually but not necessarily myeloblasts.

Bone marrow cytology

The bone marrow is usually hypercellular. Any or all lineages may be hyperplastic. Trilineage dysplasia is common. The percentage of blasts is usually increased, although a case may qualify to be categorized as RAEB on the basis of increased peripheral blood blasts alone. Erythropoiesis may be sideroblastic but because of the excess of blasts the case is categorized as RAEB not as RARS.

An iron stain may show ring sideroblasts, other abnormal sideroblasts and increased iron stores. Either an MPO or a SBB stain should be performed routinely both to confirm the lineage of the blasts and to exclude the presence of Auer rods, which would lead to the case being categorized as RAEB-t (see below).

Bone marrow histology

Bone marrow biopsy is not usually essential for diagnosis but can give useful supplementary information. The majority of cases have increased or normal cellularity with only a small number of cases being hypocellular. Dyserythropoiesis and megakaryocytic dysplasia are seen in almost all cases (Figs 3.26 and 3.30). Blasts are increased in number, but it is not uncommon for the percentage of blasts seen in the biopsy sections to be less than that observed in marrow aspirates taken at the same time.[19] ALIP is seen in most cases.

CHRONIC MYELOMONOCYTIC LEUKAEMIA

Chronic myelomonocytic leukaemia (CMML) has features both of myelodysplasia and of a myeloproliferative disorder. It is currently recommended that it be classified with the MDS. As defined by the FAB group (see Table 3.2) the peripheral blood monocyte count is greater than $1 \times 10^9/l$ but peripheral blood blasts are less than five per cent and bone marrow blasts not greater than 20 per cent. CMML needs to be distinguished not only from other MDS but also from atypical Ph-negative chronic myeloid leukaemia with which it shares some features. It has been recommended that cases in which more than 15 per cent of circulating white cells are granulocyte precursors should be categorized as atypical chronic myeloid leukaemia and cases with fewer as CMML.[26] Although a bone marrow examination is essential for the diagnosis of CMML, a careful consideration of the peripheral blood features is equally important in the differential diagnosis. A trephine biopsy offers only supplementary information.

Clinically CMML is characterized by features of anaemia and often by hepatomegaly and spleno-

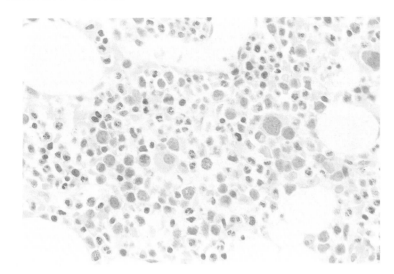

Fig. 3.30 BM trephine biopsy, RAEB, showing dysplastic megakaryocytes including micromegakaryocytes. Plastic-embedded, H&E × 390.

megaly. In a minority of patients there is tissue infiltration by monocytic cells resulting in lymphadenopathy, skin infiltration and serous effusions. Diagnosis is usually either incidental or occurs when the patient develops symptoms of anaemia or when organomegaly is noted.

Peripheral blood

There is usually anaemia, most often normocytic but sometimes macrocytic or with a dimorphic blood film. The monocyte count is, by definition, greater than $1 \times 10^9/l$. The monocytes may be morphologically normal or may show atypical features such as nuclei of bizarre shapes or increased cytoplasmic basophilia or granulation. The neutrophil count is often elevated but this is not necessary for the diagnosis. The neutrophils may be morphologically normal or a varying proportion may show dysplastic features. Granulocyte precursors are infrequent, usually less than five per cent. Occasional blasts may be present. The platelet count may be normal or low.

Bone marrow cytology

The bone marrow is hypercellular. There is hyperplasia of granulocyte precursors (Fig. 3.31).

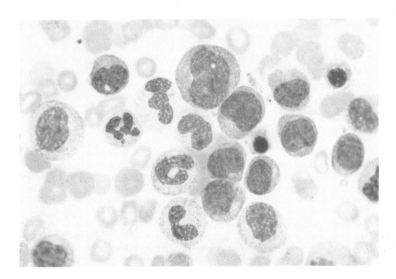

Fig. 3.31 BM aspirate, CMML, showing granulocytic hyperplasia. MGG × 940.

Hyperplasia of monocytes and their precursors is often evident but this is not always so, probably because promonocytes can be difficult to distinguish from promyelocytes and more mature monocytes leave the marrow early. The blast count in the marrow may be increased up to a level of 20 per cent. Some patients have dysplastic erythroblasts and megakaryocytes but this is not necessarily so. Sideroblastic erythropoiesis is not inconsistent with a diagnosis of CMML.

An iron stain may show abnormal sideroblasts or increased iron stores. An MPO or SBB stain should be performed in all cases with an increase of blast cells, both to confirm the lineage and to exclude the presence of Auer rods. A non-specific esterase stain such as α-naphthyl-acetate esterase is useful in identifying monocyte precursors.

Bone marrow histology

The diagnosis of CMML is usually established on peripheral blood and bone marrow aspirate features; trephine biopsy does not have a major role in diagnosis. Almost all cases have a hypercellular marrow and granulocytic hyperplasia. Some also show monocytic hyperplasia (Fig. 3.32). Some but not all cases show erythroid and megakaryocytic dysplasia. ALIP is sometimes present and there may be an absolute increase in blasts.

REFRACTORY ANAEMIA WITH EXCESS OF BLASTS IN TRANSFORMATION

As defined by the FAB group the diagnosis of refractory anaemia with excess of blasts in transformation (RAEB-t) requires that *either* peripheral blood blasts are at least five per cent *or* bone marrow blasts are greater than 20 per cent but less than 30 per cent *or* that there are Auer rods in blasts, either in the bone marrow or the peripheral blood (see Table 3.2). In practice most cases have more than 20 per cent blasts in the bone marrow whether or not they show the other features but occasional cases are categorized as RAEB-t on the basis of one of the other criteria alone.

Patients with RAEB-t are almost always symptomatic at diagnosis with bruising, bleeding, infection or symptoms of anaemia. Pallor, bruising, hepatomegaly and splenomegaly are common.

Peripheral blood

Most patients have anaemia, neutropenia and thrombocytopenia and show morphological abnormalities of all lineages. Some circulating blasts are usually present and they may contain Auer rods. There may be monocytosis, particularly in those patients where the disease represents a transformation of CMML rather than RAEB.

Bone marrow cytology

The bone marrow is usually hypercellular with trilineage myelodysplasia, an increase of blasts and sometimes Auer rods in the blasts. Sideroblastic erythropoieis is not inconsistent with a diagnosis of RAEB-t.

Bone marrow histology

Trephine biopsy is not usually essential for diagnosis but can give useful supplementary information. In addition to trilineage dysplasia there is an increase in numbers of blasts, often with ALIP. Reticulin fibrosis has been reported to be less common than in the other subtypes.[19]

THE 5q− SYNDROME

Among patients with MDS a group can be delineated with what is designated the 5q− syndrome. Patients tend to be middle-aged or elderly women with a relatively good prognosis. Haemopoietic cells show an interstitial deletion of the long arm of chromosome 5 as a single acquired chromosomal anomaly. Such patients most often have a refractory anaemia, often macrocytic, with or without ring sideroblasts and also have characteristic megakaryocytes; these are more than 30 μm in diameter but have non-lobulated nuclei (see Fig. 3.22). The platelet count is usually normal or even increased. The disease may fall into the RA or RARS categories of the FAB classification.

REFRACTORY MACROCYTOSIS

Occasional patients with myelodysplasia have refractory macrocytosis but are not anaemic and

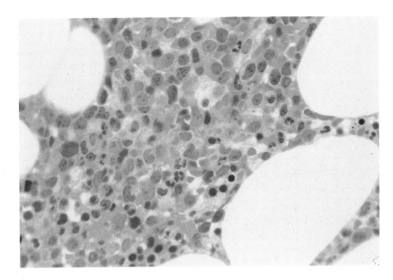

Fig. 3.32 BM trephine biopsy, CMML, showing numerous granulocyte precursors, promonocytes, monocytes and dysplastic erythroblasts. Plastic-embedded, H&E × 390.

lack features which would lead to their being assigned to any of the FAB categories of MDS. When erythropoiesis is clonal they should be recognized as having MDS and can reasonably be grouped with refractory anaemia. With long-term follow up anaemia and other features of overt MDS develop.

REFRACTORY SIDEROBLASTIC ERYTHROPOIESIS

Occasional patients are seen with primary acquired sideroblastic erythropoiesis who lack anaemia and other features which would allow them to be assigned to one of the FAB categories of MDS.[27] Nevertheless erythropoiesis is clonal and such patients should be recognized as having MDS. They can reasonably be grouped with RARS. With disease progression anaemia occurs.

SECONDARY MYELODYSPLASIA

Myelodysplasia may be secondary to deliberate or environmental exposure to mutagenic agents such as cytotoxic chemotherapy, benzene and irradiation. Such cases can be categorized according to the FAB recommendations but because they have distinctive features it is useful to consider them separately. Secondary MDS usually occurs at a younger age than primary MDS and has a much worse prognosis. Bone marrow failure

and evolution to acute leukaemia occur much earlier.

Peripheral blood

Abnormalities in the peripheral blood are usually more marked than in primary MDS. Even cases which fall into the RA and RARS categories commonly show neutropenia, thrombocytopenia, monocytosis and evidence of trilineage dysplasia.

Bone marrow cytology

The bone marrow may be hypercellular but is often hypocellular. A poor aspirate may be obtained because of associated bone marrow fibrosis. Obvious trilineage myelodysplasia is common, even in cases which meet the criteria for RA and RARS. There are usually at least some ring sideroblasts. Hypogranular neutrophils, pseudo-Pelger–Hüet neutrophils and micromega-karyocytes are also common.

Bone marrow histology

Because of the frequent difficulty experienced in obtaining a good aspirate a trephine biopsy is often important in diagnosis. The cellularity is more variable than in primary myelodysplasia. There is often a marked increase in reticulin and in contrast to primary myelodysplasia there may be collagen fibrosis. There is often a severe degree of dysplasia affecting all three lineages with numerous micromegakaryocytes.

Malignant histiocytosis

Malignant histiocytosis is a disease consequent on the proliferation in tissues of a neoplastic clone of cells of monocyte/macrophage lineage; the abnormal cells show variable phagocytic activity. This disease may be regarded as the tissue counterpart of acute monocytic leukaemia. It differs from monocytic sarcoma in that the cells of the neoplastic clone are widely distributed in peripheral tissues rather than forming localized tumours.

It appears likely that in the past a significant proportion of diagnoses of malignant histiocytosis[28,29] or of histiocytic medullary reticulosis[30] (usually regarded as a form of the same disease) were actually misdiagnoses.[31-35] The majority of cases misinterpreted as malignant histiocytosis were either reactive histiocytosis consequent on viral or other infections or reactive histiocytosis as a response to large cell anaplastic lymphoma and other T-lineage lymphomas. A less common cause of confusion is a T-cell lymphoma in which the lymphoma cells are themselves phagocytic.[36] It is important that the term malignant histiocytosis be restricted to cases in which neoplastic cells are of monocyte lineage.

The term histiocytic medullary reticulosis is probably best abandoned since the recent availability of immunophenotyping and other techniques has led to the recognition that in the great majority of cases the histiocytic proliferation and florid haemophagocytosis were consequent on a T-cell lymphoma[34,35] or a viral infection.[33] The reactive haemophagocytic syndromes are discussed further on pages 55 and 176.

The diagnosis of malignant histiocytosis rests on clinical, histological, cytochemical and immunophenotypic grounds. Neoplastic cells are primitive and although phagocytosis occurs it is not prominent.[31] Neoplastic cells can be demonstrated, by cytochemical staining or immunophenotyping, to belong to the monocyte lineage and not to the T-lymphocyte lineage, whereas in haemophagocytic syndromes consequent on a T-cell lymphoma there is an admixture of reactive mature phagocytic histiocytes and immature neoplastic cells of lymphoid lineage.[34]

Common clinical features of malignant histiocytosis are hepatomegaly, splenomegaly, lymphadenopathy, skin infiltration and systemic symptoms such as malaise, fever and weight loss.

Peripheral blood

Pancytopenia is common. Small numbers of immature cells of monocyte/macrophage lineage may be present in the blood (see Fig. 3.33).

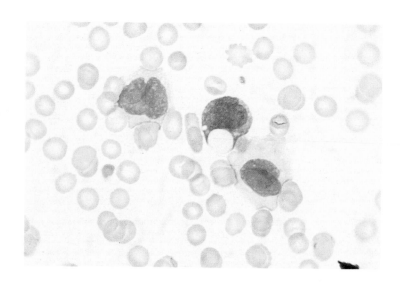

Fig. 3.33 PB, malignant histiocytosis, showing anaemia, thrombocytopenia and three abnormal cells of monocyte lineage, one of which has a phagocytic vacuole. MGG × 940.

Bone marrow cytology

At onset the bone marrow may show minimal or no infiltration by neoplastic cells. With more advanced disease there may be heavy infiltration (Fig. 3.34). The majority of neoplastic cells have the morphological features of monoblasts or 'reticulum cells'. Cells are large and usually have a round nucleus with nucleoli and a diffuse chromatin pattern. Cytoplasm is plentiful and moderately basophilic. A variable number of maturing cells with kidney-shaped nuclei and more abundant cytoplasm are also present.[31]

Some cells are phagocytic and are seen to have ingested granulocytes and their precursors, erythroblasts and platelets; however, phagocytosis is much less marked than in reactive haemophagocytosis.

Bone marrow histology

Bone marrow infiltration is more commonly detected by trephine biopsy than by bone marrow aspiration.[37] The bone marrow may appear normal at the time of diagnosis or show a mild focal infiltrate of neoplastic cells. In the later

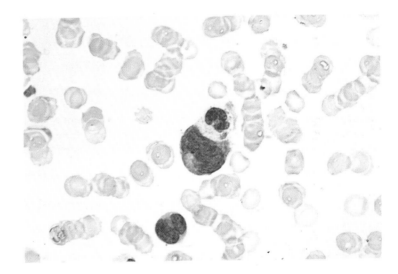

Fig. 3.34 BM aspirate, malignant histiocytosis, showing two immature cells of monocyte lineage, one of which has phagocytosed a neutrophil. MGG × 940.

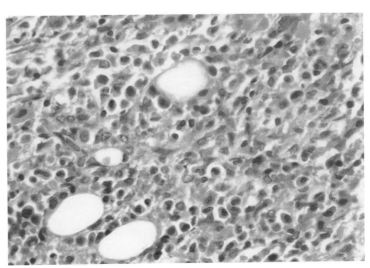

Fig. 3.35 BM trephine biopsy, malignant histiocytosis (same case as Fig. 3.34) showing a diffuse infiltrate of large cells with irregular nuclei and prominent nucleoli; haemophagocytosis is not a prominent feature. Paraffin-embedded, H&E × 390.

stages of the disease diffuse replacement of haemopoietic tissue commonly occurs (Fig. 3.35).[29,38] The infiltrate is largely composed of immature cells with large pleomorphic nuclei which may be lobulated and contain prominent nucleoli; there are moderate amounts of basophilic cytoplasm. Mitoses are usually numerous. A variable component of more mature cells of monocytic lineage may be present. Mild degrees of haemophagocytosis may be seen. However, marked haemophagocytosis is not a feature of malignant histiocytosis and when it is present a benign haemophagocytic syndrome or haemophagocytosis associated with a T-cell lymphoma should be suspected.

REFERENCES

1 Bennett JM, Catovsky D, Daniel MT, et al. (1976) Proposals for the classification of the acute leukaemias (FAB cooperative group). Br J Haematol, **33**, 451–458.

2 Bennett JM, Catovsky D, Daniel MT, et al. (1985) Proposed revised criteria for the classification of acute myeloid leukemia. Ann Intern Med, **103**, 626–629.

3 Bain BJ. Leukaemia Diagnosis; a Guide to the FAB Classification. Gower Medical Publishing, London, 1990.

4 Hayhoe FGJ and Quaglino D. Haematological Cytochemistry, 2nd edition, Churchill Livingstone, Edinburgh, 1988.

5 Islam A, Frisch B and Henderson ES (1989) Plastic embedded core biopsy: a complementary approach to bone marrow aspiration for diagnosing acute myeloid leukaemia. J Clin Pathol, **42**, 300–306.

6 Islam A, Catovsky D, Goldman JM and Galton DAG (1985) Bone marrow biopsy changes in acute leukaemia. I: observations before chemotherapy. Histopathology, **9**, 939–957.

7 Islam A, Catovsky D, Goldman J and Galton DAG (1984) Bone marrow fibre content in acute myeloid leukaemia before and after treatment. J Clin Pathol, **37**, 1259–1263.

8 Bloomfield CD and Brunning RD (1985) The revised French–American–British classification of acute myeloid leukemia: is new better? Ann Intern Med, **103**, 614–616.

9 Lorand-Metz I, Vassallo J, Aoki RY and de Souza CA (1991) Acute megakaryoblastic leukaemia: importance of bone marrow biopsy in diagnosis. Leukemia and Lymphoma, **4**, 74–75.

10 Penchansky L, Taylor SR and Krause JR (1989) Three infants with acute megakaryoblastic leukaemia simulating metastatic tumour. Cancer, **64**, 1366–1371.

11 Bennett JM, Catovsky D, Daniel MT, et al. (1991) Proposal for the recognition of minimally differentiated acute myeloid leukaemia (AML-M0). Br J Haematol, **78**, 325–329.

12 Needleman SW, Burns P, Dick FR and Armitage JO (1981) Hypoplastic acute leukemia. Cancer, **48**, 1410–1414.

13 Howe RB, Bloomfield CD and McKenna RW (1982) Hypocellular acute leukemia. Am J Med, **72**, 391–395.

14 Bennett JM, Catovsky D, Daniel MT, et al. (1982) Proposals for the classification of the myelodysplastic syndromes. Br J Haematol, **51**, 189–199.

15 Kuriyama K, Tomonaga M, Matsuo T, Ginnai I and Ichimaru M (1986) Diagnostic significance of detecting pseudo-Pelger–Hüet anomalies and micromegakaryocytes in myelodysplastic syndrome. Br J Haematol, **63**, 665–669.

16 Thiede T, Engquist L and Billstrom R (1988) Application of megakaryocytic morphology in diagnosing 5q– syndrome. Eur J Haematol, **41**, 434–437.

17 Wong KF and Chan JKC (1991) Are 'dysplastic' and hypogranular megakaryocytes specific markers for myelodysplastic syndrome? Br J Haematol, **77**, 509–514.

18 Yoshida Y, Oguma S, Uchjino H and Maekawa T (1988) Refractory myelodysplastic syndromes with hypocellular bone marrow. J Clin Pathol, **41**, 763–767.

19 Rios A, Cañizo C, Sanz MA, et al. (1990) Bone marrow biopsy in myelodysplastic syndromes: morphological characteristics and contribution to the study of prognostic factors. Br J Haematol, **75**, 26–33.

20 Frisch B and Bartl R (1986) Bone marrow histology in myelodysplastic syndromes. Scand J Haematol **36**, suppl 45, 21–37.

21 Thiele J and Fischer R (1991) Megakaryocytopoiesis in haematological disorders: diagnostic feature of bone marrow biopsies. Virchows Archiv (A), **418**, 87–97.

22 Fox SB, Lorenzen J, Heryet A, Jones M, Gatter KC and Mason DY (1990) Megakaryocytes in myelodysplasia: an immunohistochemical study on bone marrow trephines. Histopathology, **17**, 69–74.

23 Clark DM and Lampert IA (1990) Apoptosis is a common histopathological finding in myelodysplasia: the correlate of ineffective haematopoiesis. Leukemia and Lymphoma, **2**, 415–418.

24 Tricot G, de Wolf Peeters C, Hendrickx B and Verwilghen RL (1984) Bone marrow histology in myelodysplastic syndromes. Br J Haematol, **56**, 423–430.

25 Delacrétaz F, Schmidt P-M, Piguet D, Bachmann F and Costa J (1987) Histopathology of myelodysplastic syndromes: the FAB classification. *Am J Clin Pathol*, **87**, 180–186.

26 Shepherd PCA, Ganesan TS and Galton DAG (1987) Haematological classification of the chronic myeloid leukaemias. *Baillière's Clin Haematol*, **1**, 887–906.

27 Bowen DT and Jacobs A (1989) Primary acquired sideroblastic erythropoiesis in non-anaemic and minimally anaemic subjects. *J Clin Pathol*, **42**, 56–58.

28 Warnke RA, Kim H and Dorfman RF (1975) Malignant histiocytosis (histiocytic medullary reticulosis). I. Clinicopathological study of 29 cases. *Cancer*, **35**, 215–230.

29 Lampert IA, Catovsky D and Bergier N (1978) Malignant histiocytosis: a clinicopathological study of 12 cases. *Br J Haematol*, **40**, 65–77.

30 Scott RB and Robb-Smith AHT (1939) Histiocytic medullary reticulosis. *Lancet*, **ii**, 194–198.

31 Manoharan A and Catovsky D. Histiocytic medullary reticulosis revisited. In: *Haematology and Blood Transfusion*, vol 27, *Disorders of the Monocyte Macrophage System*, Schmalz IF, Huhn D and Schaefer HE (eds). Springer Verlag, Berlin, 1981.

32 Wilson MS, Weiss LM, Gatter KC, Mason DY, Dorfman RF and Warnke RA (1990) Malignant histiocytosis: a reassessment of cases previously reported in 1975 based on paraffin section immunophenotyping studies. *Cancer*, **66**, 530–536.

33 Su I-J, Lin D-T, Hsieh H-C, *et al.* (1990) Fatal primary Epstein Barr virus infection masquerading as histiocytic medullary reticulosis in young children in Taiwan. *Hematol Pathol*, **4**, 189–195.

34 Falini B, Pileri S, de Solas I, *et al.* (1990) Peripheral T-cell lymphoma associated with hemophagocytic syndrome. *Blood*, **75**, 434–444.

35 Robb-Smith AHT (1990) Before our time: half a century of histiocytic medullary reticulosis: a T-cell teaser. *Histopathology*, **17**, 279–293.

36 Kadin ME, Kamoun M and Lamberg J (1981) Erythrophagocytic T-γ lymphoma: a clinicopathological entity resembling malignant histiocytosis. *N Engl J Med*, **304**, 648–653.

37 Sonneveld P, van Lom K, Kappers-Klunne M, Prins MER and Abels J (1990) Clinico-pathological diagnosis and treatment of malignant histiocytosis. *Br J Haematol*, **75**, 511–516.

38 Ralfkiaer E, Delsol G, O'Connor NTJ, *et al.* (1990) Malignant lymphomas of true histiocytic origin. A clinical, histological, immunophenotypic and genotypic study. *J Pathol*, **160**, 9–17.

4: Myeloproliferative Disorders

The myeloproliferative disorders are a group of diseases which have in common that they are consequent on the proliferation of a clone of myeloid cells derived from a neoplastic precursor. Evidence suggests that even when differentiation is predominantly to cells of a single lineage the disorder has arisen in a multipotent myeloid stem cell or, at least in some cases, in a pluripotent stem cell capable of giving rise to cells of both myeloid and lymphoid lineages. In the myeloproliferative disorders maturation of neoplastic cells is relatively normal and cells retain some responsiveness to normal physiological controls; for this reason they may be regarded as relatively benign neoplasms. However, this group of conditions shows a greater or lesser propensity to evolve into a malignant neoplasm, resembling acute leukaemia, which rapidly leads to death. In the case of chronic granulocytic leukaemia acute transformation is very frequent and occurs at a median interval of only two to three years. Polycythaemia rubra vera, idiopathic myelofibrosis and systemic mastocytosis undergo acute transformation less often and usually after a longer chronic phase. An acute phase is least frequent in essential thrombocythaemia.

The myeloproliferative disorders differ from the myelodysplastic syndromes (MDS) in that early in the course of the disease haemopoiesis is effective with overproduction of cells of at least one lineage. Dysplastic features are either absent or not prominent. However, with disease progression haemopoiesis may become ineffective and dysplastic features may appear. Occasionally patients are seen with a condition which cannot be readily assigned to one or other category of disease because of the presence of both myeloproliferative and myelodysplastic features.

It should be noted that the correct diagnosis and classification of the myeloproliferative disorders is often more dependent on the peripheral blood features than on bone marrow cytology or histology; consideration of cytogenetic and molecular characteristics may also be necessary.

CHRONIC GRANULOCYTIC LEUKAEMIA

Chronic granulocytic leukaemia (CGL) is a rare condition resulting from the neoplastic proliferation of an early haemopoietic precursor cell that can differentiate into granulocyte, monocyte, erythroid, megakaryocyte and, under certain circumstances, lymphoid lineages. Approaching 95 per cent of patients with CGL have an acquired chromosomal abnormality in the leukaemic clone consisting of a reciprocal translocation between the long arms of chromosomes 9 and 22, t(9;22) (q34;q11); the abnormal chromosome 22 is designated the Philadelphia (Ph) chromosome. As a result of the translocation, a hybrid gene is formed from the Abelson (ABL) oncogene, carried on the long arm of chromosome 9, and the breakpoint cluster region (BCR) gene on chromosome 22. The BCR-ABL fusion gene encodes a 210 kD protein with protein kinase activity which is thought to have an important role in the pathogenesis of the disease. The majority of patients with Ph-negative CGL, which is identical to Ph-positive disease in all other respects, have been found to have a BCR-ABL fusion gene using molecular hybridization techniques, despite the absence of a 9;22 translocation.[1] This is not the case with Ph-negative atypical chronic myeloid leukaemia (see below).

CGL is very largely a disease of adult life. The overall incidence is one to 2/100 000/year with a slow increase occurring with increasing age. The disease is commoner in men than in women with

102

a male : female ratio of about 1.5 : 1. Patients may present with the symptoms of anaemia, splenic pain, or rarely leucostasis, due to a very high white cell count. However, because of the insidious onset of the disease, many patients have only minor symptoms at the time of diagnosis. Occasionally the disease is diagnosed on a routine blood count in an asymptomatic patient.

Physical examination reveals splenomegaly, although this is not usually marked until the white cell count exceeds $100 \times 10^9/l$. Hepatomegaly is also common.

Although initially the disease pursues a chronic course in which patients are often maintained in reasonably good health, the prognosis is very poor because of almost invariable transformation to an acute leukaemia which is refractory to treatment. Acute transformation is often preceded by an accelerated phase in which the disease becomes resistant to therapy.

Assessment of peripheral blood features is of major importance in the diagnosis of CGL; bone marrow cytological and histological features are of lesser importance.

Peripheral blood

The total white cell count is elevated, usually to between 20 and $500 \times 10^9/l$. The predominant cell types in the peripheral blood are neutrophils and myelocytes (Fig. 4.1); immature granulocytic cells are also present with blasts and promyelocytes usually being less than 10–15 per cent of cells.[2] Basophils are almost invariably increased and the absolute eosinophil count is increased in the great majority of patients; some eosinophil and basophil myelocytes are present. Granulocytes show normal maturation. A normocytic, normochromic anaemia is usual. The platelet count is usually normal or elevated, but does not usually exceed $1000 \times 10^9/l$. Occasional patients have thrombocytopenia. Some giant platelets are usually present and occasional bare megakaryocyte nuclei are seen.

During successful chronic phase treatment the peripheral blood count and film usually become almost normal though a degree of basophilia and occasional immature granulocytes may persist. Patients presenting with or developing extensive bone marrow fibrosis have marked anisocytosis and poikilocytosis with prominent tear-drop poikilocytes. The accelerated phase may be marked by increasing basophilia, persistent leucocytosis or the reappearance of anaemia. Acute transformation may follow an accelerated phase or the appearance of features of bone marrow fibrosis, or be heralded by the appearance of dysplastic features (such as the acquired Pelger–Hüet anomaly of neutrophils or the presence of circulating micromegakaryocytes) or there may be the abrupt appearance of increasing numbers of circulating blasts in a previously stable patient.

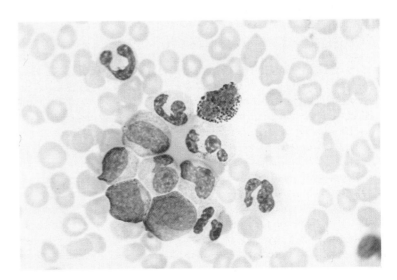

Fig. 4.1 PB, Ph-positive CGL, showing neutrophils and their precursors and one basophil. MGG × 940.

Acute transformation is myeloid in about two-thirds of cases and lymphoblastic or mixed in the remainder. Myeloblasts may show neutrophil or basophil differentiation. Megakaryoblastic transformation is not uncommon. Rarely transformation is monoblastic, eosinophilic, hypergranular promyelocytic or erythroblastic, or there are hybrid cells with both basophil and mast cell features. Often a single patient has blasts of diverse types, usually a mixture of megakaryoblasts and myeloblasts, but occasionally a mixture of lymphoblasts and blasts of myeloid lineage. As the number of blast cells in the blood increases there is a gradual disappearance of mature cells and anaemia and thrombocytopenia develop.

Bone marrow cytology

In the chronic phase of CGL the bone marrow is intensely hypercellular with granulocytic and often megakaryocytic hyperplasia (Fig. 4.2). The myeloid:erythroid ratio is greater than 10:1, usually of the order of 25:1.[1] Precursors of neutrophils, eosinophils and basophils are all increased. Cellular maturation is normal. Erythropoiesis is reduced but morphologically normal. The average size and lobulation of megakaryocytes is reduced but micromegakaryocytes with one or two small round nuclei, as seen in the MDS, are not usually a feature of the chronic phase of CGL. As a consequence of the increased

cell turnover, there is often an increase of macrophages and various storage cells (see below).

During the accelerated phase the bone marrow may show increasing basophilia, some increase of blast cells or the appearance of dysplastic features. Bone marrow aspiration may become difficult or impossible because of increasing bone marrow fibrosis.

With the onset of acute transformation the bone marrow is steadily replaced by blasts showing the usual cytological features of the lineage in question.

Bone marrow histology[3-7]

The marrow is hypercellular with loss of fat cells (Figs 4.3 and 4.4). In most cases more than 95 per cent of the marrow cavity is occupied by haemopoietic cells. There is a marked increase in granulocytic precursors with a variable degree of left shift. The normal topographic relationship of haemopoiesis is retained, with granulopoiesis occurring predominantly in the paratrabecular, peri-arterial, and pericapillary areas, although the more mature granulocytic precursors extend into the intertrabecular marrow. The increased numbers of basophils are not usually detected on histological sections because of dissolution of their granules during processing. Eosinophil precursors are increased in the majority of cases. A feature that may be helpful in distinguishing CGL

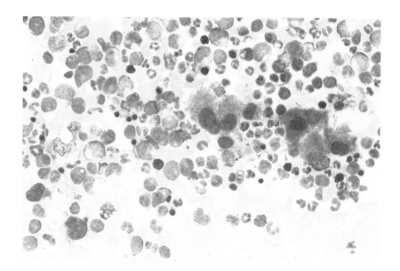

Fig. 4.2 BM aspirate, Ph-positive CGL, showing hyperplasia of all granulocytic lineages and a clump of megakaryocytes with hypolobulated nuclei. MGG × 377.

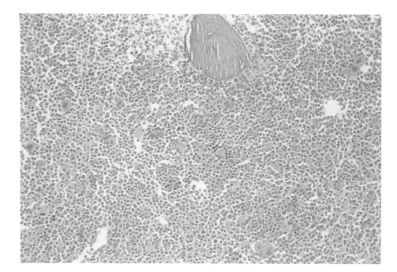

Fig. 4.3 BM trephine biopsy, CGL, showing a packed marrow with marked granulocytic hyperplasia. Plastic-embedded, H&E × 97.

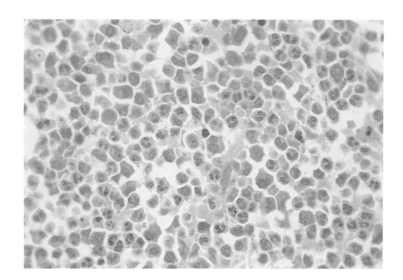

Fig. 4.4 BM trephine biopsy, CGL, showing granulocytic hyperplasia with left shift. Plastic-embedded, H&E × 390.

from a leukaemoid reaction with granulocytic hyperplasia is that in CGL there is loss of fat cells from the very earliest stages of the disease; the loss of paratrabecular fat cells is marked, whereas these are often preserved in a leukaemoid reaction.[7]

Megakaryopoiesis, and to a lesser extent erythropoiesis, occur in the peri-sinusoidal areas. There may be some megakaryocytes within sinusoids and also some near bony trabeculae.[8] Megakaryocytes are usually increased in number, often forming small clusters of cells, and in some cases this is quite a striking feature. The average size and nuclear lobe count of megakaryocytes is decreased (Figs 4.5 and 4.6). The megakaryocytic morphology is variable, with most patients having both relatively normal forms and smaller cells with small, hypolobated nuclei. It has been suggested that cases with marked megakaryocytic proliferation, often accompanied by fibrosis, should be distinguished from CGL and classified as chronic megakaryocytic granulocytic myelosis. However, this distinction is arbitrary and unnecessary since such cases, when they are

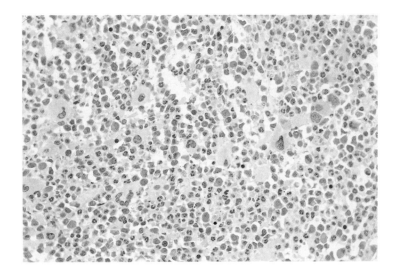

Fig. 4.5 BM trephine biopsy, CGL with prominent megakaryocytic component, showing increased numbers of megakaryocytes with hypolobulated nuclei and granulocytic hyperplasia. Plastic-embedded, H&E × 195.

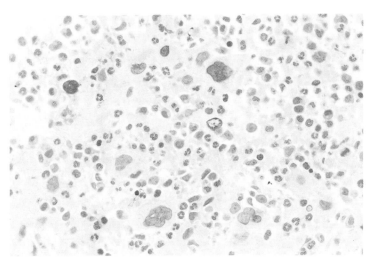

Fig. 4.6 BM trephine biopsy, CGL with prominent megakaryocytic component, showing granulocytic hyperplasia and numerous megakaryocytes with hyperchromatic, hypolobulated nuclei. Plastic-embedded, H&E × 390.

Ph-positive, do not differ in any important respect from other cases of CGL.[6,9]

Increased numbers of mast cells and plasma cells are commonly seen, usually in a perivascular position. Pseudo-Gaucher cells may be seen (see Fig. 8.15); these are macrophages which contain phagocytosed glycolipids and also haemosiderin; they are formed as a consequence of increased cell turnover. Sea-blue histiocytes may also be found (see page 236). Marrow necrosis is uncommon and when present is usually a sign of impending blast transformation.

Reticulin is usually increased, and occasionally the fibrosis is severe enough to cause confusion with primary (idiopathic) myelofibrosis[10] (see page 114). Fibrosis is more common in cases with marked megakaryocytic proliferation[5] (Fig. 4.7). It may be present at the time of diagnosis, although it is seen more often in the later stages of the disease, when it often predicts impending blast transformation. Severe fibrosis may be accompanied by osteosclerosis.

Accumulation of immature granulocytic precursors (myeloblasts and promyelocytes) in the

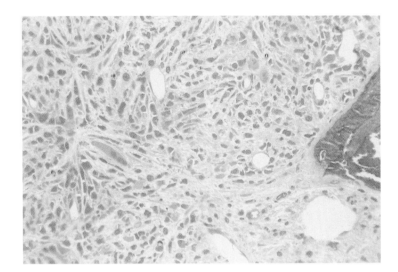

Fig. 4.7 BM trephine biopsy, CGL with fibrosis, showing marked collagen fibrosis and 'streaming' of haemopoietic cells including numerous hypolobulated megakaryocytes. Plastic-embedded, H&E × 195.

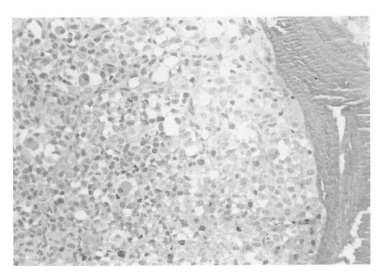

Fig. 4.8 BM trephine biopsy, CGL accelerated phase, showing accumulation of blasts in a broad paratrabecular band. Plastic-embedded, H&E × 195.

paratrabecular (Fig. 4.8) and perivascular regions often precedes transformation to an acute phase.[11]

Blast transformation[12–15] may involve part or all of a trephine biopsy. Areas of involvement contain sheets of blasts, which usually have a single prominent nucleolus and often show considerable pleomorphism. In megakaryoblastic transformation there are usually large numbers of dysplastic megakaryocytes, often with bizarre morphology, in addition to numerous megakaryoblasts. Otherwise it is often not possible to determine the lineage of blasts. Moderate or severe myelofibrosis is seen in approximately 40 per cent of cases of both myeloid and lymphoid transformation, and is an almost universal finding in megakaryoblastic transformation. Myelofibrosis may make marrow aspiration impossible so that a biopsy is necessary to establish the diagnosis of blast transformation.

ATYPICAL CHRONIC MYELOID LEUKAEMIA

Atypical chronic myeloid leukaemia[1,16,17] is a rare Ph-negative condition with a higher median age of onset and a worse prognosis than CGL.

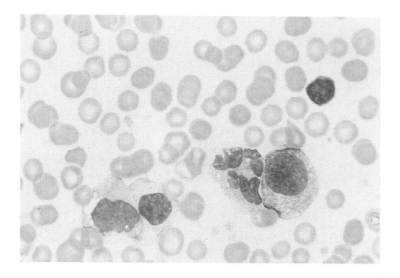

Fig. 4.9 PB, atypical CML (Ph-negative), showing a myelocyte, a bizarre tetraploid neutrophil, an abnormal monocyte, an unidentifiable cell and a lymphocyte. MGG × 940.

Common clinical features are anaemia and splenomegaly. The disorder appears to arise in a multipotent myeloid stem cell or possibly, since occasional lymphoblastic transformations have been observed, in a pluripotent stem cell.

Assessment of peripheral blood features is of major importance in the diagnosis of atypical chronic myeloid leukaemia. Bone marrow cytology and histology are of less importance.

Peripheral blood

The white cell count is elevated with an increase of neutrophils and their precursors (Fig. 4.9).

Monocytosis is more marked than in CGL while eosinophilia and basophilia are less marked and may be absent. The white cell count at presentation is, on average, not as high as in CGL while the anaemia is more severe. The platelet count is not often elevated but is commonly reduced. Maturation of cells is less normal than in CGL and dysplastic features may be present. Distinction from chronic myelomonocytic leukaemia (CMML, see page 94) is largely on the basis of the sum of promyelocytes, myelocytes and metamyelocytes being 15 per cent or higher in atypical CML but usually less than five per cent in CMML.[1]

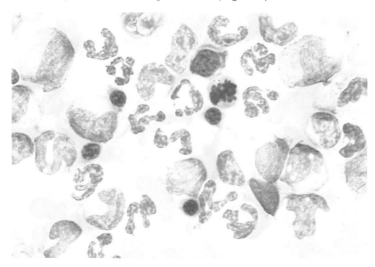

Fig. 4.10 BM aspirate, atypical CML (same patient as Fig. 4.9), showing granulocytic and monocytic hyperplasia. MGG × 940.

Bone marrow cytology

The bone marrow is hypercellular. Both granulocytic and monocytic precursors are increased (Fig. 4.10) though the cellularity is not increased to the extent that is seen in CGL and the myeloid : erythroid ratio is generally less than 10 : 1. Blasts may be increased but do not exceed 30 per cent. Megakaryocytes are decreased in about a third of cases.

Bone marrow histology

The marrow biopsy in atypical chronic myeloid leukaemia may closely resemble that of CGL, particularly when examined at low power. There is marked hypercellularity with predominance of the granulocytic series. Erythroblasts are distributed as single cells or small groups throughout the marrow with well-formed erythroblastic islands being difficult to identify. Megakaryocytes may be increased in number and are sometimes morphologically abnormal. When monocytes are increased (Fig. 4.11) this is the feature which most readily distinguishes atypical CML from CGL. The monocytes are recognized by their irregular nuclei with a diffuse chromatin pattern and moderate amounts of cytoplasm which stains pink on H&E. Atypical CML shows a variable degree of reticulin fibrosis and collagen deposition and osteosclerosis can occur. Making the distinc-

tion between atypical CML and CGL is often not possible on histological grounds alone.

POLYCYTHAEMIA RUBRA VERA

Polycythaemia rubra vera (PRV) or primary proliferative polycythaemia is a chronic myeloproliferative disorder in which the dominant feature is the excessive production of erythrocytes by the marrow with a consequent increase in the circulating red cell mass and the venous haematocrit. Frequently there is also an increase in other haemopoietic cell lines both in the marrow and in the peripheral blood and it is likely that the neoplastic clone originates from a multipotent myeloid stem cell.

Most patients present between the ages of 40 and 70 years. Many of the symptoms are related to the hyperviscosity of the blood and to the arterial or venous thromboses which occur; symptoms include headache, a feeling of fullness of the head, dizziness, tinnitus, dyspnoea, visual disturbance, Raynaud's phenomenon, claudication and gangrene. Pruritus may occur, probably consequent on histamine secretion by basophils. Up to 70 per cent of cases have been found to have splenomegaly and 40 per cent hepatomegaly.

Polycythaemia rubra vera must be distinguished from secondary polycythaemia which is usually consequent on either chronic generalized tissue hypoxia (for example, due to high

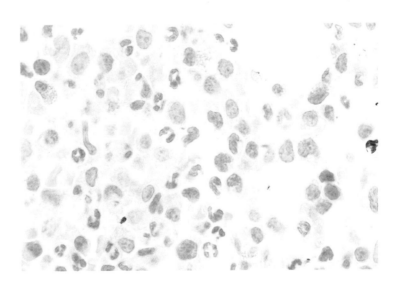

Fig. 4.11 BM trephine biopsy, atypical CML, showing granulocytic hyperplasia and numerous abnormal monocytes. Paraffin-embedded, H&E × 970.

altitude, chronic hypoxic pulmonary disease, cyanotic congenital heart disease) or on inappropriate erythropoietin production (usually a result of chronic renal hypoxia or ectopic production of erythropoietin by a tumour). In many patients with secondary polycythaemia the cause is readily apparent, but sometimes there is diagnostic difficulty and the differential diagnosis then depends on consideration of clinical, peripheral blood and bone marrow features. Hepatomegaly and splenomegaly are not a feature of secondary polycythaemia.

Polycythaemia rubra vera may enter a 'burnt out' or 'spent' phase in which there is initially a reduction of red cell production together with increased bone marrow fibrosis; with disease progression there is development of all the clinical and pathological features usually associated with idiopathic myelofibrosis. A small proportion of patients, particularly those who have been treated with alkylating agents or ^{32}P, develop acute myeloid leukaemia. The incidence of acute leukaemia is much increased in those in whom myelofibrosis has developed, but acute transformation can also occur without any warning signs or, occasionally, follows the appearance of myelodysplastic features.

Untreated polycythaemia rubra vera had a median survival of about one and a half years but with currently available treatment the median survival is about 12 years.

Peripheral blood

The blood count shows an elevation of the red cell count, haemoglobin concentration and haematocrit. As a consequence of the increased blood viscosity the blood film shows a crowding together of the red cells, an appearance described as a 'packed film'. In some patients iron stores have been exhausted and there is also microcytosis and hypochromia. The white cell count is commonly elevated due to an increase of the neutrophil count. Occasionally neutrophilia is marked. Absolute basophilia is often present. Small numbers of immature granulocytes may be present. Many patients have a moderately elevated platelet count.

In patients with secondary polycythaemia basophilia is not seen and neutrophilia and thrombocytosis are unusual. Superimposed iron deficiency is uncommon.

Bone marrow cytology

The bone marrow usually shows marked erythroid hyperplasia and often some degree of granulocytic and megakaryocytic hyperplasia (Fig. 4.12). The average size and nuclear lobulation of megakaryocytes is increased. Iron stores are often absent and the features of superimposed iron deficiency may be present.

In patients with secondary polycythaemia, hypercellularity is less; granulocytic and mega-

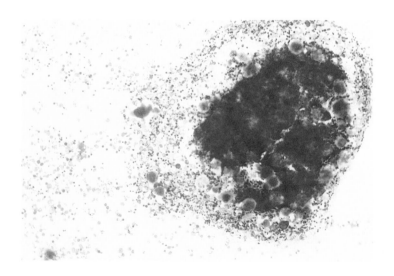

Fig. 4.12 BM aspirate, PRV, bone marrow fragment showing marked hypercellularity attributable to erythroid, granulocytic and megakaryocyte hyperplasia. MGG × 94.

karyocytic hyperplasia and superimposed iron deficiency are not usually present.

Bone marrow histology[3,18-20]

There is usually marked hypercellularity, with haemopoietic cells often filling more than 90 per cent of the marrow space. There is commonly an increase in cells of all three haemopoietic lineages. Erythropoiesis is hyperplastic but morphologically normal (Fig. 4.13). Megakaryocyte morphology is often abnormal with both large, polylobulated forms and an increased number of micromegakaryocytes being seen; the average size of megakaryocytes is considerably increased as is their nuclear lobulation. Often there is clustering of megakaryocytes (Fig. 4.13). There is an increase in emperipolesis and in mitotic figures in megakaryocytes.[8] Granulocytic hyperplasia is of the neutrophil lineage and sometimes also the eosinophil lineage. Many cases show a mild increase in reticulin with about 10 per cent of patients showing a moderate or marked increase.[20] Vascular sinusoids are usually increased in number and may be dilated. Marrow iron stores are decreased or absent.

Up to 30 per cent of cases of PRV develop severe marrow fibrosis which is morphologically indistinguishable from primary myelofibrosis (see page 114); this is more common in cases with marked megakaryocytic proliferation.

In patients with secondary polycythaemia the bone marrow is only moderately hypercellular. There is erythroid hyperplasia, but the other haemopoietic cell lines are normal. In particular the megakaryocytic abnormalities seen in polycythaemia rubra vera are not present, reticulin is normal and sinusoids are not increased. In contrast to PRV, marrow iron stores are usually normal in secondary polycythaemia.[18,19]

Typical cases of PRV can be readily distinguished on histological features from secondary polycythaemia. It should be noted, however, that this is not always the case and some patients in whom a diagnosis of PRV can be made on the basis of clinical, or clinical and cytogenetic features do not have diagnostic histopathological features.[18,20]

ESSENTIAL THROMBOCYTHAEMIA

Essential thrombocythaemia, in common with the other myeloproliferative disorders, is a disease resulting from the clonal proliferation of a multipotent myeloid stem cell but with the predominant disease features resulting from increased platelet production. The disease is seen at all ages but is predominately one of middle and old age. It is characterized by a marked thrombocytosis (usually $1-4 \times 10^{12}/l$) often resulting in haemorrhagic or thrombotic episodes or both.

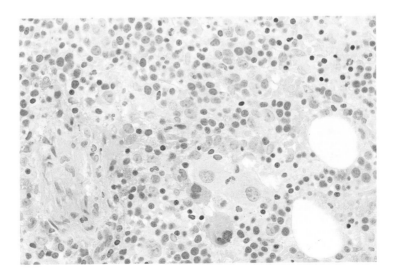

Fig. 4.13 BM trephine biopsy, PRV, showing hypercellularity, erythroid hyperplasia and a cluster of immature megakaryocytes. Plastic-embedded, H&E × 390.

Approximately 20 per cent of patients are asymptomatic and are diagnosed incidentally on routine blood counts. The proportion of patients in whom the diagnosis is made incidentally before the occurrence of symptoms is steadily increasing with the widespread use of automated blood counters. About two-thirds of symptomatic patients suffer venous or arterial thrombosis or symptoms attributable to small vessels' obstruction, such as headache, dizziness, visual disturbance, paraesthesiae and peripheral vascular insufficiency. About a third of symptomatic patients have abnormal bleeding, for example into the gastrointestinal tract and subcutaneous tissues.

Moderate splenomegaly is seen in up to 40 per cent of cases and hepatomegaly in up to 20 per cent.[21] Some patients suffer repeated splenic infarcts, resulting in splenic atrophy and hyposplenism. Pruritus occurs in a minority of patients.

Since marked thrombocytosis can occur not only in essential thrombocythaemia but also in both polycythaemia rubra vera (PRV) and chronic granulocytic leukaemia the diagnosis is in part one of exclusion. Cases with an increased red cell mass are classified as PRV rather than as essential thrombocythaemia. Similarly, cases which are found to have the Ph chromosome are better regarded as a variant of CGL, or alternatively can

be designated specifically 'Ph-positive essential thrombocythaemia'; they have a different disease course from Ph-negative essential thrombocythaemia, showing a marked propensity to either develop typical CGL or to transform into acute leukaemia.[21] It should be noted that in iron deficient patients it can be impossible to distinguish between essential thrombocythaemia and PRV on clinical or histological grounds; the distinction can only be made after a trial of iron therapy, which is not usually justified.

Essential thrombocythaemia may terminate in acute leukaemia or myelofibrosis but, if Ph-positive cases are excluded, the chronic phase of the disease is usually very long.

Peripheral blood

The blood film shows an increased number of platelets with the average platelet size being increased. There are usually some giant platelets and agranular and hypogranular platelets; platelet aggregates may also be present. Occasional bare megakaryocyte nuclei are seen. Mild leucocytosis, neutrophilia and occasional immature granulocytes may be present but the white cell count does not usually exceed $20 \times 10^9/l$. Absolute basophilia is sometimes present but the presence of more than three to five per cent of basophils is predictive of the case being Ph-positive.[21,22] In

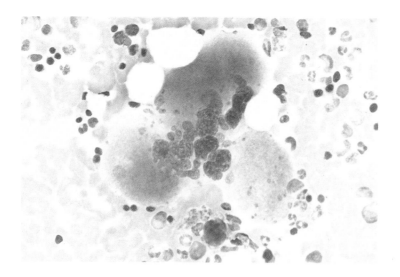

Fig. 4.14 BM aspirate, essential thrombocythaemia, showing four megakaryocytes, one of which is small while three are very large with hyperlobulated nuclei. MGG × 377.

patients who have suffered splenic infarction the usual changes of hyposplenism will be found—Howell—Jolly bodies, acanthocytes, target cells and occasional spherocytes. Patients who have suffered haemorrhagic episodes may show the features of iron deficiency.

When thrombocytosis occurs as a feature of other myeloproliferative disorders the same morphological features are seen as in essential thrombocythaemia. However, in reactive thrombocytosis the platelets are small and normally granulated and circulating megakaryocyte nuclei are not seen.

Bone marrow cytology

The bone marrow aspirate shows an increase in megakaryocytes which are generally large and well lobulated (Fig. 4.14). In some cases there is an overall increase in cellularity due to granulocytic hyperplasia.

Bone marrow histology[4,8,23]

The marrow biopsy findings are extremely variable and in some cases there may be no specific diagnostic features.[23] The marrow is usually hypercellular, although this is not as marked as in the other myeloproliferative disorders. Megakaryocytes are increased in numbers in all cases,

but the degree of hyperplasia is very variable and does not correlate closely with the platelet count. Large clusters of megakaryocytes are commonly seen (Fig. 4.15). The average size of megakaryocytes is increased as is the lobulation of their nuclei (Fig. 4.16); nuclear chromatin pattern is normal in contrast to the hyperchromatic nuclei which may be seen in primary myelofibrosis.[4] In contrast to PRV, megakaryocytes are not pleomorphic and micromegakaryocytes are not increased.[8] Some may be sited abnormally, close to the endosteum and emperipolesis and mitotic figures are increased.[8] There may be mild or moderate granulocytic and erythroid hyperplasia. A mild focal increase in reticulin sometimes occurs but if there is marked reticulin fibrosis a diagnosis of primary myelofibrosis with thrombocytosis is more likely. Although it has been suggested that, in the majority of instances, essential thrombocythaemia and PRV cannot be distinguished on histological grounds[21] other authors have considered that the lack of atypia of megakaryocytes in thrombocythaemia can allow a distinction to be made.[8]

In reactive thrombocytosis there may be some increase in megakaryocyte numbers and size and an increase in emperipolesis, but megakaryocytes are otherwise morphologically normal; they do not occur in large clusters or close to the endosteum.[8] The bone marrow reticulin is also normal.

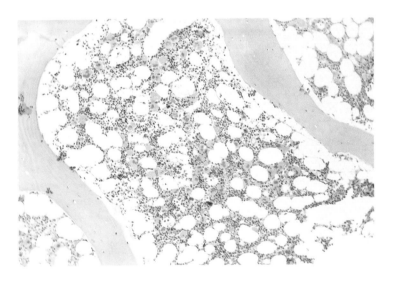

Fig. 4.15 BM trephine biopsy, essential thrombocythaemia, showing mild hypercellularity with a marked increase in megakaryocytes which are forming large clusters. Plastic-embedded, H&E × 97.

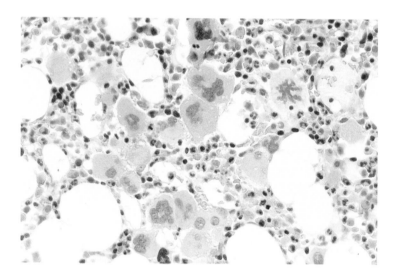

Fig. 4.16 BM trephine biopsy, essential thrombocythaemia, showing clustering of megakaryocytes. The megakaryocytes are mainly large and hyperlobulated, although some small forms are present. Plastic-embedded, H&E × 390.

PRIMARY (IDIOPATHIC) MYELOFIBROSIS (AGNOGENIC MYELOID METAPLASIA)

Primary myelofibrosis is also known as myelofibrosis with myeloid metaplasia and as agnogenic myeloid metaplasia. It is a chronic myeloproliferative disorder characterized by splenomegaly, a leucoerythroblastic anaemia and marrow fibrosis; there is extramedullary haemopoiesis, particularly in the spleen but also in the liver and sometimes in other organs such as kidney, lymph nodes, adrenals, lung, gastrointestinal tract, skin, dura and pleural and peritoneal cavities. The disease is consequent on proliferation of a clone of neoplastic cells arising from a multipotent myeloid stem cell. Proliferation of bone marrow fibroblasts with deposition of reticulin and collagen is reactive to the myeloid proliferation.

Bone marrow fibrosis indistinguishable from primary myelofibrosis may also develop secondary to polycythaemia rubra vera and, less often, essential thrombocythaemia. Chronic granulocytic leukaemia may also evolve into myelofibrosis or, less often, patients whose myeloid cells are Ph-positive may present with a condition which is indistinguishable from idiopathic myelofibrosis. Patients with preceding PRV, essential thrombocythaemia or CGL are classified as myelofibrosis secondary to these specific myeloproliferative disorders rather than as primary myelofibrosis. Similarly patients with clinical and pathological features of myelofibrosis who are found to have an increased red cell mass or the Ph chromosome are best regarded as having variants of PRV and CGL rather than primary myelofibrosis.

Primary myelofibrosis usually affects the middle-aged and elderly. It is a chronic disorder in which patients may remain relatively asymptomatic until the later stages. It is not uncommon for the diagnosis to be incidental. Some degree of splenomegaly is almost invariable and is often very marked. Slight or moderate hepatomegaly is also common. Not surprisingly, survival is longest in those patients who are asymptomatic at the time of diagnosis. Overall, approximately 50 per cent of patients will be alive five years after diagnosis.

Myelofibrosis sometimes terminates in a condition resembling chronic myeloid leukaemia with very striking myeloid proliferation and increasing hepatomegaly and splenomegaly. In 10–20 per cent of cases myelofibrosis terminates by transformation to acute leukaemia; this is usually a myeloblastic transformation but, rarely, it is lymphoblastic, suggesting that the disease may have arisen in a pluripotent rather than a multipotent stem cell. Leukaemic transformation should be suspected when there is a rapid increase in splenic size or the sudden development of anaemia or thrombocytopenia.

Acute myelofibrosis resembles chronic idio-

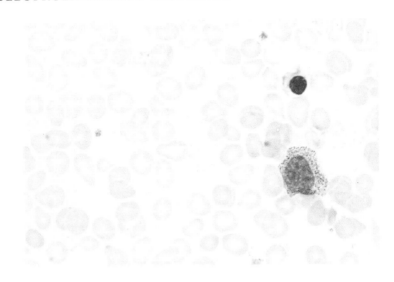

Fig. 4.17 PB, idiopathic myelofibrosis, showing anisocytosis, poikilocytosis (including tear-drop poikilocytes), a myelocyte and an erythroblast. MGG × 940.

pathic myelofibrosis in that there is marrow fibrosis as a consequence of proliferation of neoplastic myeloid cells. It has a rapidly progressive course characterized by severe pancytopenia with minimal or absent splenomegaly. It is best regarded as a variant of acute leukaemia (generally acute megakaryoblastic leukaemia) (see page 81). The fibrotic marrow usually contains large numbers of megakaryoblasts together with immature megakaryocytes; sometimes there are also myeloblasts. The fibrotic component may be reticulin only or reticulin and collagen.

Peripheral blood

The most characteristic peripheral blood findings are pancytopenia with a leucoerythroblastic blood film and with striking poikilocytosis including tear-drop poikilocytes (Fig. 4.17). There is sometimes a mild basophil leucocytosis. Granulocytes and platelets may show some dysplastic features such as hypolobulation of neutrophil nuclei, reduced granulation of eosinophils or large or hypogranular platelets. Occasional circulating micromegakaryocytes can be seen. Sometimes in the early stages of the disease when the bone marrow is hypercellular there is leucocytosis or mild thrombocytosis rather than cytopenia; with disease progression leucopenia, neutropenia and thrombocytopenia supervene.

In the final phase of myelofibrosis a progressive

rise of the white cell count can be seen with a WBC up to $100-200 \times 10^9/l$ and with the appearance in the peripheral blood of increasing numbers of blasts, promyelocytes and myelocytes. Eosinophilia and basophilia may also occur in this phase so that the blood film can be indistinguishable from that of chronic myeloid leukaemia. In other patients in whom an acute transformation occurs there is a rapid rise in the blast count with worsening anaemia, neutropenia and thrombocytopenia.

The blood film in patients with secondary myelofibrosis, for example that due to bone marrow metastases, may be virtually indistinguishable from that of chronic idiopathic myelofibrosis there being pancytopenia, a leucoerythroblastic blood film and striking poikilocytosis. However, basophilia, circulating micromegakaryocytes and dysplastic features do not occur so their presence suggests that the correct diagnosis is primary myelofibrosis.

The blood film in acute myelofibrosis is characterized by pancytopenia with occasional circulating blast cells or other immature cells. Poikilocytosis is not usually a feature.

Bone marrow cytology

As a consequence of the fibrosis, aspiration of bone marrow is often difficult in patients with myelofibrosis. In the early stages of the disease an

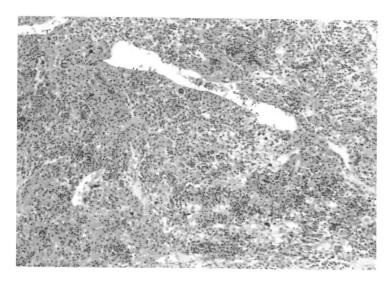

Fig. 4.18 BM trephine biopsy, idiopathic myelofibrosis (cellular phase), showing marked hypercellularity, with an increase in all three haemopoietic cell lines, and ectatic sinusoids. Paraffin-embedded, H&E × 97.

aspirate is sometimes obtained and shows very hypercellular fragments with hyperplasia of all lineages; maturation is fairly normal although there may be some dysplastic features. In the later stages of the disease there is often failure to obtain an aspirate (a 'dry tap') or attempted aspiration yields only blood (a 'blood tap'). Diagnosis then rests on the peripheral blood and trephine biopsy appearances.

Bone marrow histology

In the early stages the marrow may be diffusely hypercellular with an increase in all haemopoietic cell lines with normal maturation[24] (Figs 4.18 and 4.19). However megakaryocytes often predominate, and immature forms are usually present. The megakaryocytic morphology is extremely variable; the nuclei may be small and hypolobulated or hyperchromatic and hyperlobulated. Micromegakaryocytes are increased. Megakaryocytes may be clustered (Fig. 4.19) or sited abnormally, close to the endosteum.[8] Granulocyte precursors may show an abnormal clustering centrally in the intertrabecular spaces.[25] In hypercellular marrows there is usually only a mild to moderate increase in reticulin (Fig. 4.20). Later there is a more marked

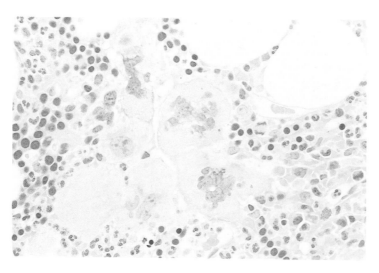

Fig. 4.19 BM trephine biopsy, idiopathic myelofibrosis (cellular phase), showing a cluster of megakaryocytes with hyperlobulated nuclei. Plastic-embedded, H&E × 390.

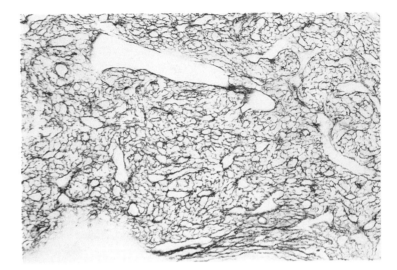

Fig. 4.20 BM trephine biopsy, idiopathic myelofibrosis (cellular phase), showing grade 3 reticulin deposition with numerous ectatic sinusoids outlined (same case as Fig. 4.18). Paraffin-embedded, Gordon—Sweet stain × 97.

increase with coarse fibres running in parallel bundles. Streaming of haemopoietic cells may be noted when reticulin is increased (Fig. 4.21). Marrow sinusoids are distended and contain foci of haemopoietic cells (Fig. 4.18); in the early stages this feature may be more easily detected on sections stained for reticulin. The interstitium may be oedematous and show an increase of lymphocytes, plasma cells, mast cells and macrophages. The incidence of benign lymphoid nodules is increased. The interstitium may also contain platelets which have been released inappropriately within the marrow rather than into sinusoids.

As the degree of fibrosis increases, granulocytic and erythroid precursors in the marrow decrease and the morphological abnormalities in the megakaryocytic series become more pronounced. In severely fibrotic marrows there is fibroblast proliferation and collagen deposition (Figs 4.22 and 4.23). Sinusoids may be obliterated by progressive fibrosis but capillaries are very numerous.[26] Fibrotic changes are often focal with marked variability within a single biopsy; one intertrabecular space may show hypercellular marrow while an adjacent one shows dense fibrosis. In severely fibrotic marrows there may also be an increase of osteoblasts with new bone formation resulting in

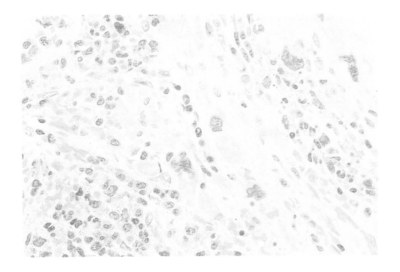

Fig. 4.21 BM trephine biopsy, idiopathic myelofibrosis (fibrotic phase), showing 'streaming' of residual haemopoietic cells, which include numerous dysplastic megakaryocytes, and collagen fibrosis. Plastic-embedded, H&E × 390.

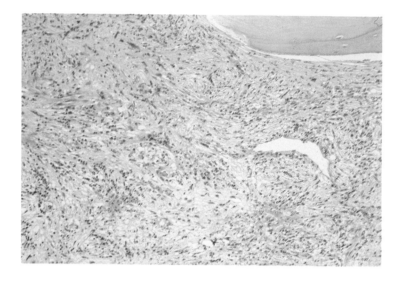

Fig. 4.22 BM trephine biopsy, idiopathic myelofibrosis (fibrotic phase), showing marked collagen fibrosis, with reduction in all haemopoietic cell lines. Paraffin-embedded, H&E × 97.

osteosclerosis (Fig. 4.23); the thickening of bone trabeculae is often marked. Bone deposition may be both by peritrabecular osteoid deposition and by metaplastic bone formation in the marrow cavity.[25] Newly deposited bone is woven bone.

It is generally considered that myelofibrosis progresses from a hypercellular phase to a hypocellular fibrotic phase and this sequence of events may be seen on serial biopsies.[24,27,28] However, the rate of progression is very variable between patients and in some studies progressive changes have not been observed.[23] In some patients sequential biopsies show a decrease rather than an increase in fibrosis; to what extent this is due to variation in the degree of fibrosis from one part of the bone marrow to another cannot be readily determined.

Distinction between primary myelofibrosis and that evolving out of other myeloproliferative disorders is not possible on histological grounds alone.

In order to distinguish between primary myelofibrosis and that secondary to non-haemopoietic neoplasia it is necessary, in patients with dense fibrosis, to look carefully for the presence of malignant cells embedded in the fibrous tissue.

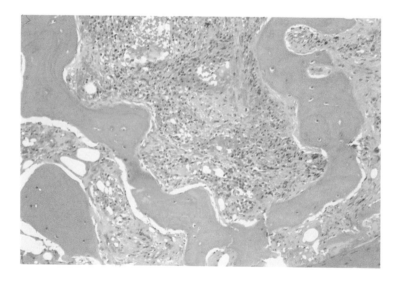

Fig. 4.23 BM trephine biopsy, osteomyelosclerosis, showing irregular thickening of bone trabeculae and marked collagen fibrosis of the intervening marrow. Paraffin-embedded, H&E × 97.

Sometimes it can be difficult to distinguish metastatic carcinoma cells from small dysplastic megakaryocytes. If necessary, immunological markers for megakaryocytes (see page 34) or for cells of epithelial origin (see page 248) can be used to confirm the nature of abnormal cells.

When acute transformation supervenes in idiopathic myelofibrosis increasing numbers of blasts are seen in the biopsy.

SYSTEMIC MASTOCYTOSIS

Mast cell proliferation may be confined to the skin or may be generalized, the latter condition being designated systemic mastocytosis or systemic mast cell disease. Systemic mastocytosis is a rare condition characterized by the neoplastic proliferation of mast cells. Mast cells are derived from a myeloid stem cell and the mast cell proliferation is often associated with granulocytic hyperplasia. Consequently systemic mastocytosis is best regarded as a myeloproliferative disorder. Various organs may be involved, including the bone marrow, liver, spleen, lymph nodes and skin; the most typical skin lesions are those of urticaria pigmentosa. Patients often have symptoms related to the release of secretory products by the neoplastic mast cells; these include abdominal pain, nausea and vomiting, diarrhoea, flushing, and bronchospasm.[29-31] Systemic mastocytosis may pursue either an indolent or an aggressive clinical course. The term 'malignant mastocytosis' is sometimes used to describe systemic mast cell disease with a rapidly progressive clinical course. Prognosis is worst in the minority of patients with overt mast cell leukaemia. Patients with an aggressive course are less likely to have skin involvement and more likely to have hepatomegaly, splenomegaly, leukocytosis, anaemia and thrombocytopenia.[32,33] Although patients can be divided into two or three groups with varying prognosis on the basis of clinical and haematological features[32,33] there is in fact a continuous spectrum of disease characteristics.

Patients with systemic mastocytosis may develop myelodysplasia, all five FAB categories of the myelodysplastic syndromes having been observed.[34] Systemic mastocytosis may also terminate in acute myeloid leukaemia, sometimes appearing *de novo* and sometimes following a period of myelodysplasia. The leukaemia is occasionally mast cell leukaemia but more often is another category of AML. Commonest are acute myeloblastic or acute myelomonocytic leukaemia (FAB categories M1, M2 and M4) but occasional cases of erythroleukaemia or megakaryoblastic leukaemia (FAB categories M6 and M7) have also been reported.[34]

Peripheral blood[31,33,35,36]

In patients with an indolent clinical course the peripheral blood is most often normal but a minority of patients show evidence of abnormal proliferation of other myeloid lineages (neutrophilia, eosinophilia, basophilia, monocytosis, thrombocytosis). Circulating mast cells are usually not noted.

In patients who pursue an aggressive clinical course peripheral blood evidence of a myeloproliferative disorder is more prominent. The majority of patients have neutrophilia, many have eosinophilia, basophilia or monocytosis and a minority have thrombocytosis. Cytopenias are also common, particularly anaemia and thrombocytopenia but sometimes leukopenia and neutropenia. Hypogranular and hypersegmented eosinophils, resembling those seen in the idiopathic hypereosinophilic syndrome, may be present.[36] In some patients the peripheral blood features cannot be distinguished from those of chronic myeloid leukaemia. Some patients have myelodysplastic features such as the acquired Pelger–Hüet anomaly of neutrophils. Occasional patients have circulating mast cells, usually in small numbers. In the few patients in whom mast cell leukaemia supervenes there are larger numbers of circulating mast cells, usually with atypical cytological features such as hypogranularity or nuclear lobulation (Fig. 4.24).

Bone marrow cytology

The bone marrow aspirate is normo- or hypercellular and contains increased numbers of mast cells (Fig. 4.25). These may be under-represented in an aspirate in comparison with a trephine because of the fibrosis provoked by mast cell

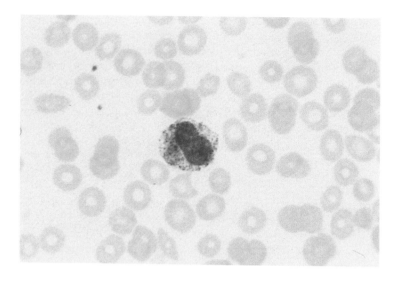

Fig. 4.24 PB, mast cell leukaemia, showing a hypogranular mast cell. MGG × 940.

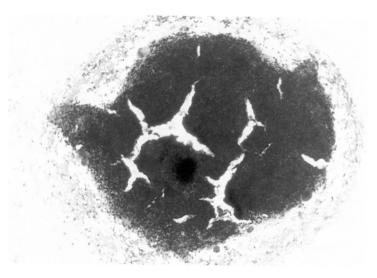

Fig. 4.25 BM aspirate, systemic mastocytosis, showing an intensely hypercellular fragment due mainly to granulocytic hyperplasia. MGG × 94.

proliferation. They may also remain in the fragments so that fragments as well as cell trails should be examined. Clusters of mast cells may be present.[35] When mast cells are cytologically normal they are easily indentifiable as oval or elongated cells with a central non-lobulated nucleus and with the cytoplasm packed with purple granules; when they are cytologically atypical they may be confused with basophils. Atypical features include nuclear lobulation (Fig. 4.26), hypogranularity (Fig. 4.27) and a primitive chromatin pattern. In patients who pursue

an indolent clinical course, the bone marrow is usually normocellular and contains a relatively small number of cytologically normal mast cells. Those patients who pursue an aggressive clinical course are more likely to show a hypercellular marrow with granulocytic hyperplasia and larger numbers of mast cells which, in some cases, are cytologically atypical. Granulocytic hyperplasia may include neutrophil, eosinophil and basophil lineages. In some cases there are myelodysplastic features such as ring sideroblasts and in some there is megakaryocytic hyperplasia. The bone

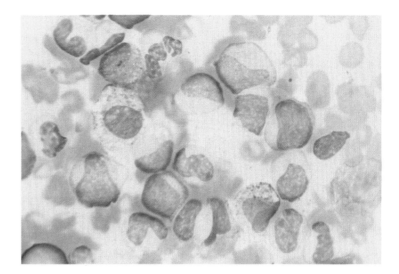

Fig. 4.26 BM aspirate, systemic mastocytosis, showing two abnormal mast cells and numerous neutrophil precursors. The mast cells are hypogranular, one has a large nucleus and the other has a lobulated nucleus. MGG × 940.

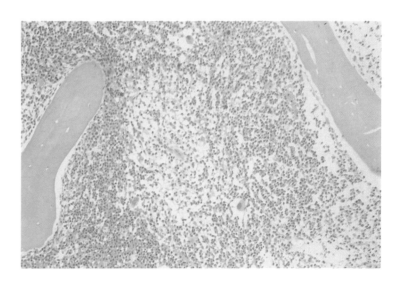

Fig. 4.27 BM trephine biopsy, systemic mastocytosis, showing marked hypercellularity with a loose focal aggregate of mast cells (centre). Paraffin-embedded, H&E × 97.

marrow appearances may be confused with those of chronic granulocytic leukaemia if the presence of large numbers of mast cells is not appreciated.

Mast cells stain with alcian blue as well as with Romanowsky stains such as Giemsa and MGG and stain metachromatically with toluidine blue; they are MPO and SBB-negative and PAS and chloroacetate esterase-positive. On immunochemistry, mast cells are positive with monoclonal antibodies of CD33, CD45 and CD68 clusters.

Bone marrow histology

The marrow biopsy is abnormal in the vast majority of cases[29,30,37] (Fig. 4.27). The most common finding is focal infiltration by mast cells in paratrabecular and perivascular areas. Eosinophils are present in variable numbers, often concentrated at the periphery of the infiltrated areas (Figs 4.28 and 4.29). Lymphocytes, plasma cells, macrophages and fibroblasts are also frequently seen in the areas of infiltration. Occasionally the lymphocytes are aggregated either at the centre or at the

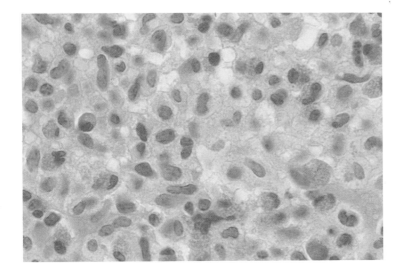

Fig. 4.28 BM trephine biopsy, systemic mastocytosis, showing numerous abnormal mast cells — with marked variation in nuclear shape and moderate amounts of pale staining cytoplasm — eosinophils, and small numbers of lymphocytes. Paraffin-embedded, H&E × 970.

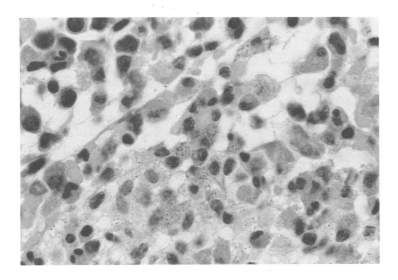

Fig. 4.29 BM trephine biopsy, systemic mastocytosis, showing basophilic granules in the cytoplasm of mast cells. Paraffin-embedded, Giemsa × 970.

periphery of a focal lesion;[30,38] immunocyto-chemical analysis has shown the lymphocytes to be a mixture of B and T cells.[39] There is usually a dense network of reticulin fibres associated with the infiltrate, and sometimes collagen deposition. There may be osteosclerosis, or evidence of increased bone turnover with osteoclasts, osteoblasts and the amount of osteoid all being increased;[38] peritrabecular fibrosis which is sometimes present may be related to increased bone turnover.

The morphology of the mast cells is variable and this may cause difficulty in their recognition, especially in H&E-stained sections. They may be either spindle shaped thus resembling fibroblasts (Fig. 4.28), or have abundant pale pink cytoplasm and irregularly shaped nuclei leading to confusion with macrophages. A Giemsa stain shows purple cytoplasmic granules (Fig. 4.29), although these are often quite scanty. With a toluidine blue stain the granules are pink (Fig. 4.30). Decalcification of specimens may lead to loss of metachromatic staining with the toluidine blue stain. Mast cells have chloroacetate esterase activity which may

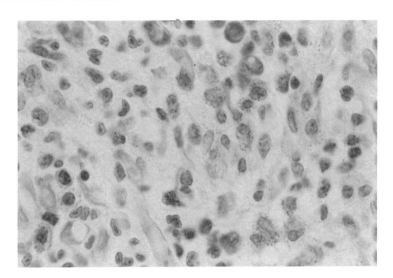

Fig. 4.30 BM trephine biopsy, systemic mastocytosis, showing purple metachromatic granules in the cytoplasm of mast cells. Paraffin-embedded, toluidine blue × 970.

be demonstrated in both paraffin and plastic-embedded sections using Leder's stain; however this stain does not work well on decalcified specimens and it should be noted that neutrophil myelocytes will also stain strongly.

Diffuse replacement of the marrow by neoplastic mast cells occur infrequently. In these cases the infiltrate is much more monomorphic than seen in the focal lesions. The mast cells are usually spindle shaped and may show nuclear atypia. There is marked reticulin fibrosis and osteosclerosis is often present. Often there are atypical mast cells in the peripheral blood allowing a diagnosis of mast cell leukaemia to be made.[37]

Lennert and Parwaresch[32] have used the marrow biopsy findings to divide patients into prognostic groups. They have described three main patterns of involvement: type I, in which there is focal infiltration, but the intervening haemopoietic marrow is normal; type II, in which there are focal lesions and marked granulocytic hyperplasia with loss of fat spaces; and type III in which there is diffuse replacement of the haemopoeitic marrow. Type I corresponds to the more benign systemic mastocytosis, type II to 'malignant mastocytosis', and type III to mast cell leukaemia. Others have also found a hypercellular bone marrow to have a poor prognostic significance.[31]

Misdiagnosis of systemic mast cell disease is not uncommon, largely because the mast cells are not recognized and are misidentified as fibroblasts, macrophages or epithelioid cells. Focal marrow lesions may be misdiagnosed as granulomas, angio-immunoblastic lymphadenopathy or focal infiltrates of lymphoplasmacytoid lymphoma. Confusion with idiopathic myelofibrosis has occurred; however, when marrow fibrosis occurs as a response to systemic mastocytosis mast cells are recognizable in the fibrous tissue, allowing the distinction from other causes of myelofibrosis to be made. In patients with a heavy mast cell infiltrate misdiagnosis as hairy cell leukaemia is possible because of the even spacing of nuclei, a feature which is typical of hairy cell leukaemia. The two crucial points in making a correct diagnosis are that Giemsa-stained sections should be routinely examined and that the cell types in any apparent granulomas should be determined. The 'pseudo-granulomas' of systemic mast cell disease commonly have eosinophils and lymphocytes associated with them and sometimes lymphoid nodules and plasma cells; the mast cells may show atypical features. Mast cells are also often associated with focal marrow infiltrates of lymphoplasmacytoid lymphoma (see page 145). However, these reactive mast cells are morphologically normal and are a minority population in the areas of infiltration. In angio-immunoblastic lymphadenopathy there may be focal or diffuse infiltration by a hetero-geneous population of cells that often includes plasma cells, lymphocytes and many eosinophils (see page 168). However immunoblasts, which are not features of systemic mastocytosis, are present and often prominent.

By definition cutaneous mastocytosis is con-fined to the skin. However, bone marrow infil-tration occasionally develops in patients who initially had mast cell infiltration apparently con-fined to the skin and in a study of paediatric cases of cutaneous mastocytosis 10 out of 15 trephine biopsies showed focal perivascular and peri-trabecular aggregates of mast cells, eosinophils and early myeloid cells.[35,40]

UNCLASSIFIABLE AND TRANSITIONAL MYELOPROLIFERATIVE DISORDERS

Occasional patients are seen who clearly have a myeloproliferative disorder but whose disease either cannot be readily classified or alternatively has characteristics of two usually distinct myelo-proliferative disorders. Patients are also seen who have a condition with characteristics both of a myeloproliferative and of a myelodysplastic disorder.

Pettit et al.[41] described a group of patients with a condition intermediate between PRV and idio-pathic myelofibrosis which they designated 'transitional myeloproliferative disorder'. In these patients the criteria for PRV were generally met but in addition there was moderate or marked splenomegaly, a leucoerythroblastic blood film, extramedullary haemopoiesis and a hypercellular marrow with increased reticulin. In the majority of patients the condition had stable characteristics for a number of years and thus did not represent a transient phase between PRV and post-polycythaemic myelofibrosis.

The Polycythemia Vera Study Group[28] have used the designation 'undifferentiated chronic myeloproliferative disorder' for another group of patients with splenomegaly and a leucoerythro-blastic blood film without an increased red cell mass, Ph chromosome or significant marrow fibrosis.

Many patients with systemic mastocytosis have evidence of involvement of other myeloid

lineages. In some patients the platelet count or white cell count is so greatly elevated that a diagnosis of essential thrombocythaemia or chronic myeloid leukaemia is considered. How-ever, it is likely that such cases represent a myelo-proliferative disorder with differentiation to several lineages, rather than the coexistence of two separate diseases. Similarly, the emergence of myelodysplasia or acute leukaemia in patients with systemic mast cell disease represents evol-ution of the neoplastic clone. There have also been several reports of the coexistence of systemic mastocytosis and polycythaemia rubra vera; whether this represents coincidence or a single neoplastic stem cell giving rise to cells of diverse lineages is not yet clear.

The existence of patients with characteristics of two myeloproliferative disorders or with fea-tures of a myeloproliferative disorder without specific features allowing assignation to a defined disease category is not surprising given that all myeloproliferative disorders are the result of pro-liferation of a multipotent myeloid stem cell with the potential for differentiation into various lineages, and since reticulin and collagen depo-sition are a common response to the proliferation of the neoplastic clone.

REFERENCES

1 Shepherd PCA, Ganesan TS and Galton DAG (1987) Haematological classification of the chronic myeloid leukaemias. *Baillière's Clin Haematol*, **1**, 887–906.
2 Spiers ASD, Bain BJ and Turner JE (1977) The periph-eral blood in chronic granulocytic leukaemia. *Scand J Haematol*, **18**, 25–38.
3 Burkhardt R, Frisch B and Bartl R (1982) Bone biopsy in haematological disorders. *J Clin Pathol*, **35**, 257–284.
4 Burkhardt R, Bartl R, Jager K, et al. (1986) Working classification of chronic myeloproliferative dis-orders based on histological, haematological, and clinical findings. *J Clin Pathol*, **39**, 237–252.
5 Lazzarino M, Morra E, Castello A, et al. (1986) Myelofibrosis in chronic granulocytic leukaemia: clinicopathological correlations and prognostic significance. *Br J Haematol*, **64**, 227–240.
6 Rozman C, Cervantes F and Feliu E (1989) Is the histological classification of chronic granulocytic leukaemia justified from the clinical point of view? *Eur J Haematol*, **42**, 150–154.

7 Schmid C, Frisch B, Beham A, Jager K and Kettner G (1990) Comparison of bone marrow histology in early chronic granulocytic leukaemia and in leukaemoid reaction. *Eur J Haematol*, **44**, 154–158.

8 Thiele J and Fischer R (1991) Megakaryocytopoiesis in haematological disorders: diagnostic features of bone marrow biopsies. An overview. *Virchows Archiv (A)*, **418**, 87–97.

9 Knox WF and Bhavnani M (1981) Histological classification of chronic granulocytic leukaemia. *Clin Lab Haematol*, **6**, 171–175.

10 Clough VC, Geary CG, Hashmi K, Davson J and Knowlson T (1979) Myelofibrosis in chronic granulocytic leukaemia. *Br J Haematol*, **42**, 515–526.

11 Islam A (1988) Prediction of impending blast cell transformation in chronic granulocytic leukaemia. *Histopathology*, **12**, 633–639.

12 Peterson LC, Bloomfield CD and Brunning RD (1976) Blast crisis as an initial or terminal manifestation of chronic myeloid leukaemia. A study of 28 patients. *Am J Med*, **60**, 209–220.

13 Islam A, Catovsky D, Goldman J and Galton DAG (1980) Histological study of chronic granulocytic leukaemia in blast transformation. *Br J Haematol*, **46**, 326.

14 Williams WC and Weiss GB (1982) Megakaryoblastic transformation of chronic myelogenous leukemia. *Cancer*, **49**, 921–926.

15 Muehleck SD, McKenna RW, Arthur DC, Parkin JL and Brunning RD (1984) Transformation of chronic myelogenous leukaemia: clinical, morphologic, and cytogenetic features. *Am J Clin Pathol*, **82**, 1–14.

16 Kantarjian HM, Keating MJ, Walter RS, *et al.* (1986) Clinical and prognostic features of Philadelphia chromosome-negative chronic myeloid leukaemia. *Cancer*, **578**, 2023–2030.

17 Martiat P, Michaux JL and Rodhain J (1991) Philadelphia-negative (Ph⁻) chronic myeloid leukemia (CML); comparison with Ph⁺CML and chronic myelomonocytic leukemia. *Blood*, **78**, 205–211.

18 Vykoupil KF, Thiele J, Stangel W, Krmpotic E and Georgii A (1980) Polycythaemia vera. I. Histopathology, ultrastructure, and cytogenetics of the bone marrow in comparison with secondary polycythaemia. *Virchows Arch (A)*, **389**, 307–324.

19 Lucie NP and Young GAR (1983) Marrow cellularity in the diagnosis of polycythaemia. *J Clin Pathol*, **36**, 180–183.

20 Ellis JT, Peterson P, Geller SA and Rappaport H (1986) Studies of the bone marrow in polycythemia vera and the evolution of myelofibrosis and second hematologic malignancies. *Semin Hematol*, **23**, 144–155.

21 Murphy S, Iland H, Rosenthal D and Laszlo J (1986) Essential thrombocythemia: an interim report from the Polycythaemia Vera Study Group. *Semin Hematol*, **23**, 177–182.

22 Stoll DB, Peterson P, Exten R, *et al.* (1988) Clinical presentation and natural history of patients with essential thrombocythemia. *Am J Hematol*, **27**, 77–83.

23 Wolf BC and Nieman RS (1985) Myelofibrosis with myeloid metaplasia: pathophysiologic implications of the correlation between bone marrow changes and progression of splenomegaly. *Blood*, **65**, 803–809.

24 Lennert K, Nagai K and Schwarze EW (1975) Pathoanatomical features of the bone marrow. *Clinics in Haematology*, **4**, 331–351.

25 Pereira A, Cervantes F, Brugues R and Rozman C (1990) Bone marrow histopathology in primary myelofibrosis: clinical and haematologic correlations and prognostic evaluation. *Eur J Haematol*, **44**, 95–99.

26 Apaja-Sarkkinen M, Autio-Harmainen H, Alavaikko M, Risteli J and Risteli L (1986) Immunohistochemical study of basement membrane proteins and type III procollagen in myelofibrosis. *Br J Haematol*, **63**, 571–580.

27 Lohmann TP and Beckman EN (1983) Progressive myelofibrosis in agnogenic myeloid metaplasia. *Arch Pathol Lab Med*, **107**, 593–594.

28 Laszlo J (1975) Myeloproliferative disorders (MPD): Myelofibrosis, myelosclerosis, extramedullary haematopoiesis, undifferentiated MPD, and haemorrhagic thrombocythaemia. *Semin. Hematol*, **12**, 75–98.

29 Webb TA, Chin-Yang L and Yam LT (1982) Systemic mast cell disease: a clinical and haematopathologic study of 26 cases. *Cancer*, **49**, 927–938.

30 Brunning RD, Parkin JL, McKenna RW, Risdall R and Rosai J (1983) Systemic mastocytosis: extracutaneous manifestations. *Am J Surg Pathol*, **7**, 425–438.

31 Travis WD, Li C-Y, Bergstralh EJ, Yam LT and Swee RG (1988) Systemic mast cell disease: analysis of 58 cases and literature review. *Medicine*, **67**, 345–368.

32 Lennert K and Parwaresch MR (1979) Mast cells and mast cell neoplasia: a review. *Histopathology*, **3**, 349–365.

33 Horny H-P, Ruck M, Wehrmann M and Kaiserling E (1990) Blood findings in generalized mastocytosis: evidence of frequent simultaneous occurrence of myeloproliferative disorders. *Br J Haematol*, **76**, 186–193.

34 Travis WD, Li C-Y, Yam LT, Bergstralh EJ and Swee RG (1988) Significance of systemic mast cell disease with associated haematologic diagnosis. *Cancer*, **62**, 965–972.

35 Parker RI (1991) Hematologic aspects of masto-

cytosis: I: bone marrow pathology in adult and pediatric systemic mast cell disease. *J Invest Dermatol*, **96**, suppl, 475–515.

36 Parker RI (1991) Hematologic aspects of mastocytosis: II: management of hematologic disorders in association with systemic mast cell disease. *J Invest Dermatol*, **96**, suppl, 525–545.

37 Horny H-P, Parwaresch MR and Lennert K (1985) Bone marrow findings in systemic mastocytosis. *Hum Pathol*, **16**, 808–814.

38 Fallon MD, Whyte MP and Teitelbaum SL (1981) Systemic mastocytosis associated with generalized osteopenia. *Hum Pathol*, **12**, 813–820.

39 Horny H-P and Kaiserling E (1987) Lymphoid cells and tissue mast cells of bone marrow lesions in systemic mastocytosis: a histological and immuno-histological study. *Br J Haematol*, **69**, 449–455.

40 Kettelhut BV, Parker RI, Travis WD and Metcalfe DD (1989) Hematopathology of the bone marrow in cutaneous mastocytosis. *Am J Clin Pathol*, **91**, 558–562.

41 Pettit JE, Lewis SM and Nicholas AW (1979) Transitional myeloproliferative disorder. *Br J Haematol*, **43**, 167–184.

5: Lymphoproliferative Disorders

In this chapter we shall discuss acute and chronic leukaemias of lymphoid lineage, Hodgkin's disease and non-Hodgkin's lymphomas. The acute and chronic lymphoid leukaemias will be classified according to the FAB classifications,[1,2] Hodgkin's disease according to the Rye classification[3] and non-Hodgkin's lymphoma (NHL) according to the Kiel classification.[4,5] The Kiel and Rye classifications are summarized in Tables 5.1 and 5.2. Where possible we shall relate the Kiel classification to other systems of lymphoma classification, in particular to Rappaport's classification,[6] since this classification was widely used for many years, and to the Working Formulation for Clinical Usage.[7] We shall also indicate where FAB categories of leukaemia can be related to specific lymphomas of the Kiel classification. Certain other lymphomas with distinctive clinicopathological features which are not specifically included in the Kiel classification will also be discussed.

PATTERNS OF INFILTRATION OF BONE MARROW IN LYMPHOPROLIFERATIVE DISORDERS

Bone marrow infiltration is frequent in lymphoproliferative disorders. Such infiltration can be detected by a variety of procedures including microscopic examination of bone marrow aspirates and trephine biopsies and the use of the techniques of molecular biology. Assessment of cytological details can be carried out on smears of aspirates, on imprints from trephine biopsies and on thin sections of plastic-embedded biopsies. Histological features can be assessed on sections of either trephine biopsies or aspirated fragments. The pattern of infiltration can only be fully

Table 5.1 The Kiel classification of malignant lymphomas[4]

B-lineage	
Low grade	Lymphocytic
	chronic lymphocytic leukaemia
	prolymphocytic leukaemia
	hairy cell leukaemia
	Lymphoplasmacytic/lymphoplasmacytoid (immunocytoma)
	lymphoplasmacytoid
	lymphoplasmacytic
	Plasmacytic
	Centroblastic/centrocytic
	follicular ± diffuse
	diffuse
	Centrocytic
High grade	Centroblastic
	Immunoblastic
	Large cell anaplastic
	Burkitt lymphoma
	Lymphoblastic
T-lineage	
Low grade	Lymphocytic
	chronic lymphocytic leukaemia
	prolymphocytic leukaemia
	Small, cerebriform cell
	mycosis fungoides
	Sézary's syndrome
	Lymphoepithelioid (Lennert's lymphoma)
	Angioimmunoblastic (angioimmunoblastic lymphadenopathy with dysproteinaemia, lymphogranulomatosis X)
	T-zone
	Pleomorphic, small cell*
High grade	Pleomorphic, medium and large cell*
	Immunoblastic*
	Large cell anaplastic
	Lymphoblastic

* HTLV-I ±.

Table 5.2 The Rye classification of Hodgkin's disease[3]

Category		Specific histological characteristics
Lymphocyte predominance	Lymphocytic and histiocytic, nodular	Typical Reed–Sternberg cells may be quite infrequent; polyploid L and H variant of Reed–Sternberg cell present; prominent proliferation of lymphocytes, histiocytes or both
	Lymphocytic and histiocytic, diffuse	
Nodular sclerosis		Typical Reed–Sternberg cells often very infrequent; lacunar cell variant of Reed–Sternberg cell present; collagen bands present
Mixed cellularity		Moderately frequent Reed–Sternberg cells; variable proliferation of reactive cells; usually some disorderly fibrosis
Lymphocyte depleted	With diffuse fibrosis	Reed–Sternberg cells frequent; extensive disorderly fibrosis; reactive cells infrequent
	Reticular variant	Reed–Sternberg cells frequent and pleomorphic variant of Reed–Sternberg cell present — either may predominate; reactive cells infrequent

assessed on sections from trephine biopsies. Any of three patterns can be seen, either alone or in combination[8-10] (Fig. 5.1). Such patterns are important in the differential diagnosis of lympho-proliferative disorders and can also be of prognostic significance. They are designated (**1**) interstitial, (**2**) focal and (**3**) diffuse.

1 Interstitial infiltration indicates the presence of individual neoplastic cells interspersed between haemopoietic and fat cells. Although there is generalized marrow involvement there is considerable sparing of normal haemopoiesis.

2 Focal infiltration indicates that there are foci of neoplastic cells separated by residual haemopoietic marrow. Focal infiltration can be further categorized as paratrabecular or random. In paratrabecular infiltration the neoplastic cells are immediately adjacent to the bony trabeculae, either in the form of a band lining a trabecula or as an aggregate with a broad base abutting on a trabecula. In random infiltration the aggregates of neo-

plastic cells have no particular relationship to bony trabeculae. Random infiltrates can be further subdivided into nodular and patchy, the former having a well-defined round border and the latter an irregular margin. A distinction should be made between random nodules or patchy aggregates which incidentally touch the bone surface and true paratrabecular infiltration.

3 Diffuse infiltration indicates extensive replacement of normal marrow elements, both haemopoietic tissue and fat, so that marrow architecture is effaced. An alternative designation is a 'packed marrow' pattern;[9] this latter term could be preferred since it is unambiguous whereas 'diffuse' could be taken to also include interstitial infiltration.

Various mixed patterns of infiltration also occur including mixed interstitial-nodular and mixed interstitial-diffuse.

A further unusual pattern of infiltration is the presence of lymphoma cells within the marrow

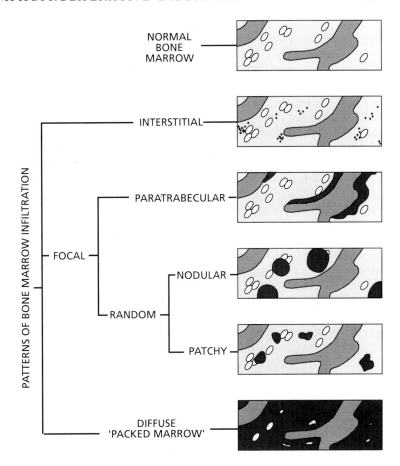

Fig. 5.1 Patterns of bone marrow infiltration observed in lymphoproliferative disorders.

sinusoids. In rare cases neoplastic lymphoid cells in the bone marrow may be confined to the sinusoids.[11,12]

Among B-lineage lymphomas bone marrow infiltration is commoner in low-grade tumours than in high-grade. Overall, infiltration is probably commoner in B-cell lymphomas than in T-cell[13,14] but the frequency of infiltration detected in T-cell lymphoma has varied widely in reported series (see page 52). The relative frequency of different patterns of infiltration varies between T and B lymphomas and between different histological categories but in general focal infiltration is more common than diffuse.[15] This is particularly so of B-cell lymphomas; diffuse infiltration is relatively more common in T-cell lymphomas than in B-cell.

Lymphomatous infiltration of the marrow needs to be distinguished from infiltration by reactive lymphocytes. Consideration should be given both to the pattern of infiltration and to cytological characteristics. Interstitial infiltration can occur in both neoplastic and reactive conditions. Paratrabecular infiltration and a 'packed marrow' (diffuse infiltration) are indicative of neoplasia. Nodular infiltrates have to be distinguished from benign nodular hyperplasia (see page 161). Caution should be exercised in diagnosing lymphoma solely on the basis of the presence of nodules of small lymphocytes since it can be difficult to identify a small number of lymphoid nodules as neoplastic purely on morphological grounds; immunohistochemistry (see below) may be needed.

Increased reticulin deposition (reticulin fibrosis), restricted to the area of marrow infiltration, is common in lymphoma.[16] Collagen fibrosis is less common.

Trephine biopsy is generally more successful at detecting marrow infiltration than is bone marrow aspiration; this is a consequence of the frequency of focal infiltration and of fibrosis. In a series of 93 cases, Foucar et al.[15] found that trephine sections and aspirate smears were both positive in 79 per cent of cases, trephine sections alone were positive in 18 per cent and smears alone were positive in three per cent. Similarly Conlan et al.[13] reported that in 102 cases of NHL with marrow involvement the trephine section, marrow clot section, and marrow aspirate smears were positive in 94, 65 and 46 per cent of cases respectively; in only six per cent of cases was the bone marrow aspirate positive when the trephine biopsy was negative. The rate of detection of bone marrow infiltration is increased when a larger volume of marrow is sampled; this can be achieved either by increasing the size of the trephine biopsy or by performing multiple biopsies.

Immunohistochemical techniques on sections of paraffin-embedded tissue (see page 36) are useful in establishing or confirming the nature of lymphoid infiltrates. Some specialized units advocate the use of frozen sections, since this allows more detailed analysis of lymphocyte phenotype, important in the detection of aberrant or unusual phenotypes which can be useful in the diagnosis of T-cell lymphomas.[11,14]

There may be discordance between the type of lymphoma seen in the marrow and that present in the lymph node or other tissues. The frequency of such discordance varies from 16 to 40 per cent in reported series.[13,17–19] In a smaller number, varying between 6 and 21 per cent there is discordance as to grade of lymphoma. Discordance is most often seen in B-cell lymphomas. Although Conlan et al.[13] observed discordance in 25 per cent of T-cell lymphomas no discordance was found in two other series of T-cell lymphomas.[20,21] One surprising and relatively common occurrence is the presence of a centroblastic/centrocytic (follicular) lymphoma in the lymph node and an immunocytoma (see page 145) in the marrow.[17,19] This may represent differentiation of tumour in the marrow site. Such a phenomenon has been reported in node-based centroblastic/centrocytic lymphomas.[22]

The clinical importance of marrow involvement varies with the category of non-Hodgkin's lymphoma. In general, in low-grade lymphomas the presence of marrow involvement does not adversely affect the clinical outlook. In patients with high-grade lymphoma at an extra-medullary site the presence of high-grade lymphoma in the marrow is a poor prognostic sign, often predictive of central nervous system involvement.[23] The presence of low-grade lymphoma in the marrow of patients with high-grade lymphoma has been considered to have no adverse effect on prognosis;[18] however, there is evidence to suggest that such patients have continuing risk of late relapse of low-grade lymphoma.[23]

Acute lymphoblastic leukaemia

Acute lymphoblastic leukaemia (ALL) is the disease resulting from the proliferation in the bone marrow of a neoplastic clone of immature lymphoid cells with the morphological features of lymphoblasts. Common clinical features are bruising, pallor, lymphadenopathy, hepatomegaly and splenomegaly. The peak incidence is in childhood but the disease occurs at all ages. ALL has been classified on the basis of morphology of bone marrow cells by the French–American–British group (FAB classification).[1] It has been further classified on the basis of morphology, immunology and cytogenetics (MIC classification).[24] We shall employ these classifications and their suggested terminology.

Immunological markers show that about three-quarters of cases of ALL are of B lineage and about one-quarter of T lineage. Within the B-lineage cases, four immunophenotypic groups are recognized which may be analogous to successive stages of maturation of normal B lymphocytes. The most immature group, designated early B-lineage ALL, expresses certain antigenic markers shared with other B-lineage cells; these antigens, recognizable with well-standardized monoclonal antibodies (McAb), include those belonging to CD19, CD22 and CD24 'clusters'. The next group, which includes the majority of cases, is designated common ALL since cases express also the common ALL antigen (CD10). The third group, designated pre-B ALL, continues to express pan-B markers and CD10 but also expresses the μ chain

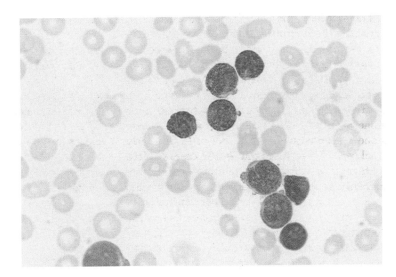

Fig. 5.2 BM aspirate, L1 ALL, showing a uniform population of small and medium-sized blasts with a high nucleo-cytoplasmic ratio. MGG × 940.

of IgM, in the cytoplasm but not on the cell surface. The fourth group, designated B-ALL, comprises a small minority of cases whose cells express surface membrane immunoglobulin (SmIg); since neoplastic cells of these cases are immunophenotypically mature and have the same cytological features as the cells of Burkitt's lymphoma it would be justifiable to classify these cases as a lymphoma presenting in a leukaemic phase but, by convention, they are classified with the acute lymphoblastic leukaemias. T-lineage ALL is divided into two or more immunopheno-typic groups. Cases with the least mature immunophenotype are designated pre-T ALL; neoplastic cells express markers characteristic of T-lymphocytes and their precursors such as CD1, CD3, CD5 and CD7 but do not express CD2 or form rosettes with sheep red blood cells. Cases whose cells have a more mature phenotype, either expressing CD2 or forming sheep red blood cell rosettes, are designated T-ALL. T-lineage ALL can also be divided into three rather than two immunophenotypic groups corresponding to the phenotype of early, intermediate and late thymocytes.

The acute lymphoblastic leukaemias are closely related to the lymphoblastic lymphomas of the Kiel classification, the majority of which are of T lineage and the minority of B lineage (see pages 160 and 177).

Peripheral blood

In the majority of cases of ALL, leukaemic lymphoblasts similar to those in the bone marrow are present in the peripheral blood; as a consequence the total white cell count is commonly increased. Normocytic normochromic anaemia and thrombocytopenia are also common.

Bone marrow cytology

The bone marrow is markedly hypercellular and is heavily infiltrated by leukaemic blasts. Normal haemopoietic cells are reduced in number but are morphologically normal. The blast cells vary in morphology between cases. The FAB morphological categories are designated L1, L2 and L3. In L1 ALL (Fig. 5.2) the blasts are fairly small and relatively uniform in appearance with a round nucleus and a regular cellular outline. The nucleo-cytoplasmic ratio is high, chromatin pattern is fairly homogeneous, and nucleoli are inconspicuous or inapparent. In L2 ALL (Fig. 5.3) the blasts are generally larger and more pleomorphic. Cytoplasm is more plentiful, the nuclei vary in shape and nucleoli may be prominent. In L3 ALL (Fig. 5.4) the cells are again large but are relatively uniform. The cells and their nuclei are usually round, the chromatin is stippled and nucleoli are prominent. The cytoplasm is strongly basophilic

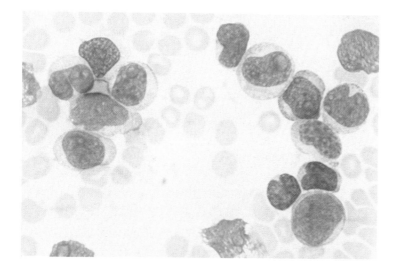

Fig. 5.3 BM aspirate, L2 ALL, showing large pleomorphic blasts. MGG × 940.

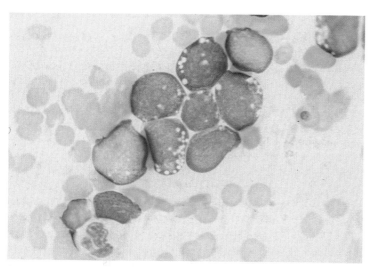

Fig. 5.4 BM aspirate, L3 ALL in a patient with AIDS, showing blasts with marked cytoplasmic basophilia and heavy cytoplasmic vacuolation. MGG × 940.

and contains prominent vacuoles. L3 morphology has been found to correlate with a mature B-cell immunophenotype. With this exception there is no correlation between immunophenotype and morphology. Bone marrow necrosis may complicate ALL and, rarely, an aspirate may contain only necrotic cells.

In T-lineage ALL there may be massive enlargement of the thymus by lymphoblasts and in lymphoblastic lymphoma the bone marrow may be infiltrated by lymphoblasts, particularly late in the course of the disease. If large groups of patients with T-lineage ALL and T lymphoblastic

lymphoma are compared some differences in the most prevalent immunophenotypes can be detected, with lymphoblastic lymphoma tending to have the more mature phenotype, but individual cases cannot be distinguished on this basis. The less common B lymphoblastic lymphoma has a similar immunophenotype to B-lineage ALL. The distinction between lymphoblastic lymphoma and ALL is therefore to some extent arbitrary. When there is any difficulty in distinguishing between the two conditions it is suggested that cases which at presentation have more than 25–30 per cent of bone marrow blasts should be

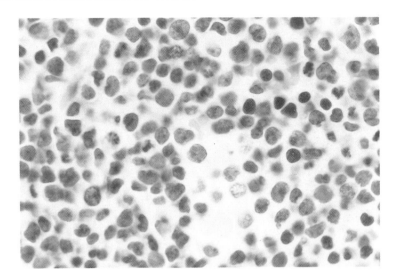

Fig. 5.5 BM trephine biopsy, L1 ALL, showing diffuse infiltration by lymphoblasts. Note the high nucleo-cytoplasmic ratio and finely stippled chromatin pattern. Plastic-embedded, H&E × 940.

classified as ALL and cases with fewer bone marrow blasts should be classified as lymphoblastic lymphoma.

Bone marrow histology

The marrow is diffusely infiltrated by lymphoblasts which replace most of the haemopoietic and fat cells. The infiltrating cells vary in size but are on average around twice the diameter of red blood cells. They are characterized by a large nucleus and minimal cytoplasm (Fig. 5.5). The chromatin is finely stippled with one or two small or medium-sized nucleoli. Some cases of T-ALL have cells with small, hyperchromatic nuclei or with nuclear clefting and folding.[25] Cytoplasmic vacuoles can sometimes be discerned with difficulty in L3 ALL (see also page 160). In general mitotic figures are more frequent in L3 ALL than in L1 and L2. Among L1 and L2 cases T-ALL have been noted to have a higher mitotic rate than other cases of ALL.[25] Bone marrow necrosis, usually patchy, occurs in some patients.

Reticulin fibrosis occurs to a varying degree in up to 57 per cent of cases of ALL and collagen fibrosis in a quarter.[26] Reticulin fibrosis regresses slowly following remission of the leukaemia. Fibrosis is responsible for occasional failure to obtain an aspirate.

The diagnosis of ALL is usually easily obtained from the cytology of bone marrow aspirates or peripheral blood films so that trephine biopsy is not usually necessary. Occasionally when there is minimal evidence of leukaemia in the peripheral blood and when bone marrow cannot be aspirated the diagnosis is dependent on a trephine biopsy. The most important differential diagnosis is that of AML. In general ALL blasts have a very high nucleo-cytoplasmic ratio and are more regular than the blasts of AML. There are no myelodysplastic features and the primitive cells do not contain granules. Myeloblasts may be positive for chloroacetate esterase and expression of leucocyte common antigen is either weak or not detectable. Lymphoblasts express leucocyte common antigen and usually also either CD3 or L26 (CD20). It may also be necessary to distinguish between ALL and infiltration of the marrow by lymphoma. Lymphoblastic lymphoma cannot be distinguished cytologically from ALL but infiltration is usually patchy with intervening areas of surviving haemopoietic tissue and fat. In other high-grade lymphomas the cells are larger and more pleomorphic than those of ALL. In low-grade lymphomas infiltration is often focal and the nuclei show at least some degree of chromatin condensation. Mitotic figures are quite uncommon.

A preleukaemic episode of marrow aplasia is a rare form of presentation of ALL, seen in about two per cent of childhood cases and in some adults.[27,28] Trephine biopsies show a hypocellular marrow; haemopoietic cells are generally reduced but there may be some sparing of megakaryocytes. Increased lymphoblasts are not detected. A common feature is the presence of reticulin fibrosis and increased numbers of fibroblasts.[27] Recovery occurs, usually spontaneously, and after an interval of some weeks ALL is manifest in the marrow and the peripheral blood. It is difficult to distinguish an aplastic preleukaemic phase of ALL from aplastic anaemia, although the presence of increased reticulin and fibroblasts may suggest that the aplastic anaemia is not the correct diagnosis.

B-LINEAGE LYMPHOMAS AND CHRONIC LEUKAEMIAS

CHRONIC LYMPHOCYTIC LEUKAEMIA

Chronic lymphocytic leukaemia (CLL) is a disease resulting from a neoplastic proliferation of mature B lymphocytes which infiltrate the bone marrow and circulate in the peripheral blood. CLL is predominantly a disease of middle and old age. Patients diagnosed in the early stages of the disease may have no abnormal physical findings. In patients with more advanced disease common clinical features are lymphadenopathy, hepatomegaly and splenomegaly. There is commonly an immune paresis, with impaired B- and T-cell function and reduced concentration of immunoglobulins.

CLL cells show weak expression of monoclonal SmIg which is commonly IgM with or without IgD. They express pan-B markers such as CD19, CD20, and CD24. The pan-B marker CD22 is expressed in the cytoplasm but weakly if at all on the cell surface. In addition CLL cells often express CD5 and CD23. They do not usually express FMC7.

Various arbitrary levels of peripheral blood lymphocyte count, for example more than 5 to $10 \times 10^9/l$, have been suggested to establish this diagnosis of CLL. The lower count is quite adequate for diagnosis if the cells are shown to be monoclonal B lymphocytes with typical morphological and immunological features.

In the Kiel classification CLL falls into the category of low-grade lymphocytic lymphoma.

In Rappaport's classification it is histologically equivalent to diffuse well-differentiated lymphocytic lymphoma and in the Working Formulation it is equivalent to malignant lymphoma, small lymphocytic.

Examination of the peripheral blood is essential in the diagnosis of CLL. A bone marrow aspirate is of little importance in comparison with a trephine biopsy which yields information important both for diagnosis and prognosis. Some non-Hodgkin's lymphomas are easily confused with CLL if a trephine biopsy is not examined.

Peripheral blood

The blood film shows a uniform population of mature, small lymphocytes with round nuclei, clumped chromatin, scanty cytoplasm and a regular cellular outline (Fig. 5.6). Broken cells, designated smear cells or smudge cells, are characteristic but not pathognomonic since they are occasionally seen in a variety of other conditions. With advanced disease there is anaemia and thrombocytopenia. Auto-immune haemolytic anaemia may complicate CLL, either early or late in the course of the disease; the blood film then shows spherocytes and the direct antiglobulin test is positive; when bone marrow reserve is adequate there is also polychromasia and the reticulocyte count is increased. Auto-immune destruction of platelets may also occur and in patients with early disease may be responsible for an isolated thrombocytopenia.

Patients with CLL may have a small proportion of cells with the morphology of prolymphocytes, that is with a prominent nucleolus and more abundant cytoplasm. If these cells constitute more than 10 per cent of lymphocytes it is likely that prolymphocytoid transformation is occurring.[29] In less than five per cent of cases CLL undergoes transformation to large cell lymphoma, designated Richter's syndrome; transformed cells are only rarely present in the peripheral blood but when present have the same cytological features as large cell lymphoma in leukaemic phase.

Bone marrow cytology

The bone marrow is hypercellular and contains increased numbers of mature lymphocytes which are uniform in appearance. Normal haemopoietic

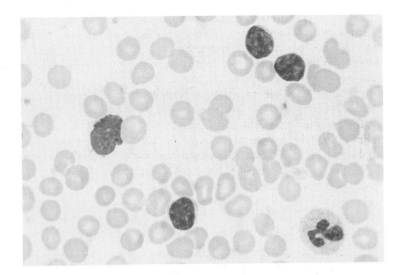

Fig. 5.6 PB film, CLL, showing a uniform population of small mature lymphocytes. One smear cell is present. MGG × 940.

cells are reduced, there being a continued fall with disease progression. Various arbitrary percentages of bone marrow lymphocytes, for example more than 30 per cent or more than 40 per cent, have been suggested as necessary to establish the diagnosis of CLL. A figure of 30 per cent is quite adequate for diagnosis if a good aspirate, not diluted with peripheral blood, is obtained and if other features are typical.

When prolymphocytoid transformation of CLL occurs increasing numbers of prolymphocytes are present in the bone marrow. Transformation to large cell lymphoma (Richter's syndrome) some-

times occurs in the bone marrow but more often occurs initially at an extramedullary site with bone marrow infiltration being a late event. When bone marrow infiltration occurs the cells usually have the morphology of pleomorphic immunoblastic lymphoma.

Bone marrow histology

In the usual case at presentation, the vast majority of the neoplastic cells in the marrow are small lymphocytes (Fig. 5.7). These cells are slightly larger than the average normal lymphocyte. They

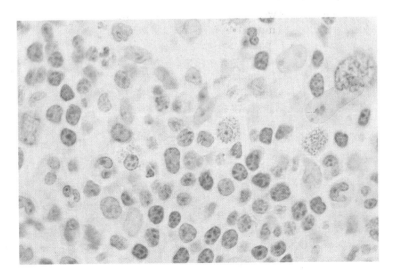

Fig. 5.7 BM trephine biopsy, CLL, mature small lymphocytes infiltrating between residual normal haemopoietic cells. BM trephine biopsy, H&E × 940.

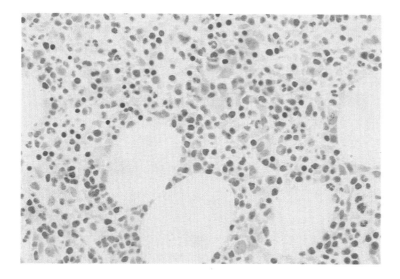

Fig. 5.8 BM trephine biopsy, CLL, interstitial infiltration. Plastic-embedded, H&E × 377.

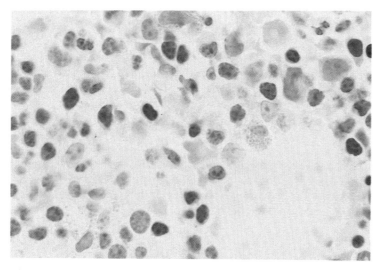

Fig. 5.9 BM trephine biopsy, CLL, interstitial infiltration. Plastic-embedded, H&E × 940.

have nuclei with coarse clumped chromatin and insignificant nucleoli; there is little cytoplasm. The nuclear outline appears somewhat irregular in paraffin- and plastic-embedded sections. In addition to the predominant small lymphocytes there are small numbers of prolymphocytes and immunoblasts. The latter are large cells with plentiful cytoplasm and a large nucleus with a prominent nucleolus. Their cytological features resemble those of lymphoid cells exposed to mitogens or to antigenic stimulation. Prolymphocytes are intermediate in size between small lymphocytes and immunoblasts; they have nuclei

with dispersed chromatin and a nucleolus which is often large and prominent. Some cases of CLL have prominent mast cells.

Four histological patterns of marrow infiltration are seen in CLL interstitial (Figs 5.8 and 5.9), nodular (Fig. 5.10), diffuse (Fig. 5.11) and mixed (see page 128).[8,30] Mixed indicates a combination of nodular and interstitial patterns. There is little if any increase in reticulin.[16]

Bone marrow trephine examination in CLL provides a valuable prognostic indicator which is partly independent of clinical stage. Most investigators have demonstrated a statistically signific-

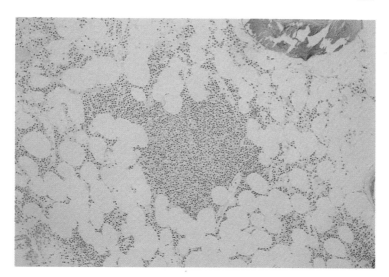

Fig. 5.10 BM trephine biopsy, CLL, nodular infiltration. Plastic-embedded, H&E × 94.

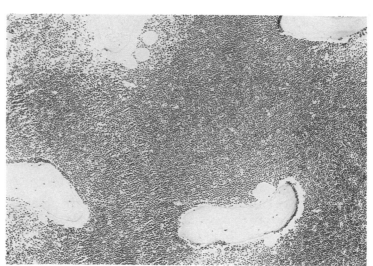

Fig. 5.11 BM trephine biopsy, CLL, diffuse infiltration ('packed marrow' pattern). Plastic-embedded, H&E × 94.

ant difference between the outcome in cases with a diffuse pattern (poor prognosis) and those with non-diffuse (nodular and interstitial) patterns (good prognosis).[8,30,31] Some workers have further found cases with a mixed pattern to have a prognosis intermediate between that of the above two groups.[8] Somewhat divergent findings were reported by Frisch and Bartl;[32] they also found the shortest survival in those with a 'packed marrow' pattern, but those with an interstitial pattern of infiltration had a shorter survival than those with a nodular infiltrate.

Attempts have been made with some success to integrate the clinical staging systems with the pattern of bone marrow infiltration. In general, within a single stage, patients in whom the bone marrow is diffusely infiltrated do worse than those with non-diffuse patterns of infiltration.[30,31]

In prolymphocytoid transformation of CLL[29] there are increased numbers of prolymphocytes and immunoblasts in the marrow. In Richter's syndrome[33,34] transformation is usually at an extramedullary site and the marrow is infiltrated only in a minority of cases; the infiltrate is of immunoblasts admixed with bizarre giant cells

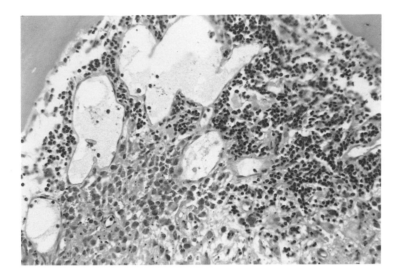

Fig. 5.12 BM trephine biopsy, Richter's transformation of CLL: part of the section shows residual mature small lymphocytes and part infiltration by pleomorphic immunoblasts. Paraffin-embedded, H&E × 390.

some of which resemble Reed–Sternberg cells (Fig. 5.12). In the majority of cases the marrow shows only the characteristic features of CLL.

LYMPHOCYTIC LYMPHOMA

Small cell lymphocytic lymphoma is a lympho-proliferative disorder which has lymph node histological features identical to those of chronic lymphocytic leukaemia but which differs from CLL in clinical and haematological features. Some patients have disease clinically confined to one lymph node group. Others have generalized lymphadenopathy which may be accompanied by hepatomegaly or splenomegaly.

In the Kiel classification this lymphoma is classified as malignant lymphoma, low-grade, small lymphocytic. Likewise in the Working Formulation and in Rappaport's classification it falls into the same category as CLL.

Peripheral blood

The lymphocyte count is normal at presentation and the peripheral blood film shows no specific abnormalities. A minority of patients develop lymphocytosis during the course of the illness, usually during the first few years after presentation.[35]

Bone marrow cytology

The bone marrow is infiltrated in the majority of patients, particularly but not exclusively those who have clinically apparent generalized disease.[35-37] Cytological features of the infiltrating cells are the same as those of CLL.

Bone marrow histology

The incidence of bone marrow involvement as determined from biopsy sections varies from 30 to 90 per cent.[15,38,39] Various patterns of infiltration have been reported. Pangalis and Kittas[38] found a nodular pattern in all of six patients with bone marrow infiltration but others[10,15,36] have observed focal, interstitial and occasionally diffuse patterns. The cytological features of the infiltrate are similar to those seen in CLL; there are predominantly small lymphocytes with round or slightly irregular contours and occasional immunoblasts.

No correlation has been found between the bone marrow findings and survival.[38,40]

B-PROLYMPHOCYTIC LEUKAEMIA

B-prolymphocytic leukaemia (PLL) is a disease consequent on the proliferation of a clone of

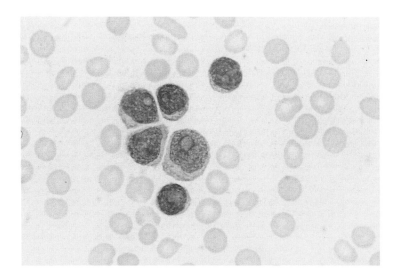

Fig. 5.13 PB film, B-PLL, showing prolymphocytes with plentiful cytoplasm and a single prominent nucleolus. MGG × 940.

mature B cells with distinctive cytological characteristics. The disease is much less common than CLL and on average occurs at an older age. About a quarter of cases of PLL are of T lineage (see page 162). There is generally marked splenomegaly but only minor lymphadenopathy.

PLL cells show strong expression of monoclonal SmIg which is usually IgM with or without IgD. Pan-B markers are expressed; the immunophenotype differs from that of CLL in that CD5 and CD23 are not usually expressed whereas CD22 and FMC7 are commonly positive.

In the Kiel classification PLL falls into the category of low-grade, lymphocytic lymphoma.

Peripheral blood examination is most important in the diagnosis of PLL; bone marrow aspiration and trephine biopsy are less important.

Peripheral blood

The white cell count is typically quite high, for example $50-100 \times 10^9$/l or even higher. Anaemia and thrombocytopenia may be present. Leukaemic cells are larger and in many cases less homogeneous than those of CLL. They vary in size with the larger cells having moderately abundant, weakly basophilic cytoplasm and a round nucleus containing a prominent nucleolus (Fig. 5.13). Smaller cells tend to have a somewhat

higher nucleo-cytoplasmic ratio and the nucleolus is less prominent.

Bone marrow cytology

The bone marrow is infiltrated by cells of similar appearance to those in the peripheral blood. Often the morphology is less characteristic than in the PB.

Bone marrow histology[41]

Recognition of prolymphocytes in tissue sections is rather difficult although techniques of plastic embedding make this easier. The cells are slightly larger than those of CLL with round nuclei. The chromatin is in coarse clumps and there is a distinct and usually prominent nucleolus (Figs 5.14 and 5.15). When biopsies are well fixed and preserved it is possible to distinguish some but not all cases of T-PLL from B-PLL by the presence of 'knobby' or convoluted nuclei. Some cases show increased eosinophils or plasma cells or sinusoidal dilatation.

The following four patterns of marrow infiltration have been found in PLL: interstitial, interstitial-nodular, interstitial-diffuse (Fig. 5.14), and diffuse (Fig. 5.15). The commonest pattern is interstitial-nodular. The pure nodular form of

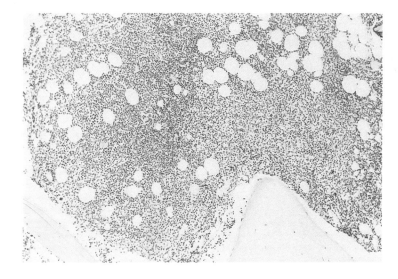

Fig. 5.14 BM trephine biopsy, B-PLL, showing interstitial/diffuse infiltration. Plastic-embedded, H&E × 94.

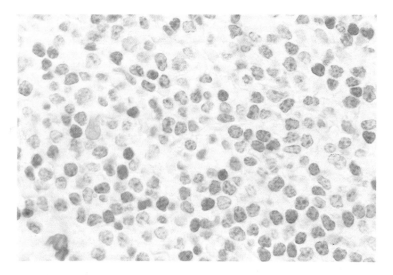

Fig. 5.15 BM trephine biopsy, B-PLL, showing diffuse infiltration by medium-sized cells, many of which have a single prominent nucleolus. Plastic-embedded, H&E × 94.

infiltration which occurs in CLL is not seen in PLL. Similar patterns of infiltration are seen in B- and T-PLL. In contrast to CLL, all cases show increased reticulin.

HAIRY CELL LEUKAEMIA

Hairy cell leukaemia is a disease consequent on the proliferation, particularly in the spleen, of a clone of cells with distinctive morphology and the immunophenotype of late B-lineage cells. The common clinical features are splenomegaly and

signs and symptoms consequent on anaemia and neutropenia.

Hairy cells almost always have tartrate-resistant acid phosphatase (TRAP) activity in the cytoplasm; such activity is very uncommon in other lymphoproliferative disorders. The cells show strong SmIg expression which in about a third of cases is IgM with or without IgD, and in the remaining two-thirds is IgA or IgG. The pan-B markers CD19, CD20 and CD22 are usually expressed but CD24 is usually negative. FMC7 is usually expressed and in addition there is ex-

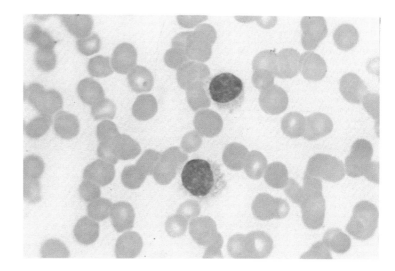

Fig. 5.16 PB film, hairy cell leukaemia, showing two hairy cells with weakly basophilic cytoplasm which has irregular hair-like projections. MGG × 940.

pression of several markers which are otherwise uncommon in chronic leukaemias of B lineage — CD11c, CD25, CD71, HC2 and several markers also expressed on plasma cells. The pattern of expression of markers suggests that the hairy cell represents a late stage in B-cell differentiation.

Hairy cell leukaemia falls into the Kiel category of malignant lymphoma, low-grade, small lymphocytic. It is not included in the Rappaport classification or the Working Formulation.

The diagnosis of hairy cell leukaemia can often be suspected from peripheral blood examination and confirmed by a bone marrow aspirate. However, hairy cells may be infrequent in the blood and the characteristic reticulin fibrosis commonly renders aspiration difficult. Examination of trephine biopsy sections therefore plays an important role in diagnosis.

Peripheral blood

Hairy cells are usually present in the peripheral blood only in small numbers and in some cases none is detected. Pancytopenia is usual. Neutropenia and monocytopenia are particularly severe. The leukaemic cells are larger than those of CLL and have abundant weakly basophilic cytoplasm with irregular cytoplasmic margins (Fig. 5.16). The nucleus may be round, oval, kidney or dumbbell shaped or bi-lobed. There is some condensa-

tion of chromatin. No nucleolus is apparent. The demonstration of TRAP activity is important in confirming the diagnosis.

Bone marrow cytology

The bone marrow is often difficult or impossible to aspirate. When an aspirate is obtained the predominant cell is a hairy cell with the same morphological features as the few leukaemic cells in the peripheral blood. When fragments can be aspirated mast cells are often very prominent within the fragments.

Bone marrow histology

The degree of marrow involvement is very extensive in all but the earliest of cases.[42-45] Infiltration is either focal or diffuse, but in this condition focal involvement is usually extensive with large confluent patches involving up to 50 per cent of the marrow. Distinct nodules or a predilection for specific areas of the marrow are not found. A third pattern of infiltration is that of interstitial infiltration in a severely hypoplastic marrow; this appearance can lead to a misdiagnosis of aplastic anaemia.[44,46]

The infiltrates consist of widely spaced mononuclear cells ranging in size from 10 to 25 μm producing a striking appearance on low power

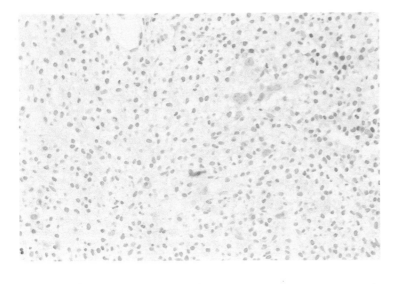

Fig. 5.17 BM trephine biopsy, hairy cell leukaemia, showing diffuse infiltration by 'hairy cells'; note the characteristic 'spaced' arrangement of the cells. Plastic-embedded, H&E × 188.

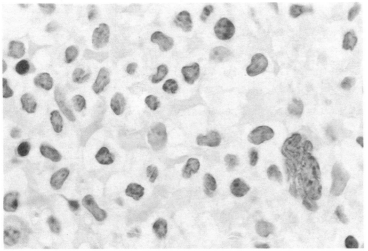

Fig. 5.18 BM trephine biopsy, hairy cell leukaemia, showing diffuse infiltration by 'hairy cells'; note the characteristic 'spaced' arrangement of the cells and the irregularity of nuclei. Plastic-embedded, H&E × 940.

examination (Figs 5.17 and 5.18). The relatively wide separation of the nuclei is due to a zone of abundant pale or water-clear cytoplasm and also in part, particularly in paraffin-embedded sections, to cytoplasmic retraction (Fig. 5.19); this appearance is accentuated by the underlying reticulin fibrosis which holds the cells apart. The tumour cell nuclei appear bland with pale, stippled chromatin; nucleoli are not prominent (Fig. 5.19). Nuclei vary in both size and in shape and may include round, oval, indented, dumb-bell shaped and bi-lobed forms. The mitotic rate is low. In some cases there are foci of hairy cells with spindled or fusiform nuclei giving the cells a fibroblastic appearance; however a fibrous or fusiform pattern may also be due to clusters of fibroblasts.[44] Red blood cells may be seen in infiltrated areas, either apparently extravasated or surrounded by a layer of hairy cells; this appearance resembles the red blood cell lakes seen in the spleen and liver.[43,44] Plasma cells, lymphocytes and mast cells are also often apparent in the area of infiltration.

Residual haemopoiesis is observed in all but the most severely infiltrated areas. Haemopoietic elements are scattered among the infiltrating

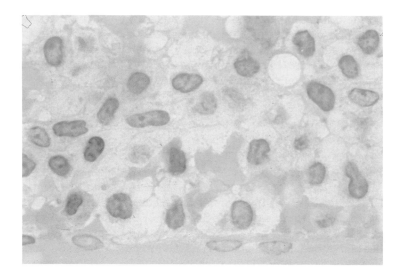

Fig. 5.19 BM trephine biopsy, hairy cell leukaemia, showing bland nuclei of various shapes surrounded by shrunken cytoplasm with irregular margins; clear spaces surround the cells. Plastic-embedded, H&E × 970.

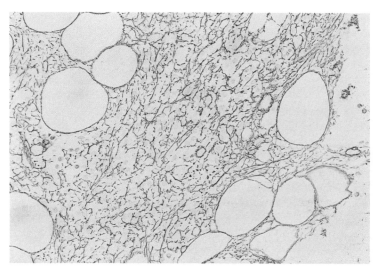

Fig. 5.20 BM trephine biopsy, hairy cell leukaemia, showing increased reticulin. Plastic-embedded, Gomori stain × 188.

hairy cells and consist of isolated erythroid clusters and megakaryocytes; granulocyte precursors are particularly sparse.[44,45]

When the marrow is hypocellular small clusters of hairy cells and residual haemopoietic cells are identified between the fat cells.

Reticulin fibrosis occurs in the areas of marrow infiltration producing a characteristic mesh-like pattern (Fig. 5.20). Collagen fibrosis is not usual.[16,47] Rare patients have osteosclerosis.[48,49]

Both the extent of infiltration[43,50] and cellular morphology have been found to be of prognostic importance in hairy cell leukaemia. A lesser degree of infiltration was found predictive of a good response to splenectomy[50] and of longer survival.[43] Nuclear form was found to be of prognostic significance with patients with small, round or ovoid nuclei having a better survival than those with intermediate-sized convoluted or large, indented nuclei;[43] it has been suggested that this prognostic relevance is related more to increasing nuclear size in these three types than to nuclear shape *per se*.[51] The presence of rod-like cytoplasmic inclusions, corresponding to ribosomal-lamella complexes, has also been found to correlate with a worse prognosis.[43]

The differential diagnosis of hairy cell leuk-aemia includes other lymphoproliferative dis-orders, idiopathic myelofibrosis and aplastic anaemia. The spacing of the hairy cells and the regular meshwork of reticulin are useful in mak-ing the distinction from other lymphoprolifer-ative disorders. In the past some cases of hairy cell leukaemia were misdiagnosed as idiopathic myelofibrosis. Since the distinctive histological features of hairy cell leukaemia are now well re-cognized this diagnostic problem should not arise. The differential diagnosis between the hypo-plastic variant of hairy cell leukaemia and aplastic anaemia depends on recognition of the infiltrating hairy cells. In difficult cases cytochemistry or immunocytochemistry (see below) may be of use.

Bone marrow histology may be modified by therapy. Splenectomy corrects hypersplenism but rarely has any effect on the bone marrow tumour burden. The two chemotherapeutic agents now most frequently employed in treatment, deoxyco-formycin and α-interferon, significantly reduce infiltration. α-interferon causes a slow but pro-gressive decline in the number of bone marrow hairy cells over a period of several months with a response being seen in the great majority of patients.[47,52,53] This is accompanied by a slow increase in haemopoietic cells, but recovery of haemopoiesis, particularly granulopoiesis, lags behind reduction of hairy cell infiltration.[47] Des-pite early optimistic reports, complete clearing of hairy cells from the marrow occurs in only a small minority of patients.[54] The loss of hairy cells can continue after the cessation of therapy but in general there is subsequently a tendency for their numbers to rise slowly.[47,53] At the end of therapy the marrow often shows reduced cellularity and occasionally it is severely hypocellular.[47,53] Deoxycoformycin is more ef-fective than α-interferon in clearing hairy cells from the marrow, complete remission being ob-served in about three-quarters of cases.[54,55] With clearing of hairy cells the increased reticulin is progressively lost but in general the loss of reticu-lin lags behind the loss of hairy cells. Reticulin fibrosis may resolve completely when complete remission is achieved. The rare osteosclerotic lesions also resolve.[48]

Cytochemistry and immunocytochemistry are of use in diagnosis and in monitoring therapy. The TRAP reaction can be useful in diagnosis but its value in monitoring therapy is reduced by the fact that interferon therapy causes a reduction of hairy cell TRAP activity.[52] Immunohisto-chemistry is helpful in identifying residual hairy cells. The two most helpful markers are 4KB5 (CD45RA) and L26 (CD20); they stain B cells in general and hairy cells can then be identified by cytological features.[56]

HAIRY CELL VARIANT LEUKAEMIA

A rare variant form of hairy cell leukaemia occurs which differs from hairy cell leukaemia in cyto-logical and haematological features and in its responsiveness to various therapeutic agents.[57] The major clinical feature is splenomegaly.

The cytochemical and immunological markers of hairy cell variant differ in some respects from those of hairy cell leukaemia. TRAP activity is usually not detected. CD11c, CD19, CD20, CD22, FMC7 and various plasma cell markers are usually positive and CD30 is usually negative but, con-trary to the usual findings in hairy cell leukaemia, CD25 and HC2 are usually negative.

Hairy cell variant falls into the Kiel category of low-grade, lymphocytic lymphoma.

Peripheral blood

Hairy cell variant differs from hairy cell leuk-aemia in that the white cell count is usually moderately to markedly elevated and numerous hairy cells are present in the peripheral blood. Anaemia and thrombocytopenia are each seen in about 50 per cent of patients but pancytopenia is generally less pronounced than in hairy cell leuk-aemia and monocytopenia and neutropenia are not usual. The cells have somewhat more cyto-plasmic basophilia than classical hairy cells but show the same irregular cytoplasmic margins. The nucleus, which shows moderate chromatin condensation, is the major distinguishing feature from hairy cell leukaemia because it contains a prominent nucleolus similar to that of pro-lymphocytic leukaemia (Fig. 5.21). Variable numbers of binucleate cells and of large cells with hyperchromatic nuclei are seen.[57]

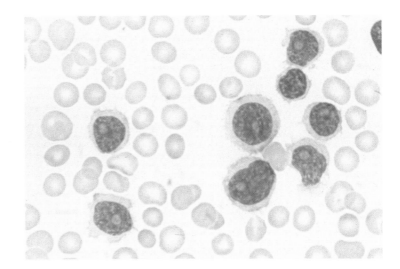

Fig. 5.21 PB film, variant form of hairy cell leukaemia; the nuclei have prominent nucleoli resembling those of prolymphocytes and the cytoplasm is weakly basophilic with hair-like projections. MGG × 940.

Bone marrow cytology

Bone marrow aspiration is usually easier than in hairy cell leukaemia. The aspirate contains numerous cells with the same features as those in the blood.

Bone marrow histology

The trephine biopsy[57] differs from that of hairy cell leukaemia. Infiltration is interstitial. Cells may be in clumps without the intercellular spaces which are characteristic of hairy cell leukaemia, or there may be a mixture of clumps of cells and spaced cells. Moderately condensed chromatin and prominent nucleoli are apparent. There is only a slight to moderate increase in reticulin fibres.

IMMUNOCYTOMA

The term 'immunocytoma' indicates a lymphoma in which neoplastic cells show some features of plasma cell differentiation. The Kiel classification divides immunocytomas into: (i) lymphoplasmacytic lymphoma, in which some of the neoplastic cells are mature plasma cells, and (ii) lymphoplasmacytoid lymphoma, in which there are neoplastic cells with characteristics between those of B lymphocytes and those of plasma cells, but in which mature plasma cells are absent. The ma-jority of haematologists do not distinguish between the two conditions and tend either to use the two terms 'lymphoplasmacytic' and 'lymphoplasmacytoid' interchangeably or to use one or other term to indicate all immunocytomas. In the Rappaport classification immunocytoma falls into the category diffuse lymphocytic lymphoma, well differentiated with plasmacytoid features. In the Working Formulation it is malignant lymphoma, low-grade, small lymphocytic with plasmacytoid features.

The neoplastic cells have cytological characteristics intermediate between those of mature B lymphocytes and those of plasma cells. They usually express both membrane and cytoplasmic immunoglobulin. Secretion of a monoclonal immunoglobulin is common; this is most often IgM but sometimes IgG, IgA, an immunoglobulin heavy chain or an immunoglobulin light chain. The diagnosis of immunocytoma is based on cytological and histological features. Clinical features are very variable. Some patients present with typical features of a lymphoma such as lymphadenopathy or splenomegaly. Others, however, present with signs and symptoms consequent on the presence of the abnormal monoclonal immunoglobulin without necessarily having any signs of lymphoma. The clinical presentations include specific syndromes such as: (i) Waldenström's macroglobulinaemia (see page 195), when there is hyperviscosity due to

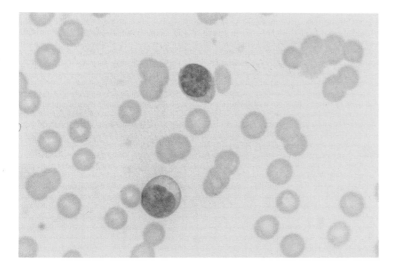

Fig. 5.22 PB film, lymphoplasmacytic lymphoma (immunocytoma), showing a lymphocyte, a plasmacytoid lymphocyte, increased rouleaux formation and increased background staining. The patient had a high concentration of an IgM paraprotein and the clinical features of Waldenström's macroglobulinaemia. MGG × 940.

production of large amounts of an IgM paraprotein (ii) cold haemagglutinin disease (CHAD), when the paraprotein is a cold agglutinin with specificity against the I, or less often the i, antigen of the erythrocyte (iii) idiopathic or essential cryoglobulinaemia, when the paraprotein is either itself a cryoglobulin or has antibody activity against another immunoglobulin, the immune complex being a cryoglobulin, and (iv) acquired angio-oedema due to C1 inhibitor deficiency, when the paraprotein has antibody activity and an immune reaction leads to consumption of C1 inhibitor with a consequent susceptibility to angio-oedema. These specific entities and several other rare conditions which may be associated with the histological features of immunocytoma are dealt with in more detail in chapter 6. Splenic lymphoma with villous lymphocytes[58] can be regarded as a specific morphological variant of immunocytoma. As has been noted previously (see page 130) a significant proportion of patients with centroblastic/centrocytic (follicular) lymphoma in lymph nodes may have a bone marrow infiltrate with the histological features of immunocytoma.

Peripheral blood

In some patients the peripheral blood film is normal. In others there are circulating plasmacytoid lymphocytes (Fig. 5.22), usually present only in small numbers. Plasmacytoid lymphocytes are slightly larger than normal lymphocytes and show various combinations of features usually associated with plasma cell differentiation such as more abundant and more basophilic cytoplasm, an eccentric nucleus, coarse chromatin clumping or the presence of a paler-staining area adjacent to the nucleus which represents the Golgi zone. In some cases there is anaemia or increased rouleaux formation and increased background staining consequent on the presence of a paraprotein. Patients whose paraprotein is a cold agglutinin show red cell agglutination unless the blood specimen has been kept warm until the blood film is made. Occasionally in patients with a cryoglobulin globular or fibrillar deposits of the paraprotein are seen in the blood film.

In cases designated splenic lymphoma with villous lymphocytes there are pleomorphic cells varying from plasma cells through plasmacytoid lymphocytes to 'villous' lymphocytes (Fig. 5.23). The latter are somewhat larger than CLL cells and have a round or oval nucleus with moderately condensed chromatin and, in about half the cases, a small nucleolus; the cytoplasm is basophilic with short villi, often at one pole of the cell. The white cell count is either normal or moderately elevated.

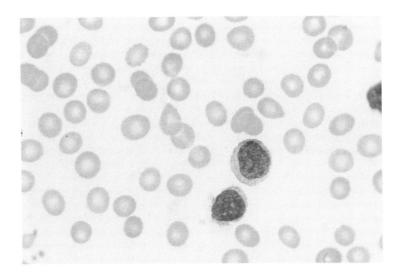

Fig. 5.23 PB film, SLVL, showing two lymphocytes one of which has 'villous' projections. MGG × 940.

Bone marrow cytology

The bone marrow aspirate may be abnormal but this is not necessarily so; even some patients with circulating neoplastic cells have an apparently normal aspirate. This is so, for example, in about 50 per cent of patients presenting with SLVL; some such patients are found to have a nodular infiltrate on trephine biopsy.[58] When present, the lymphoma cells in the bone marrow vary from infrequent to numerous. They have the same cytological features as those in the peripheral blood. Cells often contain cytoplasmic or nuclear inclusions but neither of these features is specific for a neoplastic proliferation; the inclusions are PAS-positive. There is sometimes an increase in mast cells or macrophages.

Bone marrow histology

Bone marrow involvement is frequent in immunocytomas, the reported incidence varying from 50 to more than 80 per cent of cases.[35,37,59] The patterns of infiltration seen are similar to those of CLL — interstitial, nodular, mixed (interstitial-nodular) and diffuse.[15,38,59] Paratrabecular infiltrates have also been described.[60] Many of the infiltrating cells are mature small lymphocytes. Others show evidence of plasma cell differentiation (Figs 5.24 to 5.27). In addition to the usual nuclear and cytoplasmic features of plasma cells there may be cells with intracytoplasmic or intranuclear inclusions (Russell bodies and Dutcher bodies respectively) (Figs 5.25 to 5.27). In lymphoplasmacytic lymphoma there are mature lymphocytes, plasma cells and cells with intermediate characteristics (lymphoplasmacytoid lymphocytes). In lymphoplasmacytoid lymphoma there are mature lymphocytes and plasmacytoid lymphocytes. In both types a small number of immunoblasts are present. A third subtype of immunocytoma, designated polymorphous immunocytoma, has also been recognized;[59,61] it is characterized by a wide spectrum of lymphoid cells — lymphocytes, plasma cells, lymphoplasmacytoid cells and immunoblasts — and by frequent mitoses.

An increase in mast cells usually accompanies an immunocytic infiltration. In cases with a paraprotein, bone marrow vessels can contain homogeneous PAS-positive material.[62] Reticulin fibres are frequently increased in the area of infiltration.[16]

Both the pattern of infiltration and cytological features have both been found to be related to prognosis. Diffuse infiltration is associated with advanced disease and the worst prognosis.[38,59] A nodular infiltrate is associated with the best prognosis while a mixed interstitial-nodular infiltrate is intermediate.[59] Bartl *et al.*[59] found a relationship between the pattern of infiltration and

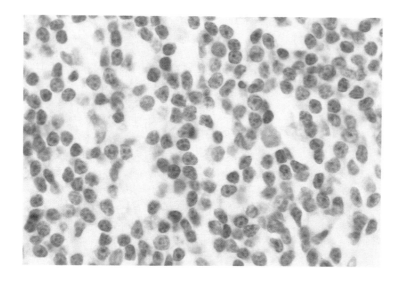

Fig. 5.24 BM trephine biopsy, SLVL, showing diffuse infiltration by mature small lymphocytes and occasional cells with plasmacytoid features. Plastic-embedded, H&E × 940.

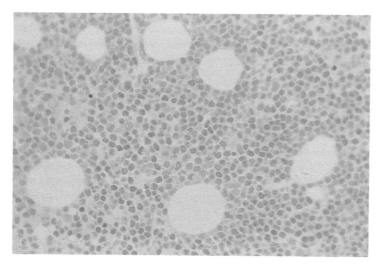

Fig. 5.25 BM trephine biopsy, lymphoplasmacytic lymphoma, showing diffuse infiltration by lymphocytes, plasmacytoid lymphocytes, and occasional plasma cells; note the cytoplasmic and intranuclear inclusions. Plastic-embedded, H&E × 390.

cytology and reported further that the worst prognosis was found in the polymorphous sub-type, an intermediate prognosis in lymphoplasmacytic lymphoma and the best prognosis in lymphoplasmacytoid lymphoma. Immunoblastic lymphoma may supervene in immunocytoma with an associated worsening of prognosis.

PLASMACYTIC LYMPHOMA

Plasmacytic lymphoma, consisting entirely of plasma cells without an admixture of lymphocytes is very rare as a node-based lymphoma;[61] it does not involve the bone marrow unless it becomes disseminated in the late stages of the disease. Cells of similar type infiltrate the bone marrow in multiple myeloma (see chapter 6).

CENTROBLASTIC/CENTROCYTIC LYMPHOMA

The terminology applied to lymphomas composed of cells considered analogous to the cells of normal lymphoid follicles has been a source of great confusion to both histopathologists and haematologists, a situation which has not been fully resolved with the introduction of the Work-

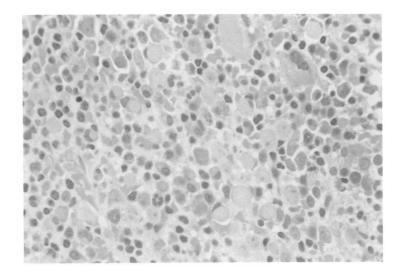

Fig. 5.26 BM trephine biopsy, lymphoplasmacytic lymphoma, showing diffuse infiltration by lymphocytes, plasmacytoid lymphocytes and plasma cells; note the large intracytoplasmic inclusions (Russell bodies) compressing nuclei giving some cells a 'signet ring' appearance. Plastic-embedded, H&E × 390.

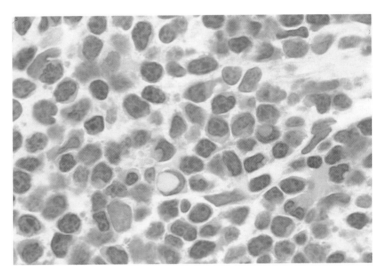

Fig. 5.27 BM trephine biopsy, lymphoplasmacytoid lymphoma, showing diffuse infiltration by lymphocytes and plasmacytoid lymphocytes; note the cytoplasmic and intranuclear inclusions. Plastic-embedded, H&E × 970.

ing Formulation. Lymphomas which exhibit a clearly follicular pattern of growth are of follicular centre origin but this is also true of lymphomas with a mixed follicular and diffuse pattern and of some lymphomas with a totally diffuse pattern of growth; the nature of the latter group can be established from a combination of cytological features, membrane markers and cytogenetic-molecular biological characteristics. A specific translocation, t(14;18)(q32;q21), is associated with a high percentage of neoplasms of follicular centre origin. In the Kiel classification cells of follicular centre origin are designated centrocytes

and centroblasts. Unfortunately one of the same terms, 'centrocyte', has been applied also to a different cell type, a small cleft cell now believed to originate in the mantle zone of the follicle[63] rather than in the follicular centre. In the Rappaport classification small and large cells of follicular origin are designated respectively poorly differentiated lymphocytes and 'histiocytes' while in the Working Formulation they are designated small cleaved (that is, cleft) cells and large cleaved or non-cleaved cells. The approximate equivalents in the three classifications are shown in Table 5.3.[4,7,64]

Table 5.3 Classification of malignant lymphomas of follicular centre cell origin (excluding Burkitt's lymphoma) according to the Kiel classification and the Working Formulation for Clinical Usage[4,7,64]

Working Formulation	Kiel classification

Low grade
B. Follicular, predominantly small cleaved cell
   Diffuse areas
   Sclerosis
 	
C. Follicular, mixed small cleaved cell and large
     cell
   Diffuse areas
   Sclerosis
	Low grade
	
	Centroblastic/centrocytic, small, follicular ±
	diffuse areas

Intermediate grade
D. Follicular, predominantly large cell
   Diffuse areas
   Sclerosis
	Low grade
	Centroblastic/centrocytic, large, follicular ±
	diffuse areas

	High grade Centroblastic, follicular

F. Diffuse, mixed small cell and large cell
   Sclerosis
   Epithelioid component
	Low grade
	Centroblastic/centrocytic, small, diffuse

G. Diffuse, large cell Cleaved cell	Centroblastic/centrocytic, large, diffuse
	High grade Centroblastic, diffuse
Non-cleaved cell Sclerosis	

Centroblastic/centrocytic lymphoma is rare in childhood and quite uncommon during adolescence. Cases occur throughout adult life. Unlike all other mature B cell lymphomas, the incidence is similar in men and women. The commonest clinical feature is lymphadenopathy, either localized or generalized. Some patients have hepatomegaly or splenomegaly. Patients with advanced disease may also have pleural effusions or ascites with neoplastic cells in the effusions. Centroblastic/centrocytic lymphoma is commonly widely disseminated (stage IV disease) at presentation. Centroblastic/centrocytic lymphoma may transform to centroblastic lymphoma or, less often, to immunoblastic lymphoma.

In the minority of patients with circulating lymphoma cells the diagnosis of centroblastic/centrocytic lymphoma can usually be suspected from the cytological and membrane marker characteristics of the peripheral blood cells; a biopsy is required for confirmation. Definitive diagnosis usually requires a lymph node biopsy, although a minority of cases with a follicular growth pattern in the bone marrow can be diagnosed by trephine biopsy. A bone marrow aspirate commonly fails to detect bone marrow infiltration, as a consequence both of the focal nature of infiltration and of increased reticulin deposition. A trephine biopsy is therefore important if accurate staging is required. However, patients with stage III and stage IV disease are often treated with the same therapeutic protocols and in this case bone marrow examination is not essential.

Peripheral blood

The blood count and film are often normal at presentation, even in patients with stage IV disease. When there is heavy bone marrow infiltration the haemoglobin concentration and platelet and neutrophil counts may be reduced. A significant minority of patients have circulating neoplastic cells. These may be infrequent or may be present in very large numbers. Morphology varies between cases. In some patients, particularly those with high counts, the cells are smaller than normal lymphocytes with a very high nucleo-cytoplasmic ratio, condensed chromatin and narrow clefts in some nuclei (Fig. 5.28). In patients with lower counts the cells are somewhat larger. Cytological features may include scanty cytoplasm, angular shape, homogeneous rather than clumped chromatin and narrow nuclear clefts. The lymphoma cells are more pleomorphic than those of CLL. Generally only small lymphocytes, corresponding to those recognized histologically as centrocytes, are present in the peripheral blood. Even cases with a large proportion of centroblasts in tissue sections usually have only centrocytes circulating.

Patients who do not have any peripheral blood abnormality at presentation may develop it during the course of the disease. In a minority of patients transformation to a large cell (centroblastic) lymphoma is associated with the appearance in the blood of large cells corresponding to centroblasts. These cells are rather pleomorphic with plentiful cytoplasm, little chromatin condensation and prominent, often peripheral nucleoli; the nuclei may be predominantly round or may be cleft.

The lymphoma cells of centroblastic/centrocytic lymphoma have strongly expressed SmIg and are positive for pan-B markers such as CD19, CD20, CD22 and CD24. They are CD5 negative, sometimes positive for CD38 and usually positive for CD10 and FMC7.

Bone marrow cytology

The bone marrow is commonly infiltrated, even when the peripheral blood is normal. However, because bone marrow infiltration is often patchy, the bone marrow aspirate may be normal even when there is infiltration detectable histologic-

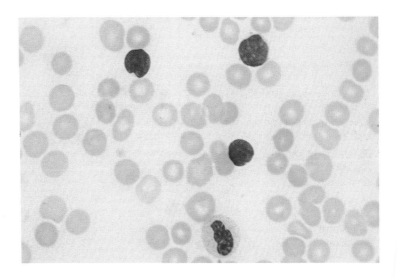

Fig. 5.28 PB film, centroblastic/ centrocytic (follicular) lymphoma, showing very small lymphocytes with dense, cleaved nuclei and very scanty cytoplasm. MGG × 940.

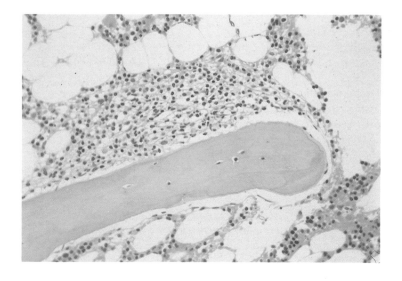

Fig. 5.29 BM trephine biopsy, centroblastic/centrocytic lymphoma showing a broad-based paratrabecular infiltrate of centrocytes; note normal bone marrow above and below. Paraffin-embedded, H&E × 195.

ally. When the aspirate is abnormal the cells may show the same morphological features as those in the peripheral blood, but they are often less easy to recognize with certainty.

Bone marrow histology

The bone marrow is infiltrated in 25–60 per cent of cases[15,36,37] with only about half of patients with bone marrow infiltration having lymphoma cells recognizable microscopically in the peripheral blood. Infiltration is predominantly focal and very rarely diffuse; the focal lesions are overwhelmingly paratrabecular in location (Fig. 5.29) but they may be random patchy or there may be a mixture of random and paratrabecular infiltrates. When infiltration is heavy individual focal lesions may coalesce and replace large areas of marrow; however the paratrabecular concentration of lymphoma can usually still be appreciated. In most series of patients a nodular pattern (Fig. 5.30), resembling that in the lymph node, has been found to be quite uncommon.[13,15,65–67] Divergent findings have been reported by Bartl *et al.*;[9] they reported 'a strictly nodular pattern frequently of follicles

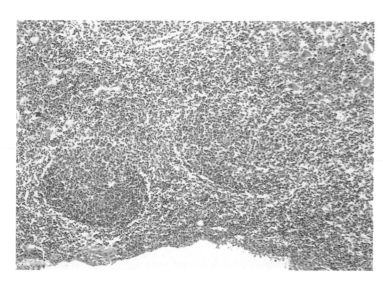

Fig. 5.30 BM trephine biopsy, centroblastic/centrocytic lymphoma, showing diffuse infiltration with formation of follicles. Paraffin-embedded, H&E × 97.

with germinal centres' and did not observe a paratrabecular pattern. This discrepancy may be because this group classified lymphomas on the sole basis of the cytology of the bone marrow infiltrate. It may be that some cases which others would have classified as centroblastic/centrocytic have been classified as centrocytic.

The predominant lymphoma cell in the bone marrow is the small cleft lymphocyte or centrocyte (Figs 5.31 and 5.32). These cells are larger than small lymphocytes with more plentiful cytoplasm and nuclei which are irregular and often angular or elongated. The nuclear chromatin is less dense and clumped than that of the small lymphocyte. The nuclear clefting may be difficult to recognize in paraffin-embedded tissue sections but can be seen in plastic-embedded sections. Smaller but variable numbers of large cells, either cleft (large centrocytes) or non-cleft (centroblasts) are present. Large centrocytes have irregular or cleft nuclei while centroblasts have round nuclei; both cell types have a moderate amount of cytoplasm and small nucleoli abutting on the nuclear membrane. There are also some large cells with large central nucleoli which resemble immunoblasts. A minority of patients have epithelioid granulomas (see Fig. 2.14). Reticulin fibres are significantly increased in infiltrated areas.[16] Dis-

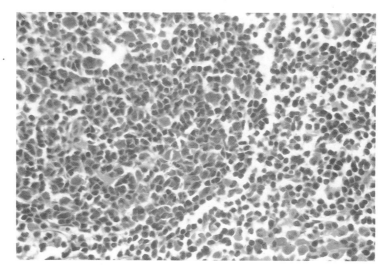

Fig. 5.31 BM trephine biopsy, centroblastic/centrocytic lymphoma (same case as Fig. 5.30), showing a follicle composed of centrocytes. Paraffin-embedded, H&E × 390.

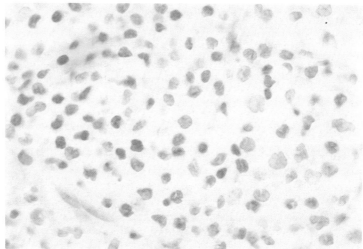

Fig. 5.32 BM trephine biopsy, centroblastic/centrocytic lymphoma, showing an infiltrate composed predominantly of centrocytes. Plastic-embedded, H&E × 940.

cordant immunocytoma or large cell lymphoma may occur in the marrow of patients with centroblastic/centrocytic lymphoma (see page 130).

Following chemotherapy the areas of previous infiltration may be recognized as hypocellular paratrabecular foci, containing reticulin with or without residual centrocytes.[67]

CENTROCYTIC LYMPHOMA

Lymphomas classified as malignant lymphoma, low grade, centrocytic in the Kiel classification appear to constitute a specific entity recognizable on the basis of histological features, membrane markers and a characteristic cytogenetic abnormality.[63] The lymphoma cells are analogous to lymphocytes of the mantle zone of the lymphoid follicle. Other groups have recognized this lymphoma and have described it under other names including lymphoma of intermediate differentiation (intermediate lymphoma) and mantle zone lymphoma.[63,68] Mantle cell lymphoma, nodular or diffuse variant, has been suggested as a unifying name.[63] This lymphoma is not recognized as a separate entity in the Rappaport classification but cases usually fall into the category of diffuse poorly differentiated lymphocytic lymphoma. In the Working Formulation cases are classified as diffuse lymphoma of small cleaved cells, a lymphoma of intermediate grade. Centrocytic lymphoma is a disease of adult life. There is a marked male predominance. Common clinical features are generalized lymphadenopathy, splenomegaly and hepatomegaly. Histological features in the lymph node include a diffuse or vaguely nodular growth pattern and a tendency for the lymphoma cells to grow in a mantle around residual normal lymphoid follicles. This lymphoma is commonly associated with a specific translocation, t(11;14)(q13;q32).

Peripheral blood cytology

In many patients the peripheral blood shows no abnormality. A leukaemic phase occurs in 20–30 per cent of patients.[68,69] A marked elevation of the white cell count occurs but is uncommon.[63,70] In many cases the cells are larger than those of CLL, varying from small to medium or large (Fig. 5.33a). They are characteristically pleomorphic; some have prominent nucleoli and some have irregular, angular or cleft nuclei;[70] in comparison with the centrocytes of follicular lymphoma cells tend to be more pleomorphic and less angular with broader nuclear clefts and more cytoplasm. Other cases have peripheral blood lymphocytes more like those of CLL, although possibly with some cleft cells, and the diagnosis is made only on lymph node biopsy.[63]

Cells express strong SmIg, usually IgM and sometimes also IgD; IgG is expressed in a minority. Cases more commonly express λ light chain than κ. Cells are positive for pan-B markers, are usually positive for both CD5 and FMC7, and may be positive for CD10.

Bone marrow cytology

The bone marrow is infiltrated in the majority of patients, including many patients who do not have lymphoma cells in the peripheral blood.[68,69] The infiltrating cells have the same morphology as those in the peripheral blood (Fig. 5.33b).

Bone marrow histology

Marrow involvement is frequent, being found in more than three-quarters of cases.[13,68,69,71] In histological sections centrocytic lymphoma is composed of small lymphoid cells of variable morphology, some with round nuclei and others with indented or cleft nuclei (Fig. 5.34). Cytologically these cells were considered to occupy an intermediate position between 'well differentiated' and 'poorly differentiated' lymphocytes, hence the designation 'lymphoma of intermediate differentiation'. Centroblasts are not seen. There may be an admixture of epithelioid macrophages.[70] Bone marrow infiltration may be paratrabecular, focal non-paratrabecular or diffuse.[9,70,72] Reticulin fibres are increased in infiltrated areas.

MISCELLANEOUS LOW-GRADE B-LINEAGE LYMPHOMAS

A lymphoma with specific histological features believed to arise from the mucosa-associated lymphoid tissue (MALT) has been designated a MALT lymphoma. Bone marrow and peripheral blood involvement are quite uncommon but have

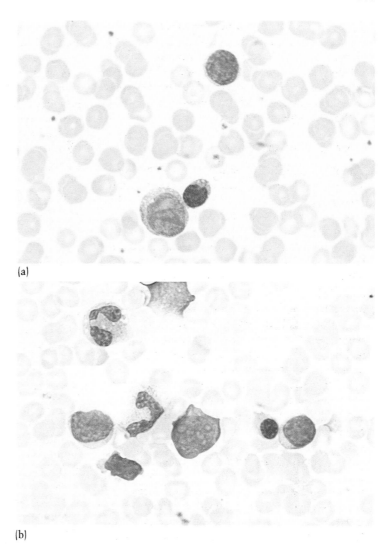

(a)

(b)

Fig. 5.33 (a) PB film, centrocytic lymphoma (mantle-zone lymphoma, lymphoma of intermediate differentiation), showing pleomorphic lymphocytes. MGG × 940. (b) BM aspirate, centrocytic lymphoma, showing pleomorphic lymphocytes varying from small, mature lymphocytes to large lymphoid cells with multiple nucleoli. MGG × 940.

been described. The lymphoma cells are morphologically similar to centrocytes. The bone marrow infiltration in a case described in detail[73] was paratrabecular and nodular with an interstitial component.

A lymphoma designated monocytoid B-cell lymphoma may have some relationship to the MALT lymphomas.[73] Peripheral blood and bone marrow involvement is similarly uncommon in this lymphoma but has been described.[74,75]

CENTROBLASTIC LYMPHOMA

Centroblastic lymphoma[64] is a high-grade lymphoma which may occur *de novo* or may represent transformation of a centroblastic/centrocytic lymphoma. In the Working Formulation centroblastic lymphoma may be classified as malignant lymphoma, follicular, predominantly large cell or as malignant lymphoma, diffuse, large cell (Table 5.3). In the Rappaport classification it is classified as nodular histiocytic or diffuse histiocytic lymphoma.

Peripheral blood

Lymphoma cells are rarely present in the peripheral blood. When centroblastic lymphoma occurs as a transformation of centroblastic/centrocytic lymphoma any circulating lymphoma

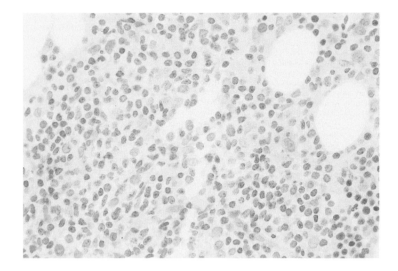

Fig. 5.34 BM trephine biopsy, centrocytic lymphoma, showing diffuse infiltration by pleomorphic small and medium-sized lymphocytes. Plastic-embedded, H&E × 377.

cells are usually centrocytes. When peripheral blood dissemination of centroblasts does occur the cells are very large and pleomorphic (Fig. 5.35). They have plentiful cytoplasm and an irregular, often lobulated nucleus containing one or more fairly prominent nucleoli.

Bone marrow cytology

Bone marrow infiltration is uncommon but is considerably more common than peripheral blood spread; in one series infiltration was detected in 15 per cent of cases. In patients with preceding centroblastic/centrocytic lymphoma the bone marrow is sometimes infiltrated by centroblasts but sometimes shows only residual low-grade lymphoma. A significant minority of patients with apparently *de novo* centroblastic lymphoma at an extramedullary site also show low-grade lymphoma of centroblastic/centrocytic type in the bone marrow;[18] the presence of low-grade lymphoma does not have the same poor prognostic significance as bone marrow infiltration by high-grade lymphoma.

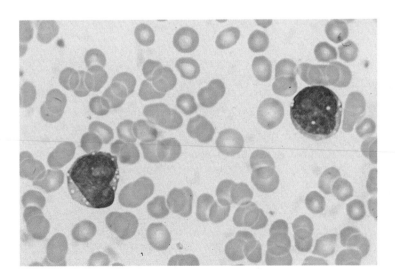

Fig. 5.35 PB film, centroblastic lymphoma, showing large lymphoma cells with a high nucleo-cytoplasmic ratio, moderately basophilic vacuolated cytoplasm and medium-sized nucleoli sited towards the periphery of the nucleus. MGG × 940.

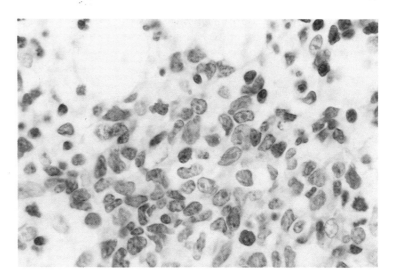

Fig. 5.36 BM trephine biopsy, centroblastic lymphoma, showing infiltration by pleomorphic centroblasts and occasional immunoblasts. Plastic-embedded, H&E × 940.

Bone marrow histology

Twenty to 30 per cent of patients with centroblastic lymphoma have infiltration of the marrow.[13,15] This may be either infiltration by centroblastic lymphoma or infiltration by discordant low-grade (centroblastic/centrocytic) lymphoma.[13,15,19] Discordance is relatively common. Low-grade lymphoma may be seen both in those with and without a previous history of low-grade lymphoma. The pattern of infiltration by centroblastic lymphoma is either focal or diffuse. The infiltrate may be composed of relatively monomorphic centroblasts or may be pleomorphic with admixed immunoblasts (Fig. 5.36), multilobulated cells and large cleft cells.

B-IMMUNOBLASTIC LYMPHOMA

Immunoblastic lymphoma of B-lineage is a high-grade lymphoma which may develop in a previously healthy subject or in a patient with immunodeficiency. The immunodeficiency may be either congenital or consequent on infection by the HIV virus or on immunosuppressive therapy. The EB virus is implicated in the pathogenesis of many but not all cases in immunodeficient subjects. The congenital immunodeficiency underlying immunoblastic lymphoma may be either a generalized failure of the immune system or a specific inability to deal with the EB virus. The frequency of iatrogenic cases is related to the intensity of immunosuppression. They have been particularly common following cardiac transplantation but have also occurred following renal and bone marrow transplantation. Several cases have been observed following bone marrow transplantation in which the lymphoma developed in donor cells. Immunoblastic lymphoma may also occur following transformation of a low-grade lymphoproliferative disease such as chronic lymphocytic leukaemia or immunocytoma. Immunoblastic lymphoma occurs at all ages. Because of the relationship to underlying immune deficiency this lymphoma forms a significant proportion of childhood lymphomas. Immunoblastic lymphoma of T-lineage also occurs (see page 175). The term 'immunoblastic sarcoma' is synonymous with immunoblastic lymphoma. In the Working Formulation this lymphoma is classified as malignant lymphoma, diffuse, large cell and in the Rappaport classification as diffuse histiocytic lymphoma.

Peripheral blood

Neoplastic cells are rarely present in the peripheral blood. When present they are very large with plentiful, strongly basophilic cytoplasm and a large nucleus containing a prominent central nucleolus. In patients with underlying immune deficiency there may be marked lymphopenia or, in patients with AIDS, pancytopenia.

Bone marrow cytology

The bone marrow is not commonly infiltrated; in one series the marrow was infiltrated in less than a quarter of patients.[37] When lymphoma cells are present they have the same morphological features as described above (Fig. 5.37). A significant minority of patients with immunoblastic lymphoma at an extramedullary site show low-grade lymphoma in the bone marrow, usually of centroblastic/centrocytic type but occasionally small lymphocytic with plasmacytoid differentiation;[18] this does not have the same grave prognostic import as marrow infiltration by immunoblasts.

Bone marrow histology

The neoplastic cells of immunoblastic lymphoma are distinguished from centroblasts by virtue of their larger size, more plentiful cytoplasm and the presence of a very large, prominent and usually central nucleolus (Fig. 5.38). Some cases have marked nuclear lobulation. Binucleated and multinucleated forms may be present. Some cells may show signs of plasma cell differentiation but it is often not possible to distinguish between

T- and B-lineage immunoblasts on morphology alone.[76]

The marrow is infiltrated in 15–20 per cent of cases.[13,37] The pattern of bone marrow infiltration may be focal random, focal paratrabecular or diffuse.[13,15,62] In some patients there is marrow infiltration by discordant low-grade lymphoma.

LARGE CELL ANAPLASTIC LYMPHOMA

Large cell anaplastic lymphoma is a high-grade lymphoma which is more commonly of T-lineage than B and will therefore be discussed under T-cell lymphomas (see page 175).

BURKITT'S LYMPHOMA

Burkitt or Burkitt's lymphoma is a high-grade lymphoma, the clinical features of which differ, depending on whether cases are endemic or sporadic. Endemic Burkitt's lymphoma occurs in tropical Africa and in New Guinea and is particularly a disease of childhood; tumour formation in the jaw is usually the most prominent clinical feature. Sporadic Burkitt's lymphoma is worldwide in distribution and occurs at all ages; the commonest clinical features are abdominal tumour formation and malignant pleural or peritoneal effusions. Cases of Burkitt's lymphoma among patients with AIDS resemble sporadic

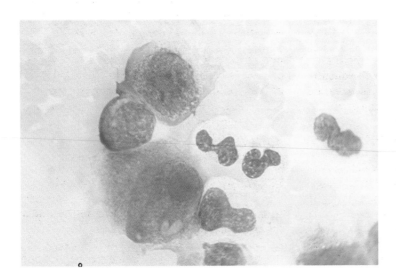

Fig. 5.37 BM aspirate, B-lineage immunoblastic lymphoma in a patient with AIDS, showing lymphoma cells varying from medium-sized to very large; note the basophilic cytoplasm and, in the largest cell, a giant nucleolus. MGG × 940.

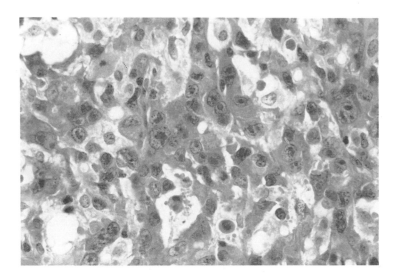

Fig. 5.38 BM trephine biopsy, B-immunoblastic lymphoma in a patient with AIDS (same case as Fig. 5.37), showing diffuse infiltration by pleomorphic immunoblasts; note the prominent central nucleoli. Paraffin-embedded, H&E × 390.

cases but meningeal lymphoma appears to be particularly common. The EB virus is an important pathogenetic factor in endemic Burkitt's lymphoma and in a significant proportion of AIDS-related cases but is not often implicated in sporadic cases. In the Working Formulation Burkitt's lymphoma is categorized as malignant lymphoma, high-grade, small non-cleaved cells. In Rappaport's classification it is categorized as undifferentiated lymphoma.

Peripheral blood cytology

In the majority of patients with Burkitt's lymphoma the peripheral blood shows no abnormality. Even when the bone marrow is infiltrated, circulating lymphoma cells are present in less than half of patients. Some patients whose peripheral blood is initially normal subsequently show circulating lymphoma cells with disease progression or relapse. The morphological features of lymphoma cells are identical to those of leukaemic cells in the L3 category of acute lymphoblastic leukaemia (see page 131). When patients present with numerous circulating neoplastic cells but no localized tumour formation is present the disease is usually categorized as L3 ALL rather than as Burkitt's lymphoma. Cases with intermediate characteristics occur and classification is then somewhat arbitrary. Peripheral blood dissemination appears to be particu-

larly common in patients with underlying AIDS. Such patients are also commonly pancytopenic even in the absence of bone marrow infiltration.

Bone marrow cytology

The bone marrow is usually normal at presentation. The frequency of bone marrow infiltration has varied from five to 20 per cent in different series. The frequency of infiltration appears to be similar in endemic (African)[77,78] and in non-endemic[79-81] cases. Our impression is that bone marrow infiltration is more common in AIDS-related Burkitt's lymphoma than in other cases. When bone marrow infiltration occurs it is usually heavy and is readily detected by either an aspirate or a trephine biopsy. However, because of their striking cytological features, a low percentage of infiltrating cells may be detected in an aspirate when the trephine biopsy is normal.[82] Some patients without infiltration of the marrow have an increase in lymphocytes.[80]

Bone marrow histology

Infiltration may be interstitial, nodular or diffuse.[80-82] Cells are very uniform in appearance; they have a round or ovoid nuclear outline and a distinct, narrow rim of cytoplasm (Fig. 5.39). Clefted or folded nuclei are rare. Nucleoli are usually brightly eosinophilic and distinct but not

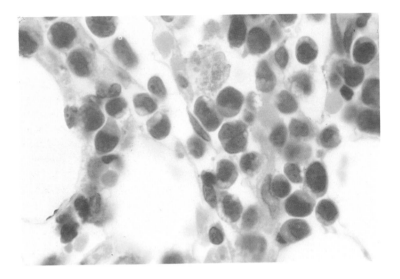

Fig. 5.39 BM trephine biopsy, Burkitt's lymphoma in a patient with AIDS, showing diffuse infiltration by lymphoblasts; note the prominent cytoplasmic vacuoles. Paraffin-embedded, H&E × 970.

usually large. The mitotic rate is high. Cytoplasmic vacuoles can sometimes be detected if specifically sought (Fig. 5.39). Tingible body macrophages, a characteristic feature in other tissues causing the so-called 'starry sky' appearance, are generally absent. Bone marrow necrosis may occur both before treatment is given and to an even greater extent after chemotherapy. Increased reticulin is frequent.

LYMPHOBLASTIC LYMPHOMA (B-LINEAGE)

Lymphoblastic lymphoma is a high-grade lymphoma. Only 10–15 per cent of cases are of B-lineage. They are predominantly adults, childhood cases being almost always T-lineage.[83] Clinical features are lymphadenopathy, either localized or generalized, with or without hepatomegaly and splenomegaly. Lytic bone lesions are common.

Peripheral blood

The peripheral blood is usually normal. When lymphoblasts are present they are identical to those of acute lymphoblastic leukaemia.

Bone marrow cytology

The bone marrow is often normal. When there is infiltration the cells cannot be distinguished on cytological details from those of ALL. By convention cases with fewer than 25 or 30 per cent of bone marrow lymphoblasts are categorized as lymphoblastic lymphoma and cases with a heavier infiltration as ALL. The distinction is to some extent arbitrary since the cells are not only morphologically but also immunophenotypically indistinguishable from those of ALL.

Bone marrow histology

Histological features are similar to those of T-lymphoblastic lymphomas (see page 177).

LYMPHOPROLIFERATIVE DISORDERS OF T-LINEAGE

The terminology of T-lineage lymphoproliferative disorders is particularly confused, with histopathologists and haematologists often failing to recognize the same entities. It is also often difficult to harmonize different histopathological classifications. In the past cases have sometimes been described using undefined terms and without reference to a clear system of classification. A single disease entity may be described under multiple designations or, conversely, a single term may be used to denote different diseases. The term T-chronic lymphocytic leukaemia has, for example, been used as a loose generic term and also to indicate conditions as diverse as large granular lymphocyte leukaemia and the small cell variant of prolymphocytic leukaemia.

There are several further problems with the classification of T-lineage lymphomas. First, it has proved difficult to devise a reproducible classification, probably as a consequence of the extreme histological diversity of T-cell lymphomas.[5] Secondly, prognosis does not show a very close relationship with whether cases are categorized histologically as low-grade or high-grade. Some cases falling into low-grade categories have a prognosis as poor as most high-grade lymphomas. Thirdly, a single category of lymphoma may include different disease entities and, conversely, cases representing a single disease entity may fall into more than one histological category. Cases of leukaemia/lymphoma associated with the HTLV-I virus, for example, clearly constitute a clinicopathological entity but despite this they fall into more than one histological category of the Kiel classification, including at least one category of low-grade lymphoma and two categories of high-grade lymphoma (see Table 5.1). Since the histopathological characteristics do not appear to be closely related to the prognosis or to other features of the disease, these cases will be discussed as a group and separately from the other T-lineage lymphomas. The converse problem occurs with the Kiel category of T-lineage, low-grade, lymphocytic lymphoma which includes under the designation 'chronic lymphocytic leukaemia' both leukaemia of large granular lymphocytes (LGL leukaemia) and two other conditions, at least one of which appears to be more closely related to prolymphocytic leukaemia. LGL leukaemia clearly differs from the other T lymphocytic lymphomas, as is recognized in the FAB[2] and MIC[84] classifications. We will discuss this group of lymphomas using the definitions and terminology of the FAB and MIC groups. The term 'peripheral T-cell lymphoma' also requires consideration although it is not part of the Kiel classification. This designation embraces all T-lineage neoplasms with the exception of acute lymphoblastic leukaemia and lymphoblastic lymphoma which have a pre-thymic or thymic phenotype;[5] however, the term is sometimes used in a more restricted sense with cutaneous T-cell lymphomas being excluded.[20] The Working Formulation does not distinguish between B-cell and T-cell lymphomas. The only T-cell neoplasm which is specifically identified is mycosis fungoides; other T-cell lymphomas are aggregated with the more common B-cell lymphomas to form rather heterogeneous groups.

The common patterns of bone marrow infiltration in T-cell lymphoma differ from those most characteristic of B-cell lymphomas. Infiltration is usually interstitial, random focal, nodular or diffuse. Nodular infiltration differs from that seen in B-cell lymphomas and in benign lymphoid hyperplasia in that the nodules often have rather ill-defined margins. Paratrabecular infiltration occurs[11,20] but is quite uncommon. T-cell lymphomas also differ from B-cell in that various reactive changes are more frequent; such changes include eosinophilia, vascular proliferation, polyclonal plasma cell proliferation, macrophage proliferation, haemophagocytosis, epithelioid cell and granuloma formation and reactive follicular hyperplasia.

The frequency with which marrow infiltration has been reported in peripheral T-cell lymphoma has varied from 10 per cent[85] to 80 per cent.[20] This wide disparity may be attributable in part to the occurrence of histologically equivocal lesions which require immunophenotyping for confirmation[11] and in part to a variable mixture, in any series of patients, of different disease entities with different probabilities of bone marrow spread.

Diagnosis and classification of T-lineage lymphomas and leukaemias is not always possible on lymph node histology alone. The immunophenotype and the cytological features of peripheral blood and bone marrow cells can be of critical importance in diagnosis. Histological features in a trephine biopsy are generally of less importance than lymph node histology and peripheral blood cytology. However, in some cases a firm diagnosis can be established from the bone marrow when other diagnostic tissue is not available.[11,20] In other patients lesions are suggestive of non-Hodgkin's lymphoma but are non-diagnostic unless supplemented by analysis of immunophenotype. The differential diagnosis includes Hodgkin's disease, the acquired immune deficiency syndrome, auto-immune diseases, malignant histiocytosis and virus-associated haemophagocytosis. The problems in

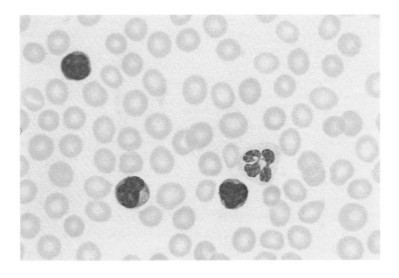

Fig. 5.40 PB film, T-PLL, showing dense irregular nuclei and, in one cell, a prominent medium-sized nucleolus. MGG × 940.

the differential diagnosis of angio-immunoblastic lymphadenopathy and related conditions are discussed on page 168.

T-prolymphocytic leukaemia

The FAB group[2] has recommended that the term T-prolymphocytic leukaemia (T-PLL) be used to cover not only cases of low-grade T-lineage lymphoma in which cells have morphological features quite similar to those of B-PLL but also other cases with smaller cells which differ more from those of B-PLL; others, including the Kiel group,[5] have preferred to classify the latter group as T-CLL but the FAB terminology is justified by the observation that, despite some variation in morphology, all these cases have many features in common, specifically their clinical and immunophenotypic profiles and characteristic cytogenetic abnormality.[2] T-PLL falls into the Kiel category of T-lineage, low-grade, lymphocytic lymphoma.

T-PLL is mainly a disease of the elderly. Patients commonly present with marked splenomegaly. Other features may include lymphadenopathy, skin infiltration and serous effusions.

Peripheral blood

The white cell count is usually high. In some cases the circulating neoplastic cells are similar in size to normal small lymphocytes while in others they are considerably larger, similar in size to B-PLL cells.[86] When cells are large there is usually relatively abundant cytoplasm and the nuclei contain a prominent central nucleolus. Some cases are cytologically indistinguishable from B-PLL cells. In others the cytoplasm is more basophilic and the nucleus is irregular. In cases with predominantly small cells the nucleo-cytoplasmic ratio is higher and the nucleolus is smaller and less prominent (Fig. 5.40); the nucleus is often irregular ('knobby') and there may also be cytoplasmic blebs. In T-PLL, cells are characteristically CD4 positive and express pan-T and mature T-cell markers such as CD2, CD3 and CD5. They also express CD7, thus differing from most other leukaemias of mature T cells.

Bone marrow cytology

The bone marrow is infiltrated by cells of the same appearance as those in the blood but the morphology is usually less well preserved.

Bone marrow histology

The patterns of infiltration seen are similar to those of B-PLL (see page 139). In some cases irregular nuclei and scanty cytoplasm suggest T lineage (Fig. 5.41) but many cases are indistinguishable from B-PLL. Reticulin fibrosis appears to be commoner than in B-PLL.[41]

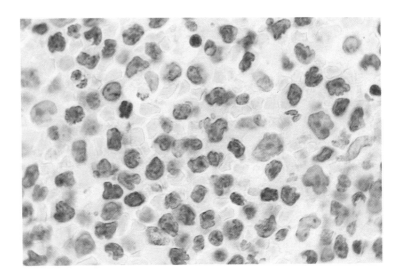

Fig. 5.41 BM trephine biopsy, T-PLL, showing large and small prolymphocytes with prominent nucleoli, particularly in the larger cells; note highly irregular nuclei. Plastic-embedded, H&E × 940.

LARGE GRANULAR LYMPHOCYTE LEUKAEMIA

The condition designated T-CLL by the FAB group[2] has neoplastic cells which are morphologically similar to normal large granular lymphocytes. Because of the varied ways in which the term T-CLL has been employed the term 'large granular lymphocyte leukaemia' (LGL leukaemia) seems preferable for this condition, as suggested by the MIC group.[84] LGL leukaemia falls into the Kiel category of T-lineage, low-grade, lymphocytic lymphoma. It should be noted, however, that although in most cases the cells are CD8 positive and have other T-cell markers there are some morphologically identical cases in which cells share some markers with natural killer cells but lack T-cell markers.

Patients with LGL leukaemia show a variable degree of lymphadenopathy, hepatomegaly and splenomegaly. A minority of patients have skin infiltration or polyarthritis.

Peripheral blood

The white cell count is increased due to an increased number of large granular lymphocytes.[87,88] In occasional patients the total white cell count is not increased although there is an increase in the number of large granular lymphocytes. The neoplastic cells are morphologically very similar to normal large granular lymphocytes (Fig. 5.42).

They have a round or oval nucleus with moderately condensed chromatin; the cytoplasm is voluminous and weakly basophilic and contains fine or coarse azurophilic granules. Smear cells are rare. Some patients have isolated neutropenia or thrombocytopenia or, less often, anaemia. These cytopenias are out of proportion to the degree of bone marrow infiltration and appear to have an immune basis. Macrocytosis is sometimes present.

Neoplastic cells are usually positive for CD2, CD3, CD5 and are most often negative for CD7.[89] They are usually CD8 positive and CD4 negative. Cells are commonly positive for CD57, a natural killer cell marker, but only a minority of cases are positive for other natural killer cell markers such as CD11b and CD16.

Bone marrow cytology

The bone marrow shows a variable infiltration by cells with the same morphology as those in the blood. In the early stages infiltration may be minimal. In patients with marked neutropenia the bone marrow usually shows immature granulocytic cells in normal numbers but mature neutrophils are lacking. Patients with thrombocytopenia usually have normal numbers of megakaryocytes. When anaemia is marked the marrow may show either a lack of maturing erythroblasts or megaloblastic erythropoiesis.

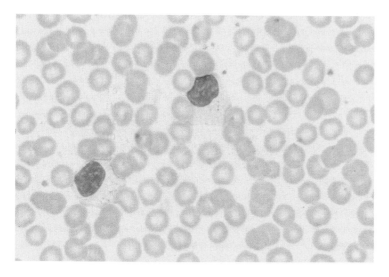

Fig. 5.42 PB film, large granular lymphocyte leukaemia, showing two large granular lymphocytes. MGG × 940.

Bone marrow histology

The marrow is infiltrated in almost all cases. However, the bone marrow infiltrate in LGL leukaemia does not have distinctive features and can be confused with that of various low-grade B-cell lymphoproliferative disorders. It is essential that peripheral blood and films of bone marrow be examined simultaneously if the nature of the infiltrate is to be recognized.

Infiltration is usually interstitial, random focal or diffuse but in occasional instances has been nodular.[90–92] The infiltrates are composed of small and medium-sized lymphocytes (Fig. 5.43), the nuclei of which have irregular contours, condensed nuclear chromatin and inconspicuous nucleoli.[92] There is a thin rim of cytoplasm in which granules are not visible. Some cases have plasmacytosis.[92] Neutropenic cases often show apparent maturation arrest at the myelocyte stage. Patients with thrombocytopenia have adequate or increased numbers of megakaryocytes.

LYMPHOMA OF SMALL CEREBRIFORM CELLS
(CUTANEOUS T-CELL LYMPHOMAS)

Low-grade, T-cell lymphoma of small cerebriform cells is manifest clinically as cutaneous lymph-

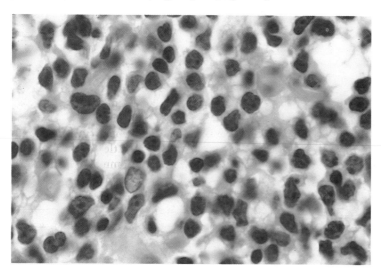

Fig. 5.43 BM trephine biopsy, large granular lymphocyte leukaemia, showing diffuse infiltration by somewhat pleomorphic small and medium-sized lymphocytes. Paraffin-embedded, H&E × 970.

oma, either mycosis fungoides or Sézary's syndrome. In both conditions there is infiltration of the dermis and the epidermis by neoplastic cells. The epidermal infiltrate is focal; the intraepidermal accumulations of lymphocytes are known as Pautrier's abscesses or micro-abscesses. Pautrier's abscesses are highly characteristic of lymphoma of small cerebriform cells but they are not pathognomonic since they may also occur in HTLV-I-associated leukaemia/lymphoma. Sézary's syndrome is characterized by generalized erythroderma, consequent on infiltration of the skin by lymphoma cells, together with circulating neoplastic cells which may be numerous or scanty; these features are detectable at the time of presentation. In mycosis fungoides the initial manifestation is usually the presence of patchy erythematous lesions but subsequently there is formation of plaques, nodules and fungating tumours. Spread to lymph nodes occurs late in the disease. Circulating neoplastic cells are sometimes but not always apparent in mycosis fungoides. There is some overlap between the conditions classified respectively as Sézary's syndrome and as mycosis fungoides and they are best regarded as different manifestations of a single disease; the circulating neoplastic cells of both arë referred to as Sézary cells. Rare patients lack clinically detectable skin lesions but have circulating neoplastic cells with the cytological features of Sézary cells, a condition which has been designated Sézary cell leukaemia.

Sézary cells are usually CD4 positive and express pan-T and mature-T markers including CD2, CD3 and CD5; they are sometimes CD7 positive.[89]

Peripheral blood

The likelihood of Sézary cells being present in the peripheral blood can be related to the nature of the skin lesions. In one study circulating neoplastic cells were not detectable in patients with localized skin plaques but were present in nine per cent of patients with generalized skin plaques, 27 per cent of those with skin tumours and 90 per cent of those with erythroderma.[93] Sézary cells vary in size from that of a normal small lymphocyte to two or three times this size. Individual patients may have predominantly small cells or predominantly large cells. Sézary cells have a high nucleo-cytoplasmic ratio. The chromatin is highly condensed, sometimes hyperchromatic. The nucleus is described as 'convoluted' or 'cerebriform'; names indicative of the intertwined lobes resembling the convolutions of the brain (Fig. 5.44). This causes the surface of the nucleus to appear grooved. Lobes are often more readily discernible in large Sézary cells than in small. Nucleoli are usually unapparent but can sometimes be detected in large cells. Cytoplasm is scanty in small cells but more abundant in large cells; it is agranular and may contain vacuoles which are found to be PAS-positive. When Sézary cells are infrequent and similar in size to normal lymphocytes they can be difficult to identify with certainty. Ultrastructural examination is very useful in those cases in which the characteristic cytological features cannot be discerned by light microscopy; demonstration of the characteristic form of the nucleus confirms the diagnosis.

Some patients have eosinophilia.[94] Except when disease is very advanced, anaemia and cytopenia are not usually a feature of Sézary's syndrome or of mycosis fungoides.

Bone marrow cytology

The bone marrow is often normal, even in a high proportion of patients with circulating neoplastic cells.[94] A variable degree of infiltration by Sézary cells can occur, particularly in the advanced stages of the disease.

Bone marrow histology

Bone marrow involvement is uncommon in cutaneous T-cell lymphomas. In mycosis fungoides infiltration is mainly seen in those with extensive extra-cutaneous disease but even at autopsy it is present in little over a quarter of patients.[95] Infiltration is commoner in Sézary's syndrome than in mycosis fungoides.[96] In the majority of cases infiltration is focal but occasionally it is diffuse. The hyperchromatic convoluted nucleus is the most helpful cytological feature differentiating Sézary cells from other lymphoma cells in histological sections. In some cases the

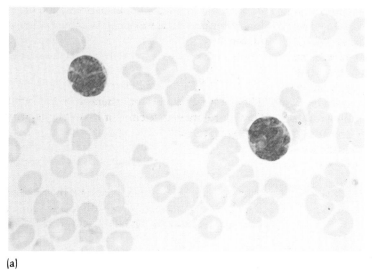

(a)

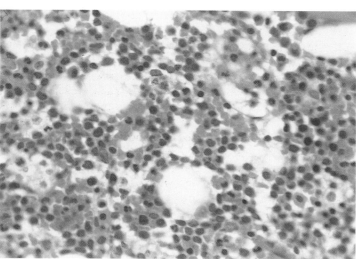

(b)

Fig. 5.44 (a) PB film, Sézary syndrome, showing two cells with convoluted nuclei and scanty cytoplasm. MGG × 940. (b) BM trephine biopsy, lymphoma of small cerebriform cells, showing heavy interstitial infiltration. Paraffin-embedded, H&E × 390.

infiltrate is pleomorphic and includes bizarre multinucleated cells. There is a moderate increase in reticulin.

Other low-grade T-cell lymphomas

The remaining four categories of low-grade T-cell lymphoma in the Kiel classification have often been grouped together as node-based peripheral T-cell lymphomas.[11,20] All are most often neoplasms of mature CD4-positive cells but express aberrant phenotypes which differ from those of normal peripheral blood T-cells. All have a considerably worse prognosis than that of low-grade B-cell lymphomas or lymphomas of small cerebriform cells. Occasional shifts between these histological types have been observed.[85] Although they have distinct histological features in lymph nodes[5,85,97,98] and differ somewhat in their clinical features[85] the bone marrow features have many similarities. Precise diagnosis usually depends on lymph node histology and immunophenotyping with bone marrow cytology and histology playing a subsidiary role. Prominent reactive changes in the bone marrow are usual. Lymphoma cells may be only a minor part of an abnormal infiltrate which may include non-neoplastic lymphocytes, plasma cells and haemophagocytic macrophages. Neutrophilic and eosinophilic hyperplasia are common and dysplastic changes are sometimes noted in haemopoietic lineages so that confusion with a myeloproliferative or even a myelodysplastic disorder has occurred.[99] Stromal changes include increased vascularity, foci of haemorrhage and necrosis, and reticulin fibrosis.

LYMPHOEPITHELIOID LYMPHOMA (LENNERT'S LYMPHOMA)

Lymphoepithelioid lymphoma (Lennert's lymphoma) is a T-cell lymphoma in which there is prominent reactive epithelioid cell proliferation. The neoplastic cells are small lymphocytes with irregular nuclei; they are usually CD4 positive and positive for mature T and pan-T markers such as CD2 and CD3.[5,85,97] The histological and cytological features are described in detail in the references cited.

Lymphoepithelioid lymphoma is predominantly a disease of the middle-aged and elderly. It is characterized clinically by lymphadenopathy, which is often generalized, and in a minority of patients by hepatomegaly, splenomegaly or rash.[85,98] Transformation to a large cell lymphoma occurs in a minority of patients; the prominent epithelioid component is then no longer present.[97]

Peripheral blood

There are no specific peripheral blood features. Some patients are anaemic or have lymphopenia or eosinophilia.[98]

Bone marrow cytology

The bone marrow aspirate may contain abnormal lymphoid cells which are small to medium in size and may have irregular nuclei.

Bone marrow histology

The bone marrow is infiltrated in only a minority of patients.[11,21,85] Involvement may be interstitial, focal or diffuse. We have observed paratrabecular involvement but this is quite uncommon. The infiltrate in the marrow is similar to that seen in the lymph nodes. There are small lymphocytes with round or irregular nuclei and a coarse chromatin pattern and a variable admixture of medium-sized lymphocytes, some immunoblasts, and possibly reactive cells including eosinophils and plasma cells (Figs 5.45 and 5.46). There may be clusters of epithelioid cells (Fig. 5.46). Reticulin is increased in the areas of neoplastic infiltration.

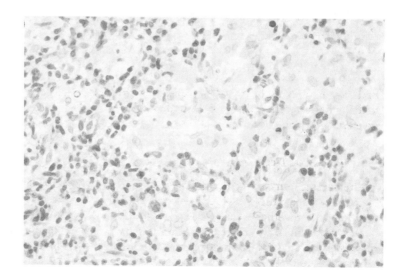

Fig. 5.45 BM trephine biopsy, Lennert's lymphoma, showing a pleomorphic lymphoid infiltrate and an admixture of epithelioid macrophages. Plastic-embedded, H&E × 188.

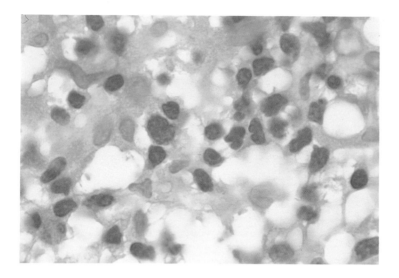

Fig. 5.46 BM trephine biopsy, Lennert's lymphoma (same case as Fig. 5.45), showing epithelioid macrophages and medium-sized lymphoid cells with irregular nuclei. Plastic-embedded, H&E × 970.

ANGIO-IMMUNOBLASTIC LYMPHOMA

The nature of the condition variously described under the names angio-immunoblastic lymph-adenopathy with dysproteinaemia (AILD), immunoblastic lymphadenopathy and lympho-granulomatosis X remains uncertain. Initially this condition was regarded as an abnormal immune reaction but evidence, derived from cytogenetic and DNA analysis, that there was an underlying clonal and probably neoplastic proliferation of T cells subsequently emerged. It is now clear that many if not all cases represent a lymphoma of CD4-positive T cells. Some pathologists consider that all cases are actually lymphomas from the beginning while others regard some cases as lymphomas and others as a reactive process with a propensity to lymphomatous transformation. It has been proposed that cases with demonstrable clonal proliferation of T cells should be classified as lymphomas and cases lacking such evidence should not. However, not all T-cell lymphomas have demonstrable rearrangement of the T-cell receptor β gene;[11,85] this may be because in some cases the proportion of neoplastic cells is very low or because T-cell receptor δ and γ genes are rearranged rather than T-cell receptor β genes. Further, although there is some correlation be-tween demonstrable gene rearrangement and cytological evidence of atypia this correlation is not perfect,[85] and although there is an early dif-ference in survival curves the curves ultimately come together.[85] A final judgement as to whether all cases of AILD, or only the majority, represent lymphoma must await further evidence.

The diagnosis of angio-immunoblastic lymph-oma rests on lymph node histology. Typically there is effacement of nodal architecture with disappearance of germinal centres, a marked pro-liferation of venules and an infiltrate which is composed of a variable mixture of lymphocytes, plasma cells, immunoblasts, epithelioid cells and proliferating dendritic reticulum cells.[5,85,98] Many cases have extracellular PAS-positive material.

Characteristic clinical features are fever and lymphadenopathy, auto-immune haemolytic anaemia and other auto-immune phenomena, allergic reactions to drugs and hypergamma-globulinaemia.

Transformation to a high-grade T-cell lym-phoma occurs in 10–15 per cent of patients.

Peripheral blood

There is usually normocytic normochromic anaemia with increased rouleaux formation and an elevated ESR. Occasionally the anaemia is leucoerythroblastic. Complicating auto-immune haemolytic anaemia is common. Some patients have lymphopenia, thrombocytopenia, neutro-philia, eosinophilia or basophilia.[98,100] Plasma cells, plasmacytoid lymphocytes and atypical lymphocytes resembling those seen in viral infections or immunological reactions may be present.

Bone marrow cytology

The bone marrow aspirate may show non-specific changes such as the features of the anaemia of chronic disease. There may be an infiltrate of small lymphocytes, sometimes with irregular nuclei, and of atypical lymphoid cells including immunoblasts. Inflammatory cells including eosinophils and plasma cells may be increased.

Bone marrow histology

The reported incidence of bone marrow infiltration varies widely, from 10 per cent[85] to 60 per cent.[101] The lesions are usually focal (patchy or nodular), either single or multiple. Distribution is usually random but is sometimes paratrabecular.[21] Diffuse infiltration can occur. The infiltrate is composed of lymphocytes, plasma cells, immunoblasts, macrophages and sometimes eosinophils or neutrophils (Figs 5.47 to 5.49). The lymphocytes have somewhat irregular nuclei and may be small and medium sized or medium sized and large. In some cases there are lymphocytes

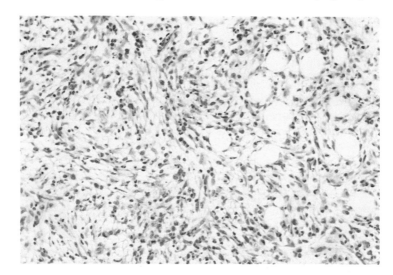

Fig. 5.47 BM trephine biopsy, angio-immunoblastic lymphoma, showing a pleomorphic lymphoid infiltrate and irregular fibrosis. Paraffin-embedded, H&E × 97.

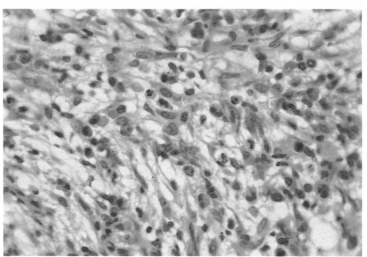

Fig. 5.48 BM trephine biopsy, angio-immunoblastic lymphoma (same case as Fig. 5.47), showing that the infiltrate is composed of medium-sized lymphocytes admixed with fibroblasts, eosinophils, immunoblasts and plasma cells. Paraffin-embedded, H&E × 390.

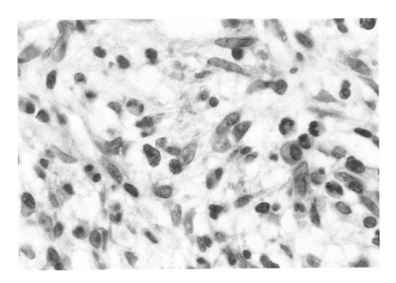

Fig. 5.49 BM trephine biopsy, angio-immunoblastic lymphoma (same case as Fig. 5.47), showing fibroblasts, eosinophils and medium-sized lymphocytes with irregular nuclei. Paraffin-embedded, H&E × 970.

resembling Hodgkin's cells or Reed—Sternberg cells and immunoblasts with clear cytoplasm.[21] Because of the presence of epithelioid macrophages focal lesions may resemble granulomas. Some cases have hyperplastic capillaries which are occasionally arborizing. Extracellular PAS-positive material is seen in only a minority of cases. Reticulin is usually increased.

Although angio-immunoblastic lymphoma may sometimes be suspected on bone marrow examination the diagnosis generally requires a lymph node biopsy. Two features which are particularly characteristic of the lymph node lesions, arborizing capillaries and PAS-positive extracellular deposits, are much less apparent and sometimes inapparent on a bone marrow biopsy. A similar pleomorphic infiltrate can occur in the bone marrow in Hodgkin's disease and in inflammatory and auto-immune conditions. The lesions of systemic mastocytosis are sometimes confused with angio-immunoblastic lymphoma if a Giemsa or toluidine blue stain is not performed.

T-ZONE LYMPHOMA

T-zone lymphoma is a T-cell lymphoma in which lymph node infiltration by small and medium-sized T-cells is initially in the paracortex with sparing of the germinal centres. Later infiltration is diffuse.[5] The neoplastic cells are usually positive for CD2, CD3 and CD4.[85]

The most common clinical presentation is with generalized lymphadenopathy.[85] A smaller number of patients have hepatosplenomegaly or rash. Progression to a high-grade lymphoma may occur.

Peripheral blood

There are no specific abnormalities in the peripheral blood.

Bone marrow cytology

The bone marrow is infiltrated by abnormal small lymphocytes in a minority of patients. There may be an admixture of inflammatory cells.

Bone marrow histology

The bone marrow has been reported to be infiltrated in less than 10 per cent of patients. There are no specific bone marrow features which distinguish this lymphoma from other low-grade peripheral T-cell lymphomas. There is some admixture of small lymphocytes with lymphoid cells showing abundant water-clear cytoplasm, with immunoblasts and with reactive cells.

PLEOMORPHIC, SMALL CELL LYMPHOMA

Pleomorphic, small cell lymphoma commonly presents with lymphadenopathy with or without skin infiltration. Some patients have hepatomegaly or splenomegaly. Diagnosis is generally based on lymph node histology. In some cases, pleomorphic, small cell lymphoma is associated with the HTLV-I virus; they will be discussed separately (see below).

The neoplastic cells are most often CD4 positive and express pan-T and mature-T markers such as CD3 and CD2.

Peripheral blood

The peripheral blood is usually normal. When neoplastic cells are present they are variable in size but larger than normal lymphocytes. They are pleomorphic with regard to size and shape of the cell and nuclear characteristics. Some nuclei are lobulated and some contain nucleoli. There may be a minority of cells resembling Sézary cells but in general the cells have more abundant cytoplasm than Sézary cells and the nuclei are not so tightly infolded.

Bone marrow cytology

The bone marrow may be normal or may show a variable degree of infiltration by neoplastic cells and inflammatory cells.

Bone marrow histology

Bone marrow infiltration may be interstitial or mixed nodular and interstitial.[11,21] The infiltrate consists predominantly of small cells with a small number of medium-sized cells; some nuclei have an irregular configuration. Cytoplasm is usually scant.

ADULT T-CELL LEUKAEMIA/LYMPHOMA

Adult T-cell leukaemia/lymphoma (ATLL) is a T-cell neoplasm occurring in subjects whose T-cells have earlier been infected by the retrovirus HTLV-I I (human T-cell leukaemia virus I). The virus is integrated into host T-cells at random sites but is integrated at a consistent site in the neoplastic clone of an individual case. The lifetime risk of leukaemia/lymphoma in patients infected by the virus has been estimated at about one in 60–80. Cases of ATLL have mainly been observed in certain areas of known endemicity of the virus,

specifically Japan and the West Indies, and in countries which have received immigrants from these two areas. More recently cases have been reported from South America with a smaller number of cases being recognized in patients from Central and West Africa, the Middle East, Taiwan and other parts of the world.[89,102–104] It is likely that co-factors are necessary for the development of ATLL; these may differ in Japan and the West Indies since the disease usually has a later age of onset in Japan.

ATLL may present as a lymphoma, without bone marrow and peripheral blood involvement, or as a leukaemia/lymphoma with both tissue infiltration and peripheral blood and bone marrow involvement. The majority of cases have an acute course but chronic and smouldering forms are recognized. Cytologically and histologically ATLL is very variable. The majority of cases fall into three Kiel categories: (i) pleomorphic, small cell (ii) pleomorphic, medium and large cell, and (iii) immunoblastic. A number of Japanese patients with lymphomas classified as Lennert's lymphoma, T-zone lymphoma and angio-immunoblastic lymphoma have also been found to be HTLV-I positive.[85] Suchi et al.[5] have reported that a smouldering course is more likely in those with histologically low-grade lymphoma but Jaffe et al.[103] did not observe any relationship between histological grade and outcome. The histological features of the lymph nodes in ATLL do not differ from those seen in lymphomas in the same histological category which are unrelated to the virus. The clinical and haematological features are, however, different. It is recommended that cases should be classified histologically but also designated ATLL and recognized as a discrete entity.

ATLL occurs in adults. Prominent clinical features are lymphadenopathy, skin infiltration and bone lesions associated with hypercalcaemia. Some patients have splenomegaly and hepatomegaly. The prognosis is generally poor with a median survival of less than a year.

ATLL cells are usually positive for CD2, CD3 and CD5. They are most often CD4 positive and differ from the cells of other types of mature T-cell lymphoma in that CD25 is positive in the majority of cases.

Examination of the peripheral blood is very

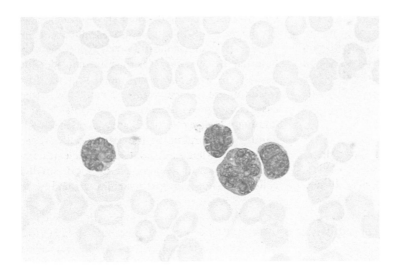

Fig. 5.50 PB film, ATLL, showing highly pleomorphic cells, the largest of which has a 'clover-leaf' or 'flower-like' lobulated nucleus containing prominent medium-sized nucleoli. MGG × 940.

important in diagnosis. Bone marrow aspiration and trephine biopsy are of lesser importance.

Peripheral blood

About three-quarters of patients have circulating lymphoma cells. These are distinctive.[89,102] They are extremely pleomorphic, varying in size, shape, nucleo-cytoplasmic ratio and degree of chromatin condensation (Fig. 5.50). Cytoplasm varies from scanty to moderately abundant and is sometimes basophilic. Some cells have nucleoli and a primitive chromatin pattern while others, usually the majority, have condensed, sometimes hyperchromatic, chromatin. Nuclei are very variable in shape but some are deeply lobulated, resembling clover leaves or flowers. Some cerebriform cells may be present, but the degree of pleomorphism usually permits the distinction from Sézary's syndrome.

Because the marrow is not usually heavily infiltrated there may be little anaemia or thrombocytopenia at presentation. Eosinophilia is not infrequent.[104]

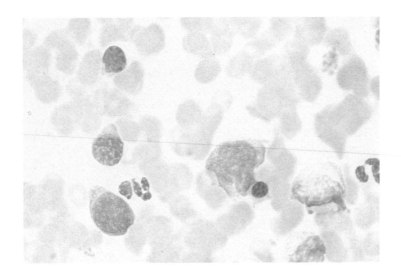

Fig. 5.51 BM aspirate, ATLL, showing an infiltrate of lymphoid cells; there is considerable variation in size: the largest cell has a lobulated nucleus. MGG × 940.

Bone marrow cytology

Patients who have leukaemia at presentation show a variable degree of bone marrow infiltration by cells similar to those described above (Fig. 5.51).

Bone marrow histology

The bone marrow is infiltrated in about three-quarters of cases. The pattern of marrow involvement may be interstitial, random focal or diffuse.

Occasionally it is paratrabecular. At presentation the degree of infiltration is often slight.

The nature of the infiltrate varies considerably between cases. Many cases show considerable variation in cell size with nuclei varying from medium size to large (Figs 5.52 and 5.53). Other cases have predominantly small cells or predominantly large cells. Cells are characteristically highly pleomorphic. In the larger cells, nuclei tend to be vesicular with a distinct nuclear membrane and two to five distinct nucleoli; smaller cells often show chromatin condensation. Nuclei

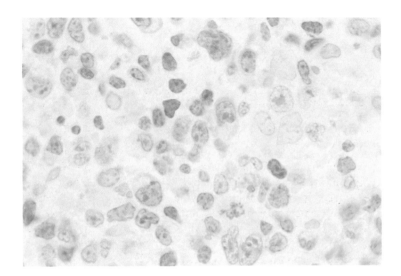

Fig. 5.52 BM trephine biopsy, ATLL, showing diffuse infiltration by highly pleomorphic small, medium and large lymphoid cells. Plastic-embedded, H&E × 940.

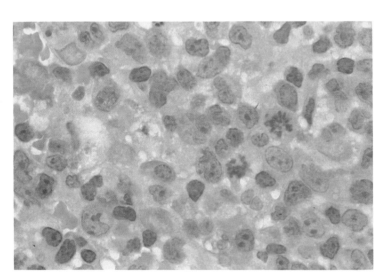

Fig. 5.53 BM trephine biopsy, ATLL, showing diffuse infiltration by highly pleomorphic medium and large lymphoid cells. Note the high mitotic rate. Plastic-embedded, H&E × 970.

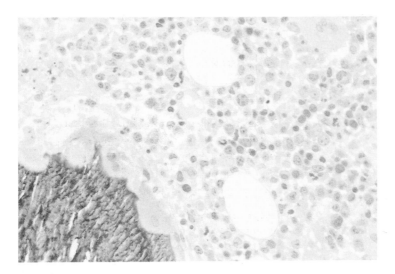

Fig. 5.54 BM trephine biopsy, ATLL, showing heavy infiltration by pleomorphic medium and large lymphocytes; note the numerous osteoclasts in Howship's lacunae giving the bone trabecula a serrated appearance. Plastic-embedded, H&E × 377.

vary in shape, being round, oval, indented, deeply lobulated or convoluted. Giant cells may be present; some of these resemble Reed–Sternberg cells while others have nuclear convolutions, coarsely aggregated chromatin and prominent nucleoli.[5] The mitotic rate is high (Fig. 5.53). In addition to the neoplastic cells there are often large numbers of eosinophils and plasma cells. Marrow vascularity may be increased.

A characteristic but not invariable feature of ATLL is extensive bone resorption with large numbers of Howship's lacunae and numerous mononucleated and multinucleated osteoclasts (Fig. 5.54). There may be associated bone re-modelling with a variable increase of osteoblast activity and paratrabecular fibrosis.[103,105] In some cases increased osteoclasts are apparent when there is no detectable infiltration in the biopsy sections.[104]

PLEOMORPHIC, MEDIUM AND LARGE CELL LYMPHOMA

Cases of pleomorphic, medium and large cell lymphoma usually present with localized or generalized lymphadenopathy. When disease is generalized there may also be hepatomegaly and splenomegaly. Some cases have skin infiltration.

Some cases of pleomorphic, medium and large cell lymphoma are associated with the HTLV-I virus (see above).

Peripheral blood

The peripheral blood is usually normal. In a minority of cases there are circulating neoplastic cells which may be medium or large, or a mixture of both. Cells are highly pleomorphic. The nucleus may be round, oval or lobulated with either a diffuse chromatin pattern or with some chromatin condensation. One or more variably sited, prominent nucleoli are commonly present. The cytoplasm is usually moderately basophilic. There are no specific cytological features which allow this lymphoma to be distinguished from large cell lymphomas of B-lineage. Immunological markers are therefore important in making a correct diagnosis. The immunophenotype is very variable but there is expression of one or more T-lineage markers.

Bone marrow cytology

The bone marrow is often normal but may show a variable degree of infiltration.

Bone marrow histology

In one series infiltration was seen in five of 11 patients at diagnosis.[21] Infiltration may be interstitial with focal accentuation, focal patchy, nodular or diffuse. Heavy infiltration is common. The tumour cells are of variable size with very atypical nuclear configurations, variously described as convoluted, hyperconvoluted, cerebriform or multilobulated. Either medium sized or large cells may predominate. Necrosis is frequently seen, and some cases have vascular hyperplasia. A localized increase in reticulin is found in the infiltrated area.

T-IMMUNOBLASTIC LYMPHOMA

T-immunoblastic lymphoma may occur *de novo* or evolve from a low-grade lymphoma. Some cases are associated with the HTLV-I virus (see above).

Peripheral blood

Peripheral blood involvement is rare.[76] When it occurs the lymphoma cells are very large with abundant basophilic cytoplasm. The nucleus is large and round and has a large, centrally placed nucleolus.

Bone marrow cytology

Bone marrow infiltration is uncommon. When an infiltrate is present the cells have the same characteristics as described for the peripheral blood (Fig. 5.55). It is often impossible to distinguish between T-lineage and B-lineage immunoblastic lymphoma by cytology alone. Both may have strongly basophilic cytoplasm and a prominent paranuclear Golgi zone. An admixture with maturing plasma cells or centroblasts, however, suggests that the lymphoma is of B-lineage.

Bone marrow histology

The pattern of infiltration may be interstitial or diffuse. Reticulin may be increased in the area of infiltration.

LARGE CELL ANAPLASTIC LYMPHOMA

Large cell anaplastic lymphoma is a high-grade lymphoma which may be of either B-lineage or T-lineage, T-lineage being commoner.[106] In some cases lineage is difficult to define. Lymphomas of this type have clinical, histological and cell marker characteristics in common regardless of lineage. They have a wide age-range, occurring in children, adolescents and adults. Cases commonly present with generalized lymphadenopathy, skin infiltration and systemic symptoms. All cases so far described have expressed a membrane antigen recognized by Ki-1 and by other antibodies of the CD30 cluster. This lymphoma is sometimes known as Ki-1 positive large cell lymphoma. The designation large cell anaplastic lymphoma is preferred for the following reasons: (i) an alternative antibody of this cluster, Ber-H2, which can be applied to paraffin-embedded

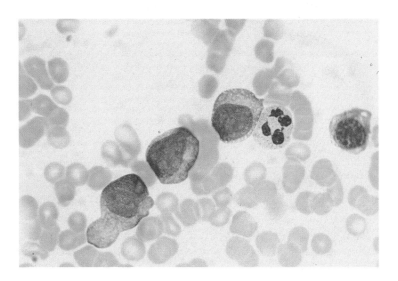

Fig. 5.55 BM aspirate, T-immunoblastic lymphoma, showing large cells with plentiful basophilic cytoplasm and prominent nucleoli. MGG × 940.

sections, is commonly employed in diagnosis instead of Ki-1, and (ii) a reaction with a single antibody is seldom sufficiently specific to justify classification of a lymphoma on this basis and this is so with large cell anaplastic lymphoma and CD30 antibodies; plasma cells are CD30-positive, Reed–Sternberg cells are commonly positive and other non-Hodgkin's lymphomas may also show some reactivity.

Peripheral blood

Circulation of lymphoma cells in the peripheral blood is uncommon. When it occurs the lymphoma cells are large and pleomorphic. Pancytopenia may occur, consequent not only on bone marrow infiltration but also on associated histiocytic proliferation and haemophagocytosis.

Bone marrow cytology

When bone marrow infiltration occurs lymphoma cells are often infrequent (Fig. 5.56), usually less than five per cent of marrow cells.[107] Neoplastic cells are large and pleomorphic, some being as large as megakaryocytes. They have weakly to strongly basophilic cytoplasm which may be finely vacuolated;[106,107] a Golgi zone may be apparent. Nuclei have irregular folds, a coarse open chromatin pattern and multiple prominent nucleoli.[107] Some cases have occasional phago-

cytic neoplastic cells. Associated histiocytic proliferation and haemophagocytosis are common and may overshadow a subtle lymphomatous infiltrate to the extent that a midiagnosis of malignant histiocytosis (see page 98) is not uncommon. Prominent haemophagocytosis may occur when there are few detectable lymphoma cells in the bone marrow.[107] Histiocytes are predominantly mature.

Bone marrow histology

Bone marrow involvement has been reported in seven to 30 per cent of cases:[106–108] it appears to be more frequent in older patients.[108] The pattern of infiltration may be interstitial, focal (sometimes with very small clusters of lymphoma cells) or diffuse.

Cytological features are variable. In most cases tumour cells are very pleomorphic and include multinucleated giant cells and cells with lobated, wreath-shaped or embryo-shaped nuclei, sometimes abutting on the cell membrane[108] (Fig. 5.57). There may be cells resembling immunoblasts and others resembling Reed–Sternberg cells. In other cases tumour cells are less pleomorphic. The mitotic rate is high.[21] Reticulin is increased in the infiltrated area.

Neoplastic cells express CD30, epithelial membrane antigen (EMA), and usually HLA-DR and activation antigens such as CD25 and CD71

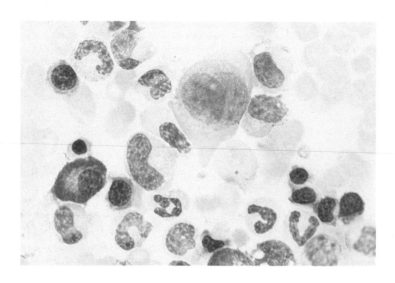

Fig. 5.56 BM aspirate, large cell anaplastic lymphoma, showing a single large bi-nucleate lymphoma cell. MGG × 940.

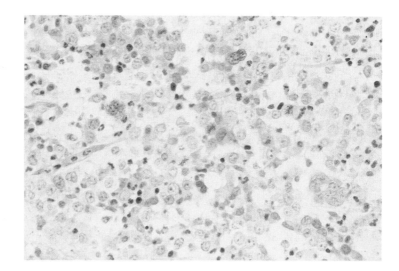

Fig. 5.57 BM trephine biopsy, large cell anaplastic lymphoma, showing highly pleomorphic lymphoma cells including multinucleated giant cells. Paraffin-embedded, H&E × 377.

(anti-transferrin). Leucocyte common antigen is expressed in only 50 per cent of cases. The CD30 antibody, Ber-H2, has been found very useful in identifying small clusters of lymphoma cells.[107]

The differential diagnosis of large cell anaplastic lymphoma includes metastatic carcinoma and amelanotic melanoma.

T-LYMPHOBLASTIC LYMPHOMA

Lymphoblastic lymphoma is much commoner in childhood than in adult life. About 80 per cent of lymphoblastic lymphomas, including the great majority of childhood lymphoblastic lymphoma, are of T-lineage.[83,109] There is a male preponderance. Thymic infiltration is very common and may be associated with pleural and pericardial effusions and superior vena cava obstruction. There may also be lymphadenopathy, hepatomegaly or splenomegaly.

Peripheral blood

The peripheral blood is often normal. Some patients have small numbers of circulating neoplastic cells which are morphologically the same as those of acute lymphoblastic leukaemia. Cells with convoluted nuclei are sometimes present but T-lymphoblasts cannot be distinguished reliably from B-lymphoblasts on morphological grounds. The presence of focal acid phosphatase activity supports T-lineage but assessment of immunological markers is necessary for a definitive diagnosis. The neoplastic cells of T-lineage lymphoblastic lymphoma have a similar immunophenotype to that of T-lineage ALL lymphoblasts. They differ from other T-lineage lymphomas in that terminal deoxynucleotidyl transferase is positive.

Bone marrow cytology

The bone marrow is often normal. Some patients have variable infiltration by lymphoblasts. By convention cases with more than 25–30 per cent of lymphoblasts in the marrow are classified as ALL rather than as lymphoblastic lymphoma. Patients in whom the bone marrow is initially normal may later, if there is disease progression, show infiltration.

Bone marrow histology

The bone marrow is infiltrated at diagnosis in approximately 60 per cent of cases.[15] Infiltration is initially focal but with disease progression focal deposits spread and coalesce to produce a diffuse pattern of infiltration. Before the routine use of chemotherapy bone marrow infiltration usually supervened in those who initially had a normal marrow. The cytological features are almost identical to those of acute lymphoblastic leukaemia.[10] Lymphoblasts are of small or medium size, slightly larger than the small lymphocyte, with scanty cytoplasm and relatively large deeply staining nuclei. Nucleoli are usually relatively small and insignificant and the chromatin is finely stippled. Mitotic figures are frequent and nuclear convolutions can be identified in some cases. A tendency to perivascular infiltration by lymphoblasts may be pronounced.[62] When marrow involvement is minimal the lymphoblasts may be difficult to identify in trephine sections and may more easily be detected in aspirates.

Hodgkin's disease

The term Hodgkin's disease covers a group of lymphomas with common clinical and histological features. The disease is consequent on the proliferation of neoplastic cells of lymph node origin but still of uncertain lineage. The neoplastic cells include distinctive polyploid cells designated Reed−Sternberg cells. These are giant cells which may be binucleated or multinucleated or have lobated nuclei; they have huge inclusion-like nucleoli and abundant cytoplasm.[110] Also present are large cells of a similar appearance but with a single round nucleus and a very large nucleolus, designated mononuclear Hodgkin's cells. In addition specific histological subtypes of Hodgkin's disease are associated with specific variant forms of Reed−Sternberg cells. The diagnosis of Hodgkin's disease requires not only the presence of characteristic neoplastic cells but also an appropriate cellular background since cells morphologically resembling Reed−Sternberg cells may be seen in other lymphomas and in reactive conditions such as infectious mononucleosis. There is a prominent inflammatory response so that the neoplastic cells are mixed with a variable number of lymphocytes, macrophages, eosinophils, plasma cells and fibroblasts. Some histological subtypes have prominent fibrosis.

The classification of Hodgkin's disease is summarized in Table 5.2.[3,110] Hodgkin's disease occurs at all ages but the sex distribution and the median age of onset differ between different histological categories. It remains to be established whether neoplastic cells in the various histological types of Hodgkin's disease are of the same lineage.

The most prominent clinical feature is usually lymphadenopathy, most often cervical lymphadenopathy. Mediastinal lymphadenopathy is also common. Patients with advanced disease may have hepatomegaly and splenomegaly. Systemic symptoms such as a fever, sweating and weight loss are common in those with advanced disease.

Examination of the bone marrow occasionally leads to the diagnosis of Hodgkin's disease, particularly in patients with lymphocyte-depleted Hodgkin's disease presenting with unexplained fever and pancytopenia.[111] More often bone marrow examination is done as part of a staging procedure. The recognition of infiltration usually requires a trephine biopsy. Detection rate is higher with bilateral biopsies or a single large biopsy.[112] Diagnostic cells are rarely present in films of aspirates although histological sections of aspirated fragments occasionally yield a diagnosis. Not all patients with Hodgkin's disease necessarily require investigation of the bone marrow as part of the staging procedure since a combination of clinical and laboratory features can be used as criteria to select those likely to have infiltration.[113] In one study the results of trephine biopsy were found to influence the management in less than one per cent of patients.[114]

Peripheral blood

The peripheral blood shows non-specific abnormalities. There may be anaemia, either normocytic normochromic or, less often, hypochromic microcytic. Rouleaux formation is often increased as is the erythrocyte sedimentation rate. Some patients have neutrophilia or eosinophilia. Occasional patients have lymphocytosis. Lymphopenia is common, with severe lymphopenia being seen in patients with advanced disease or with unfavourable histological categories. In patients with bone marrow infiltration anaemia, leucopenia and pancytopenia are common but a leucoerythroblastic blood film is relatively un-

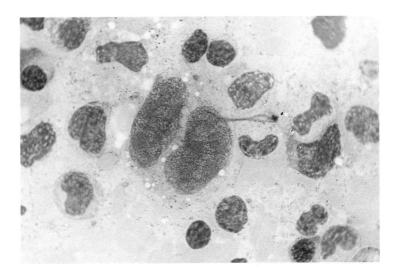

Fig. 5.58 BM aspirate, Hodgkin's disease in a patient with AIDS, showing a Reed–Sternberg cell, a binucleated giant cell with prominent inclusion-like nucleoli. MGG × 940.

common. The neoplastic cells of Hodgkin's disease rarely circulate in the peripheral blood but occasional instances of this phenomenon have been reported.

Bone marrow cytology

The bone marrow aspirate usually shows only reactive changes. The marrow is often hypercellular due to granulocytic (neutrophilic and eosinophilic) hyperplasia. Macrophages and plasma cells are often increased. Erythropoiesis is depressed and may show the features of the anaemia of chronic disease. Megakaryocytes are present in normal or increased numbers.

Even when the marrow is infiltrated it is uncommon for neoplastic cells to be present in the aspirate. When Reed–Sternberg cells are present they are very striking because of their large size, paired nuclei and large, prominent, usually centrally placed nucleoli (Fig. 5.58). With an MGG stain both they and any mononuclear Hodgkin's cells have moderately basophilic cytoplasm and the round, inclusion-like nucleoli stain deep blue.

Bone marrow histology

Bone marrow infiltration is present in five to 15 per cent of patients. Infiltration is more frequent in males, in older patients, in carriers of the HIV virus, in those with unfavourable histological types and in those with other evidence of advanced stage disease.[113,115] Infiltration is rare in lymphocyte predominant disease, and uncommon in nodular sclerosing disease whereas in lymphocyte-depleted Hodgkin's disease it has been observed in up to 50–60 per cent of cases.[114]

With an H&E stain Reed–Sternberg cells and mononuclear Hodgkin's cells have acidophilic or amphophilic cytoplasm, a prominent nuclear membrane and an eosinophilic inclusion-like nucleolus (Figs 5.59 to 5.62). The features of the various variant forms of Reed–Sternberg cells have been described in detail.[110] The criteria to establish the presence of bone marrow infiltration differ according to whether or not a tissue diagnosis of Hodgkin's disease has already been established. Recommendations were drawn up at the Ann Arbor conference in 1971.[110,116] Primary diagnosis requires the presence of Reed–Sternberg cells (Fig. 5.61) in an appropriate cellular background. The only exceptions to this diagnostic requirement are in nodular sclerosing Hodgkin's disease and the nodular variant of lymphocyte predominant Hodgkin's disease in which the presence of variant forms of Reed–Sternberg cells (Fig. 5.62) (see Table 5.2) in an appropriate cellular background may be considered sufficient to establish a diagnosis.[117] If the diagnosis of Hodgkin's disease has already

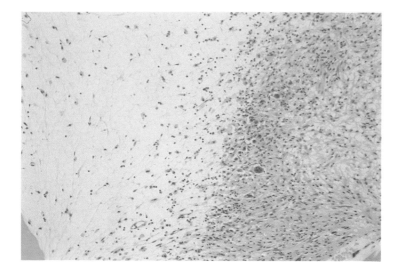

Fig. 5.59 BM trephine biopsy, nodular sclerosing Hodgkin's disease, showing an abnormal infiltrate (right) and bone marrow hypoplasia (left). Paraffin-embedded, H&E × 39.

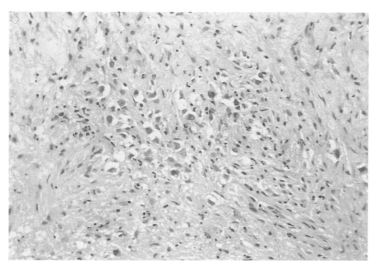

Fig. 5.60 BM trephine biopsy, nodular sclerosing Hodgkin's disease (same case as Fig. 5.59), showing fibrosis and a mixed infiltrate of mononuclear Hodgkin's cells, eosinophils and small lymphocytes. Paraffin-embedded, H&E × 195.

been established in another tissue and a bone marrow biopsy is being done for the purpose of staging the criteria for infiltration are less stringent. In this context the presence of mononuclear Hodgkin's cells in an appropriate cellular background is sufficient;[116] the presence of atypical 'histiocytes' or 'reticulum cells' or the presence of necrosis or focal or diffuse fibrosis with appropriate inflammatory cells is suggestive of Hodgkin's disease but not diagnostic.

In Hodgkin's disease the pattern of infiltration is sometimes focal but more often diffuse. Focal lesions are mainly randomly distributed although some are paratrabecular.[112,118] Focal infiltration is most common in lymphocyte predominant and nodular sclerosing Hodgkin's disease whereas lymphocyte depleted Hodgkin's disease is characterized by diffuse infiltration. Focal lesions tend to be highly cellular with a mixed infiltrate of small lymphocytes with variable numbers of eosinophils, plasma cells, macrophages and Reed–Sternberg cells and their variants. When infiltration is diffuse the pattern is more variable.[112,118–120] Four patterns may be recognized: (i) in the majority of patients the marrow is hypercellular with a mixed cellular infiltrate as

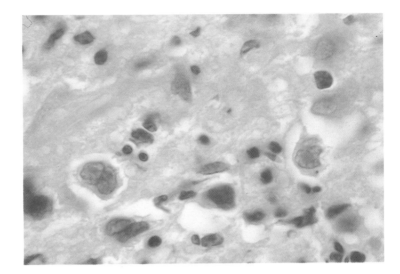

Fig. 5.61 BM trephine biopsy, nodular sclerosing Hodgkin's disease (same case Fig. 5.59), showing a Reed–Sternberg cell (left) and a mononuclear Hodgkin's cell (right). Paraffin-embedded, H&E × 970.

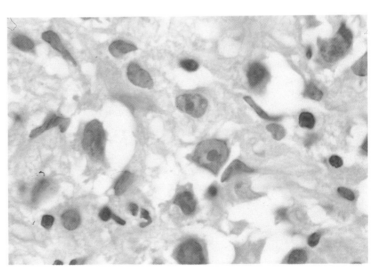

Fig. 5.62 BM trephine biopsy, nodular sclerosing Hodgkin's disease (same case as Fig. 5.59), showing a lacunar cell (left) and two mononuclear Hodgkin's cells (centre). Paraffin-embedded, H&E × 970.

above (ii) in other patients the bone marrow is very hypercellular with a predominant population of Reed–Sternberg cells and variant forms, reactive cells are not numerous (iii) in a third pattern there is a variable degree of fibrosis and in some areas the bone marrow is replaced by dense fibrous tissue with a few macrophages and lymphocytes while in other areas there are foci of neoplastic cells embedded in collagen, and (iv) in the fourth pattern the bone marrow is generally hypocellular with loose, sparsely cellular connective tissue through which are scattered more cellular foci containing lymphocytes, macro-

phages, Reed–Sternberg cells and variant forms. Various combinations of these patterns may be seen in the same biopsy or in different biopsy specimens from the same patient. Amorphous eosinophilic background material may be apparent. Necrosis is occasionally detected prior to treatment[120] but is more common in treated patients. Reticulin is increased in areas of infiltration and collagen is often present. There is sometimes osteolysis or osteosclerosis; increased bone remodelling is usual.[112]

When infiltration is focal the residual bone marrow is usually hypercellular as a consequence of granulocytic hyperplasia. Both eosinophils and neutrophils may be increased, both at the margin of infiltrates and diffusely in non-involved marrow. Non-infiltrated marrow may also show increased megakaryocytes and plasma cells.

Histological appearances in the bone marrow may differ from those in lymph nodes. Classification of the disease should therefore be based on lymph node histology when possible.

The bone marrow of patients in whom bone marrow infiltration is not detected may also show reactive changes. These may include increased granulopoiesis (neutrophilic and eosinophilic), plasmacytosis, lymphoid infiltration including formation of lymphoid aggregates, increased macrophages, increased phagocytosis, oedema, extravasation of erythrocytes, increased storage iron and the presence of sarcoid-like granulomas;[112,118] asteroid bodies may be seen in the giant cells of the granulomas. Bone marrow hypoplasia has been observed in some patients with lymphocyte depleted Hodgkin's disease in whom infiltration was not detected.[111]

In Hodgkin's disease the lymphoid infiltrate does not usually show features of cellular atypia. An exception has been noted in some patients with the nodular variant of lymphocyte-predominant Hodgkin's disease who have been reported to have paratrabecular nodules of small cleft cells indistinguishable from those seen in follicular lymphoma;[117] large atypical cells were rare or not detected.

Following successful treatment of Hodgkin's disease the lymphomatous infiltrate disappears and reactive changes including fibrosis regress. When only reticulin fibrosis is present complete regression occurs. When there has been collagen deposition some patients show complete regression and others partial.

The differential diagnosis of infiltration of the marrow by Hodgkin's disease includes idiopathic myelofibrosis, myelofibrosis secondary to metastatic carcinoma and infiltration by a peripheral T-cell lymphoma. A particular problem occurs in recognizing infiltration when there is a very pronounced fibroblastic response.[121] Idiopathic myelofibrosis is easily simulated since such patients often have splenomegaly, pancytopenia and radiologically demonstrable osteosclerosis.

Both megakaryocytes and carcinoma cells can be confused with Reed—Sternberg cells. When atypical mononuclear cells or inflammatory cells are recognized in fibrous tissue but specific diagnostic features of Hodgkin's disease are lacking diagnosis may require marrow biopsy at another site or biopsy of another tissue. The distinction between peripheral T-cell lymphoma and Hodgkin's disease may prove difficult in the marrow, as in other tissues, since several types of T-cell lymphoma may have large neoplastic cells which are difficult to distinguish from Reed—Sternberg cells and their variants and a mixed inflammatory response is also common. The most useful histological criterion is the presence in Hodgkin's disease of a hiatus between the neoplastic cells and the reactive small lymphocytes. In contrast, although bizarre giant cells resembling Reed—Sternberg cells can occur in peripheral T-cell lymphomas, they are accompanied by atypical small and intermediate-sized lymphocytes. Cytochemistry and immunocytochemistry may be useful in problem cases. Classical Reed—Sternberg cells and their mononuclear variants are usually positive for CD30 (Ber-H2 monoclonal antibody) and for CD15 (Leu-M1 monoclonal antibody) but negative for leucocyte common antigen. The L and H variant Reed—Sternberg cell (see Table 5.2), however, is CD15-negative and leucocyte common antigen-positive. T cells are positive for leucocyte common antigen and with CD3 antibodies. Megakaryocytes have amylase-sensitive PAS-positivity and can be identified with certainty with a monoclonal antibody directed at platelet glycoprotein III or with the *Ulex europeus* lectin. Staining for cytokeratin is useful in identifying carcinoma cells.

REFERENCES

1 Bennett JM, Catovsky D, Daniel MT, *et al.* (1976) Proposals for the classification of the acute leukaemias. *Br J Haematol*, **33**, 451–458.

2 Bennett JM, Catovsky D, Daniel MT, *et al.* (1989) Proposals for the classification of the chronic (mature) B and T lymphoid leukaemias. *J Clin Pathol*, **42**, 567–584.

3 Lukes RJ, Craver LH, Hall TC, Rappaport H and Ruben P (1966) Report of the nomenclature committee. *Cancer Res*, **26**, 1311.

4 Stansfeld AG, Diebold J, Kapanci Y, et al. (1988) Updated Kiel classification for lymphomas. Lancet, i, 292–293 and 373.

5 Suchi T, Lennert K, Tu L-Y, et al. (1987) Histopathology and immunopathology of peripheral T cell lymphomas; a proposal for their classification. J Clin Pathol, 40, 995–1015.

6 Rappaport H. Tumors of the hematopoietic system. In: Atlas of Tumor Pathology, sect. 3, fasc. 8. Armed Forces Institute of Pathology, Washington DC, 1966.

7 Writing committee of NCI non-Hodgkin's lymphoma classification project (1982) Non-Hodgkin's lymphoma pathologic classification project: National Cancer Institute sponsored study of non-Hodgkin's lymphoma. Summary and description of a working formulation. Cancer, 49, 2112–2135.

8 Rozman C, Hernandez-Nieto L, Montserrat E and Brugues R (1981) Prognostic significance of bone-marrow patterns in chronic lymphocytic leukaemia. Br J Haematol, 47, 529–537.

9 Bartl R, Frisch B, Burkhardt R, Jäger K, Pappenberger R and Hoffman-Fezer G (1984) Lymphoproliferations in the bone marrow: identification and evolution, classification and staging. J Clin Pathol, 37, 233–254.

10 McKenna RW and Hernandez JA (1988) Bone marrow in malignant lymphoma. Hematol Oncol Clin North Am, 2, 617–635.

11 Gaulard P, Kanavaros P, Farcet J-P, et al. (1991) Bone marrow histologic and immunohistochemical findings in peripheral T-cell lymphoma: a study of 38 cases. Hum Pathol, 22, 331–338.

12 Tateyama H, Eimoto T, Tada T, Kamiya M, Fujiyoshi Y and Kajiura S (1991) Congenital angiotropic lymphoma (intravascular lymphomatosis) of the T-cell type. Cancer, 67, 2131–2136.

13 Conlan M, Bast M, Armitage JO and Weisenburger DD (1990) Bone marrow involvement by non-Hodgkin's lymphoma: the clinical significance of morphologic discordance between the lymph node and bone marrow. J Clin Oncol, 8, 1163–72.

14 Thaler J, Dietze O, Denz H, et al. (1991) Bone marrow diagnosis in lymphoproliferative disorders: comparison of results obtained from conventional histomorphology and immunohistology. Histopathology, 18, 495–504.

15 Foucar K, McKenna RW, Frizzera G and Brunning RD (1982) Bone marrow and blood involvement by lymphoma in relationship to the Lukes–Collins classification. Cancer, 49, 888–897.

16 Thiele J, Langohr J, Skorupka M and Fischer R (1990) Reticulin fibre content of bone marrow infiltrates of malignant non-Hodgkin's lymphomas (B-cell type, low malignancy)—a morphometric evaluation before and after therapy. Virchows Archiv (A) 417, 485–492.

17 Bartl R, Hansmann M-L, Frisch B and Burkhardt R (1988) Comparative histology of malignant lymphomas in lymph node and bone marrow. Br J Haematol, 69, 229–237.

18 Fisher DE, Jacobson JO, Ault KA and Harris NL (1989) Diffuse large cell lymphoma with discordant bone marrow histology: clinical features and biological implications. Cancer, 64, 1879–1887.

19 Kluin PM, Van Krieken JH, Kleiverda K and Kluin-Nelemans HC (1990) Discordant morphologic characteristics of B-cell lymphomas in bone marrow and lymph node biopsies. Am J Clin Pathol, 94, 59–66.

20 Hanson CA, Brunning RD, Gajl-Peczalska KJ, Frizzera G and McKenna R (1986) Bone marrow manifestations of peripheral T-cell lymphoma. Am J Clin Pathol, 86, 449–460.

21 Caulet S, Delmer A, Audouin J, et al. (1990) Histopathological study of bone marrow biopsies in 30 cases of T-cell lymphoma with clinical, biological and survival correlations. Hematol Oncol, 8, 156–168.

22 Frizzera G, Anaya JS and Banks PM (1986) Neoplastic plasma cells in follicular lymphomas: clinical and pathologic findings in six cases. Virchows Arch (A), 409, 149–162.

23 Robertson LE, Redman JR, Butler JJ, et al. (1991) Discordant bone marrow involvement in diffuse large-cell lymphoma: a distinct clinical-pathologic entity associated with a continuous risk of relapse. J Clin Oncol, 9, 236–242.

24 First MIC Cooperative Study Group (1986) Morphologic, immunologic and cytogenetic (MIC) working classification of acute lymphoblastic leukemias. Cancer Genet Cytogenet, 23, 189–197.

25 McKenna RW, Parkin J and Brunning RD (1979) Morphologic and ultrastructural characteristics of T-cell acute lymphoblastic leukemia. Cancer, 44, 1290–1297.

26 Hann IM, Evans DIK, Marsden HB, Jones PM and Palmer MK (1978) Bone marrow fibrosis in acute lymphoblastic leukaemia of childhood. J Clin Pathol, 31, 313–315.

27 Breatnach F, Chessells JM and Greaves MF (1981) The aplastic presentation of childhood leukaemia: a feature of common-ALL. Br J Haematol, 49, 387–393.

28 Dharmasena F, Littlewood T, Gordon-Smith EC, Catovsky D and Galton DAG (1986) Adult acute lymphoblastic leukaemia presenting with bone marrow aplasia. Clin Lab Haematol, 8, 361–364.

29 Enno A, Catovsky D, O'Brien M, Cherchi M, Kumaran TO and Galton DAG (1979) 'Prolymphocytoid' transformation of chronic lymphocytic leukaemia. Br J Haematol, 41, 9–18.

30 Rozman C, Monserrat E, Rodríguez-Fernàndez JM, et al. (1984) Bone marrow histologic pattern — the best single prognostic parameter in chronic lymphocytic leukemia: a multivariate survival analysis of 329 cases. Blood, 64, 642–648.

31 Geisler C, Ralfkiær E, Hansen MM, Hou-Jensen K and Larsen SO (1986) The bone marrow histological pattern has independent prognostic value in early stage chronic lymphocytic leukaemia. Br J Haematol, 62, 47–54.

32 Frisch B and Bartl R (1988) Histologic classification and staging of chronic lymphocytic leukemia: a retrospective and prospective study of 503 cases. Acta Haematol (Basel), 79, 140–152.

33 Trump DL, Mann RB, Phelps R, Roberts H and Conley CL (1980) Richter's syndrome: diffuse histiocytic lymphoma in patients with chronic lymphocytic leukemia: a report of 5 cases and review of the literature. Am J Med, 68, 539–548.

34 Foucar K and Rydell RE (1980) Richter's syndrome in chronic lymphocytic leukemia. Cancer, 46, 118–134.

35 Pangalis GA, Nathwani BN and Rappaport H (1977) Malignant lymphoma, well differentiated lymphocytic: its relationship with chronic lymphocytic leukemia and macroglobulinemia of Waldenström. Cancer, 39, 999–1010.

36 Dick F, Bloomfield CE and Brunning RD (1974) Incidence, cytology and histopathology of non-Hodgkin's lymphomas in the bone marrow. Cancer, 33, 1382–1398.

37 Mazza P, Gherlinzoni F, Kemna G, et al. (1987) Clinicopathological study on non-Hodgkin's lymphomas. Haematologica, 72, 351–357.

38 Pangalis GA and Kittas C. Bone marrow involvement in chronic lymphocytic leukemia, small lymphocytic (well differentiated) and lymphoplasmacytic (macroglobulinemia of Waldenström) non-Hodgkin's lymphomas. In: Chronic Lymphocytic Leukemia, Polliack A and Catovsky D (eds). Harwood Academic Publishers, Chur, 1988.

39 Adelstein DJ, Henry MB, Bowman LS and Hines JD (1991) Diffuse well differentiated lymphocytic lymphoma: a clinical study of 22 patients. Oncology, 48, 48–53.

40 Pangalis GA, Roussou PA, Kittas C, et al. (1984) Patterns of bone marrow involvement in chronic lymphocytic leukemia and small lymphocytic (well differentiated) non-Hodgkin's lymphoma. Cancer, 54, 702–708.

41 Hernandez Nieto L, Lampert IA and Catovsky D (1989) Bone marrow histological patterns in B-cell and T-cell prolymphocytic leukemia. Hematol Pathol, 3, 79–84.

42 Vykoupil KF, Thiele J and Georgii A (1976) Hairy cell leukemia: bone marrow findings in 24 patients. Virchows Arch (A), 370, 273–289.

43 Bartl R, Frisch B, Hill W, Burkhardt R, Sommerfeld W and Sund M (1983) Bone marrow histology in hairy cell leukemia: identification of subtypes and their prognostic significance. Am J Clin Pathol, 79, 531–545.

44 Burke JS and Rappaport H (1984) The diagnosis and differential diagnosis of hairy cell leukemia in bone marrow and spleen. Semin Oncol, 11, 334–346.

45 Naeim F (1988) Hairy cell leukemia: characteristics of the neoplastic cells. Hum Pathol, 19, 375–388.

46 Lee WMF and Beckstead JH (1982) Hairy cell leukemia with bone marrow hypoplasia. Cancer, 50, 2207–2210.

47 Flandrin G, Sigaux F, Castaigne S, et al. (1986) Treatment of hairy cell leukemia with recombinant alpha interferon. I. Quantitative study of bone marrow changes during the first months of treatment. Blood, 67, 817–820.

48 Verhoef CEG, De Wolf-Peeters C, Zachee P and Boogaerts MA (1990) Regression of diffuse osteosclerosis in hairy cell leukaemia after treatment with interferon. Br J Haematol, 76, 150–151.

49 Van der Molen LA, Urba WJ, Longo DJ, Lawrence J, Gralnick H and Steis RG (1989) Diffuse osteosclerosis in hairy cell leukemia. Blood, 74, 2066–2069.

50 Golomb HM and Vardiman JW (1983) Response to splenectomy in 65 patients with hairy cell leukemia: an evaluation of spleen weight and bone marrow involvement. Blood, 61, 349–352.

51 Katayama I (1988) Bone marrow in hairy cell leukemia. Hematol Oncol Clin North Am, 2, 585–602.

52 Naeim F and Jacobs AD (1985) Bone marrow changes in patients with hairy cell leukemia treated by recombinant alpha$_2$-interferon. Hum Pathol, 16, 1200–1205.

53 Ratain MJ, Golomb HM, Bardawil RG, et al. (1987) Durability of responses to interferon alpha-2b in advanced hairy cell leukemia. Blood, 69, 872–877.

54 Doane LL, Ratain MJ and Golomb HM (1990) Hairy cell leukemia: current management. Hematol Oncol Clin North Am, 4, 489–502.

55 Catovsky D, Golde DW and Golomb HM (1990) The third international workshop on hairy cell leukemia, Laguna Miguel, California, 19–20 Oct 1989. Br J Haematol, 74, 378–379.

56 Falini B, Pileri SA, Flenghi L, et al. (1990) Selection of a panel of monoclonal antibodies for monitoring residual disease in peripheral blood and bone marrow of interferon-treated hairy cell leukaemia patients. Br J Haematol, 76, 460–468.

57 Sainati L, Matutes E, Mulligan S, et al. (1990) A variant form of hairy cell leukemia resistant to α interferon: clinical and phenotypic characteristics. Blood, 76, 157–162.

58 Melo JV, Hedge U, Parreira A, Thompson I, Lampert

I and Catovsky D (1987) Splenic B lymphoma with circulating villous lymphocytes: differential diagnosis of B cell leukaemia with large spleens. *J Clin Pathol*, **40**, 329–342.

59 Bartl R, Frisch B, Mahl G, *et al.* (1983) Bone marrow histology in Waldenström's macroglobulinaemia: clinical relevance of subtype recognition. *Scand J Haematol*, **31**, 359–375.

60 Brunning RD. Bone Marrow. In: *Ackerman's Surgical Pathology*, Rosai, J (ed). CV Mosby, St Louis, 1989.

61 Stansfeld AG. *Lymph Node Biopsy Interpretation.* Churchill Livingstone, Edinburgh, 1985.

62 Frisch B, Lewis SM, Burkhardt and Bartl R. *Biopsy Pathology of Bone and Bone Marrow.* Chapman and Hall, London, 1985.

63 Raffeld M and Jaffe ES (1991) bcl-1, t(11;14), and mantle-cell derived lymphomas. *Blood*, **78**, 259–263.

64 Hui PK, Feller AC and Lennert K (1988) High-grade non-Hodgkin's lymphoma of B-cell type. I. Histopathology. *Histopathology*, **12**, 127–143.

65 Kim H and Dorfman RF (1974) Morphological studies of 84 untreated patients subjected to laparotomy for the staging of non-Hodgkin's lymphomas. *Cancer*, **33**, 657–674.

66 Vykoupil KF and Georgii A. Non Hodgkins lymphomas in bone marrow: diagnosis according to the Kiel classification and their growth patterns and relations to survival. In: *Pathology of the Bone Marrow*, Lennert K and Hübner K (eds). Gustav Fischer Verlag, Stuttgart, 1984.

67 Osborne BM and Butler JJ (1989) Hypocellular paratrabecular foci of treated small cleaved cell lymphoma in bone marrow biopsies. *Am J Surg Pathol*, **13**, 382–388.

68 Jaffe ES, Bookman MA and Longo DL (1987) Lymphocytic lymphoma of intermediate differentiation – mantle zone lymphoma: a distinct subtype of B-cell lymphoma. *Hum Pathol*, **18**, 877–880.

69 Perry DA, Bast MA, Armitage JO and Weisenburger DD (1990) Diffuse intermediate lymphocytic lymphoma: a clinicopathological study and comparison with small lymphocytic lymphoma and diffuse small cleaved cell lymphoma. *Cancer*, **66**, 1995–2000.

70 Pombo de Oliveira MS, Jaffe ES and Catovsky D (1989) Leukaemic phase of mantle zone (intermediate) lymphoma: its characterisation in 11 cases. *J Clin Pathol*, **42**, 962–972.

71 Swerdlow SH, Habeshaw JA, Murray LJ, Dhaliwal HS, Lister TA and Stansfeld AG (1983) Centrocytic lymphoma: a distinct clinicopathologic and immunologic entity. A multiparameter study of 18 cases at diagnosis and relapse. *Am J Pathol*, **113**, 181–197.

72 Weisenberger DD, Kim H and Rappaport H (1982) Mantle-zone lymphoma: a follicular variant of intermediate lymphocytic lymphoma. *Cancer*, **49**, 1429–1438.

73 Griesser H, Kaiser U, Augener W, Tiemann M and Lennert K (1990) B-cell lymphoma of the mucosa-associated lymphatic tissue (MALT) presenting with bone marrow and peripheral blood involvement. *Leuk Res*, **14**, 617–622.

74 Carbone A, Gloghini A, Pinto A, Attadia V, Zagonel V and Volpe R (1989) Monocytoid B-cell lymphoma with bone marrow and peripheral blood involvement at presentation. *Am J Clin Pathol*, **92**, 228–236.

75 Traweek ST and Sheibani K (1990) Regarding the article entitled 'Monocytoid B-cell lymphoma with bone marrow and peripheral blood involvement at presentation'. *Am J Clin Pathol*, **94**, 117.

76 Bain BJ, Matutes E, Robinson D, *et al.* (1991) Leukaemia as a manifestation of large cell lymphoma. *Br J Haematol*, **77**, 301–310.

77 Wright DH and Pike PA (1968) Bone marrow involvement of Burkitt's tumour. *Br J Haematol*, **15**, 409–416.

78 Bluming AZ, Ziegler JL and Carbone PP (1972) Bone marrow involvement in Burkitt's lymphoma – results of a prospective study. *Br J Haematol*, **22**, 369–376.

79 Arseneau JC, Canellos GP, Banks PM, Berard CW, Gralnick HR and De Vita VT (1975) American Burkitt's lymphoma: a clinicopathologic study of 30 cases. I Clinical factors relating to prolonged survival. *Am J Med*, **58**, 314–321.

80 Banks PM, Arseneau JC, Gralnick HR, Canellos GP, De Vita VT and Berard CW (1975) American Burkitt's lymphoma: a clinicopathologic study of 30 cases. II Pathologic correlations. *Am J Med*, **58**, 322–329.

81 Levine AM, Pavlock Z, Pockros AW, *et al.* (1983) Small non cleaved follicular center cell (FCC) lymphoma: Burkitt and non-Burkitt variants in the United States. I Clinical features. *Cancer*, **52**, 1073–1079.

82 Brunning RD, McKenna RW, Bloomfield CD, Coccia P and Gajl-Peczalska KJ (1977) Bone marrow involvement in Burkitt's lymphoma. *Cancer*, **40**, 1771–1779.

83 Picozzi VJ and Coleman CN (1990) Lymphoblastic lymphoma. *Semin Oncol*, **17**, 96–103.

84 Bennett J, Juliusson G and Mecucci C (1990) A conference on the morphologic, immunologic and cytogenetic classification of the chronic (mature) B and T lymphoid leukaemias (MIC IV). *Br J Haematol*, **74**, 240.

85 Nakamura S and Suchi T (1991) A clinicopathologic study of node-based, low-grade, peripheral T-cell lymphoma: angioimmunoblastic lymphoma, T-zone lymphoma, and lymphoepithelioid lymph-

oma. *Cancer*, **67**, 2565–2578.

86 Matutes E, Garcia Talavera J, O'Brien M and Catovsky D (1986) The morphological spectrum of T-prolymphocytic leukaemia. *Br J Haematol*, **41**, 111–124.

87 Reynolds CW and Foon KA (1984) T-γ-lymphoproliferative disease and related disorders in humans and experimental animals: a review of the clinical, cellular and functional characteristics. *Blood*, **64**, 1146–1158.

88 Loughran TP Jr, Kadin ME, Starkebaum G, *et al.* (1985) Leukemia of large granular lymphocytes: association with clonal chromosomal abnormalities and autoimmune neutropenia, thrombocytopenia, and hemolytic anemia. *Ann Intern Med*, **102**, 169–175.

89 Matutes E and Catovsky D (1991) Mature T-cell leukemias and leukemia/lymphoma syndromes: review of our experience of 175 cases. *Leukemia and Lymphoma*, **4**, 81–91.

90 Brouet J, Sasportes M, Flandrin G, *et al.* (1975) Chronic lymphocytic leukaemia of T-cell origin. Immunological and clinical evaluation in eleven patients. *Lancet*, **ii**, 890–893.

91 Palutke M, Eisenberg L, Kaplan J, *et al.* (1983) Natural killer and suppressor T-cell chronic lymphocytic leukemia. *Blood*, **62**, 627–634.

92 Agnarsson BA, Loughran TP, Starkebaum G and Kadin ME (1989) The pathology of large granular lymphocyte leukemia. *Hum Pathol*, **20**, 643–651.

93 Schechter GP, Sausville EA, Fischmann, *et al.* (1987) Evaluation of circulating malignant cells provides prognostic information in cutaneous T cell lymphoma. *Blood*, **69**, 841–849.

94 Sausville EA, Eddy JL, Makuch RW, *et al.* (1988) Histopathologic staging at initial diagnosis of mycosis fungoides and the Sézary syndrome. *Ann Intern Med*, **109**, 372–382.

95 Rappaport H and Thomas LB (1974) Mycosis fungoides: the pathology of extracutaneous involvement. *Cancer*, **34**, 1198–1229.

96 Carbone A, Tirelli U, Volpe R, Sulfaro S and Manconi R (1986) Assessment of bone marrow histology in patients with cutaneous T-cell lymphoma (CTCL) at presentation and during follow up. *Br J Haematol*, **62**, 789–790.

97 Patsouris E, Noël H and Lennert K (1988) Histological and immunohistological findings in lymphoepithelioid cell lymphoma (Lennert's lymphoma). *Am J Surg Pathol*, **12**, 341–350.

98 Patsouris E, Noël H and Lennert K (1989) Angioimmunoblastic lymphadenopathy-type of T-cell lymphoma with a high content of epithelioid cells: histopathology and comparison with lymphoepithelioid cell lymphoma. *Am J Surg Pathol*, **13**, 260–275.

99 Auger MJ, Nash JRG and Mackie MJ (1986) Marrow involvement with T cell lymphoma initially presenting with abnormal myelopoiesis. *J Clin Pathol*, **39**, 134–137.

100 Knecht H (1989) Angioimmunoblastic lymphadenopathy: ten years' experience and state of current knowledge. *Semin Hematol*, **26**, 209–215.

101 Schnaidt U, Vykoupil KF, Thiele J and Georgii A (1980) Angioimmunoblastic lymphadenopathy: histopathology of bone marrow involvement. *Virchows Arch (A)*, **389**, 369–380.

102 Uchiyama T, Yodoi J, Sagawa K, Takatsuki K and Uchino H (1977) Adult T-cell leukemia: clinical and hematological features of 16 cases. *Blood*, **50**, 481–492.

103 Jaffe E, Cossman J, Blattner WA, *et al.* (1984) The pathologic spectrum of adult T-cell leukemia/lymphoma in the United States. *Am J Surg Pathol*, **8**, 263–275.

104 Shih L-Y, Kuo T-T, Dunn P and Liaw S-J (1991) Human T-cell lymphotrophic virus type I associated adult T-cell leukaemia/lymphoma in Taiwan Chinese. *Br J Haematol*, **79**, 156–161.

105 Swerdlow SH, Habeshaw JA, Rohatiner AZS, Lister TA and Stansfeld AG (1984) Caribbean T-cell lymphoma/leukemia. *Cancer*, **54**, 687–696.

106 Agnarsson BA and Kadin ME (1988) Ki-1 positive large cell lymphoma: a morphologic and immunologic study of 19 cases. *Am J Surg Pathol*, **12**, 264–274.

107 Wong KF, Chan JKC, Ng CS, Chu YC, Lam PWY and Yuen HL (1991) Anaplastic large cell Ki-1 lymphoma involving bone marrow: marrow findings and association with reactive hemophagocytosis. *Am J Hematol*, **37**, 112–119.

108 Chott A, Kaserer K, Augustin I, *et al.* (1990) Ki-1-positive large cell lymphoma: a clinicopathological study of 41 cases. *Am J Surg Pathol*, **14**, 438–448.

109 Weiss LM, Bindl JM, Picozzi VJ, Link MP and Warnke RA (1986) Lymphoblastic lymphoma: an immunophenotypic study of 26 cases with comparison of T cell acute lymphoblastic leukemia. *Blood*, **67**, 474–478.

110 Lukes RJ (1971) Criteria for involvement of lymph node, bone marrow, spleen, and liver in Hodgkin's disease. *Cancer Res*, **31**, 1755–1767.

111 Neiman RS, Rosen PJ, Lukes RJ (1973) Lymphocyte-depletion Hodgkin's disease: a clinicopathological entity. *New Engl J Med*, **288**, 751–755.

112 Bartl R, Frisch B, Burkhardt R, Huhn D and Pappenberger R (1982) Assessment of bone marrow histology in Hodgkin's disease: correlation with clinical factors. *Br J Haematol*, **51**, 345–360.

113 Ellis ME, Diehl LF, Granger E and Elson E (1989) Trephine needle biopsy in the initial staging of Hodgkin disease: sensitivity and specificity of the

Ann Arbor staging procedure criteria. *Am J Hematol*, **30**, 115–120.

114 MacIntyre EA, Vaughan Hudson B, Linch DC, Vaughan Hudson G and Jelliffe AM (1987) The value of staging bone marrow trephine biopsy in Hodgkin's disease. *Eur J Haematol*, **39**, 66–70.

115 Rosenberg SA (1971) Hodgkin's disease of the bone marrow. *Cancer Res*, **31**, 1733–1736.

116 Rappaport H, Berard CW, Butler JJ, Dorfman RF, Lukes RJ and Thomas LB (1971) Report on the committee on histopathological criteria contributing to staging in Hodgkin's disease. *Cancer Res*, **31**, 1864–1865.

117 Banks PM (1990) The pathology of Hodgkin's disease. *Semin Oncol*, **17**, 683–695.

118 O'Carroll DI, McKenna RW and Brunning RD (1976) Bone marrow manifestations of Hodgkin's disease. *Cancer*, **38**, 1717–1728.

119 Myers CE, Chabner BA, deVita VT and Gralnick HR (1974) Bone marrow involvement in Hodgkin's disease: pathology and response to MOPP chemotherapy. *Blood*, **44**, 197–204.

120 Kinney MC, Greer JP, Stein RS, Collins RD and Cousar JB (1986) Lymphocyte-depletion Hodgkin's disease: histopathologic diagnosis of marrow involvement. *Am J Surg Pathol*, **10**, 219–226.

121 Meadows LM, Rosse WR, Moore JO, Crawford J, Laszlo J and Kaufman RE (1989) Hodgkin's disease presenting as myelofibrosis. *Cancer*, **64**, 1720–1726.

6: Multiple Myeloma and Other Plasma Cell Dyscrasias

Multiple myeloma or myelomatosis is a disease resulting from the proliferation in the bone marrow of a clone of neoplastic cells which are closely related, both morphologically and functionally, to plasma cells. In the great majority of cases the neoplastic cells secrete a protein which is either a complete immunoglobulin or an immunoglobulin light chain. Clinical features result either fairly directly from the effects of the neoplastic proliferation or indirectly from effects of the protein, often designated a paraprotein, which the myeloma cells produce. The nature of this disease, in which cells of the abnormal clone are widely, randomly and diffusely distributed in the red marrow, is better reflected by the term 'myelomatosis' than by the more commonly used 'multiple myeloma'. It might be preferable if the latter term was restricted to those rare cases, more closely related to solitary myeloma, in which there are several isolated lesions but intervening bone marrow is normal. However, use of the term 'multiple myeloma' for the disease we are describing is so commonly used that we will retain it.

Multiple myeloma is a disease predominantly of the middle-aged and elderly. It has an incidence of $2-4/100\,000/$year. The disease is commoner in Blacks than in Caucasians and somewhat commoner in men than in women. Common clinical features are anaemia, bone pain, pathological fractures, hypercalcaemia and renal failure. A minority of patients have hepatomegaly or lymphadenopathy. Splenomegaly is occasionally present. Patients with symptomatic bone lesions usually have either generalized osteoporosis or discrete osteolytic lesions, but occasional patients have osteosclerosis. The paraprotein secreted is IgG in about 60 per cent of cases and IgA in about 20 per cent; some patients secrete excess monoclonal light chain (Bence Jones protein) in addition to immunoglobulin and in about 15–20 per cent of patients only light chain is produced (Bence Jones myeloma). A minority of patients produce an IgM, IgD or IgE paraprotein. Any paraprotein secreted will, since it arises from a single clone of cells, contain only a single light chain type, either $\varkappa$ or λ. Monoclonal immunoglobulins, being of high molecular weight, are usually detected only or mainly in the serum whereas, unless there is coexisting renal failure, the low molecular weight Bence Jones protein is detected only in the urine.

Myeloma cells give negative reactions for most pan-B markers but usually express several markers (detectable with monoclonal antibodies) which are also expressed by normal plasma cells such as PC-1, PCA-1, BU11 and CD38. SmIg is absent but monoclonal immunoglobulin, of the same type as is secreted, is present in the cytoplasm.

Multiple myeloma has a median survival of three to four years. It usually terminates in refractory disease, sometimes with a leukaemic phase. In some cases there is transformation to immunoblastic lymphoma. A significant minority of patients (about 10 per cent of those who survive five to 10 years after treatment) succumb to a secondary myelodysplastic syndrome or to acute myeloid leukaemia which are likely to be consequent on the prior administration of alkylating agents.

Peripheral blood

The great majority of patients have anaemia which is either normocytic, normochromic or, less often, macrocytic. In most patients there is increased rouleaux formation and increased background basophilic staining due to the presence in the blood of the paraprotein, but these features do not occur in the minority of patients whose cells secrete only Bence Jones protein. The blood film is occasionally leuco-erythroblastic and it is often possible to find a small number of plasma cells or plasmacytoid lymphocytes. In patients with more advanced disease there may be thrombocytopenia and neutropenia.

Bone marrow cytology

The bone marrow features are very variable.

Plasma cells are usually increased, often constituting between 30 and 90 per cent of bone marrow nucleated cells. The myeloma cells may be morphologically fairly normal showing the eccentric nucleus, clumped chromatin and Golgi zone typical of a normal plasma cell, or may be moderately or severely dysplastic. A common cytological abnormality is nucleo-cytoplasmic asynchrony; the cytoplasm is mature but the nucleus either has a diffuse chromatin pattern or contains a prominent nucleolus (Figs 6.1 and 6.2). Other cytological abnormalities include marked pleomorphism, voluminous cytoplasm which may be entirely eosinophilic or have 'flaming'

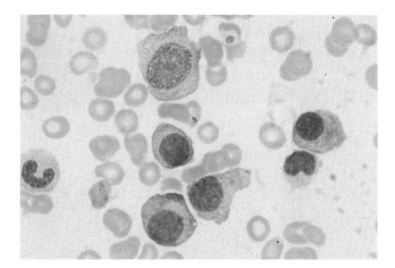

Fig. 6.1 BM aspirate, multiple myeloma, showing a range of cells from a plasmablast to mature plasma cells. MGG × 940.

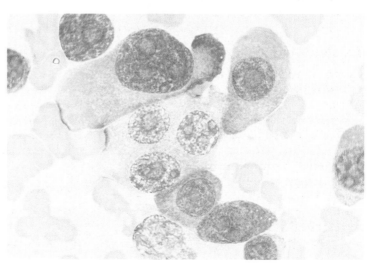

Fig. 6.2 BM aspirate, multiple myeloma, showing plasmablasts, one of which is tri-nucleated. MGG × 940.

eosinophilic margins (Fig. 6.3), increased size of cells, a high nucleo-cytoplasmic ratio, multi-nuclearity (Fig. 6.3), nuclear lobulation (Fig. 6.4), phagocytosis by myeloma cells (Fig. 6.4), uniform cytoplasmic basophilia without a distinct Golgi zone and the presence of mitotic figures. Cytoplasmic and nuclear inclusions may be present (Figs 6.5 and 6.6).

It is not always possible to make a diagnosis of multiple myeloma on bone marrow morphology alone. Multiple myeloma characteristically affects the bone marrow in a patchy manner and an aspirate from a patient with multiple myeloma will not necessarily contain a large number of plasma cells; nor will the morphology of the myeloma cells necessarily be very abnormal. Non-diagnostic aspirates are obtained in about five per cent of patients. There is no particular percentage of plasma cells which reliably separates multiple myeloma from reactive plasmacytosis or from benign monoclonal gammopathy (see below). It is necessary, in doubtful cases, to assess not only the bone marrow cytology and histology but also the clinical, radiological and biochemical features.

The bone marrow aspirate is of value not only

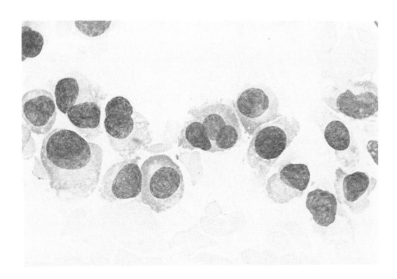

Fig. 6.3 BM aspirate, multiple myeloma, showing bi- and tri-nucleated myeloma cells and myeloma cells with flaming cytoplasm. MGG × 940.

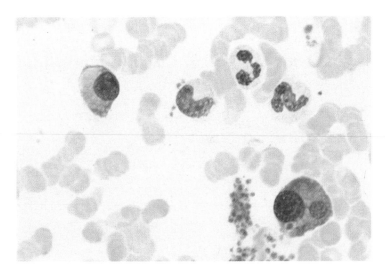

Fig. 6.4 BM aspirate, multiple myeloma, showing one myeloma cell with a bi-lobed nucleus and another which has ingested an erythrocyte. MGG × 940.

in the diagnosis of multiple myeloma but also in determining the prognosis. Both the percentage of plasma cells in the aspirate[1,2] and their degree of dysplasia[2-4] correlate with prognosis.

Bone marrow histology

A bone marrow biopsy can be of use both in the diagnosis of multiple myeloma and in assessing the prognosis. Non-diagnostic biopsies are obtained in five to 10 per cent of cases, either because of early disease or because the pattern of infiltration is nodular rather than diffuse and the biopsy has included only non-infiltrated marrow.[5] Because a larger volume of tissue is sampled than in an aspirate and because the pattern of infiltration can be ascertained, a biopsy may confirm a diagnosis of multiple myeloma when the aspirate has not done so; however, on occasions, more diagnostic information is obtained from the aspirate than from the trephine biopsy so the two investigations should be regarded as complementary. Three major patterns of infiltration are seen: (i) interstitial, with or without paratrabecular seams of plasma cells (ii) nodular, and (iii) a packed marrow.[5] When infiltration is interstitial,

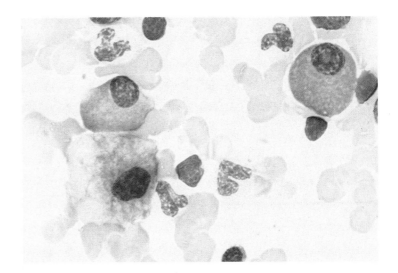

Fig. 6.5 BM aspirate, multiple myeloma, showing three myeloma cells, one of which has its cytoplasm distended by secretory products. MGG × 940.

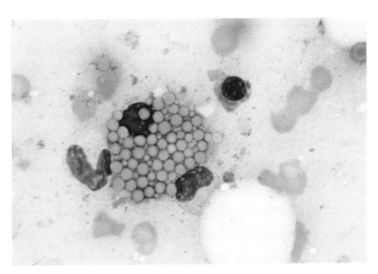

Fig. 6.6 BM aspirate, multiple myeloma, showing a Mott cell. MGG × 970.

myeloma cells are dispersed among haemopoietic and fat cells (Fig. 6.7) whereas in a 'packed marrow' (Fig. 6.8) the normal architecture of the marrow is obliterated. In reactive plasmacytosis infiltration is interstitial and large accumulations of plasma cells are not seen. Some histopathologists have considered that plasma cells sited around capillaries are indicative of reactive plasmacytosis rather than multiple myeloma[5] but others have observed this feature also in multiple myeloma.[6] Myeloma cells show varying degrees of dysplasia. In some cases myeloma cells are morphologically very similar to normal plasma cells while in others they have nucleoli or are pleomorphic (Fig. 6.9) or frankly blastic with a diffuse chromatin pattern and a prominent nucleolus (Fig. 6.10).

Bone changes associated with multiple myeloma are either diffuse osteoporosis with thinning of all trabeculae, or osteolytic lesions with resorption of bone by osteoclasts. Diffuse osteoporosis has been found to be associated with a packed marrow pattern of infiltration while osteolytic lesions are found particularly in those

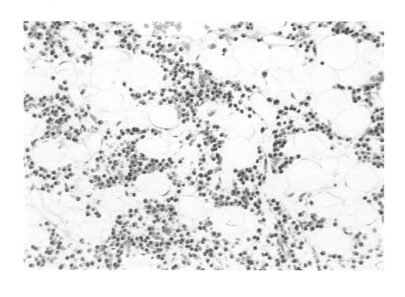

Fig. 6.7 BM trephine biopsy, multiple myeloma, showing focal and interstitial infiltration of the marrow by plasma cells. Paraffin-embedded, H&E × 195.

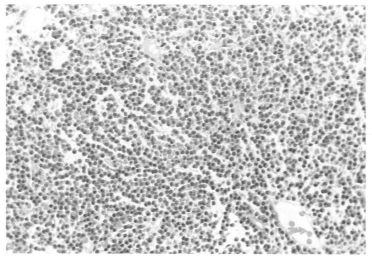

Fig. 6.8 BM trephine biopsy, multiple myeloma, showing diffuse infiltration by plasma cells (packed marrow). Paraffin-embedded. H&E × 195.

with nodular infiltration.[5] Non-specific changes which may be associated with multiple myeloma include reduced haemopoiesis, even in the absence of heavy infiltration, increased reticulin deposition, a lymphoid infiltrate and, occasionally, the presence of granulomas (see Fig. 2.15).

The prognosis in myeloma can be related to: (i) the extent of plasma cell infiltration (the histological stage) (ii) the pattern of infiltration, and (iii) the cytological features of the cells (the histological grade).[5] Bartl et al.[5] found that a nodular pattern of infiltration correlated with more aggressive disease and with a worse prognosis than was seen when the pattern of infiltration was interstitial with or without paratrabecular seams of plasma cells; a packed marrow pattern indicated a worse prognosis than either of the other patterns. They and a number of other investigators have been able to relate prognosis also to the degree of dysplasia of the myeloma cells.[7,8] They have suggested a classification that divides myeloma into three groups: (i) low grade, in which the plasma cells are mature with minimal dysplasia (ii) intermediate grade, in which the plasma

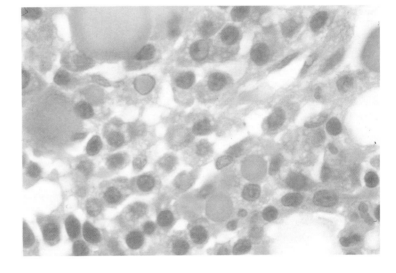

Fig. 6.9 BM trephine biopsy, multiple myeloma, showing plasma cells with moderate nuclear pleomorphism and numerous eosinophilic intranuclear (Dutcher) and intracytoplasmic (Russell) inclusion bodies. Paraffin-embedded, H&E × 970.

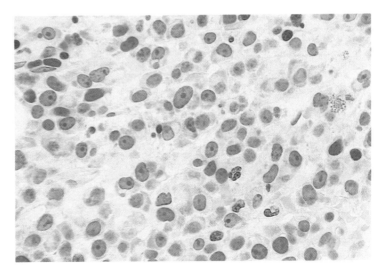

Fig. 6.10 BM trephine biopsy, multiple myeloma (plasmablastic), showing plasmablasts with marked variation in nuclear size and shape and prominent central nucleoli. Plastic-embedded, H&E × 940.

cells are dysplastic but not frankly blastic, and (iii) high grade, comprising plasmablasts. The three grades have median survivals of 60, 32 and 10 months respectively.[4,5]

Plasmablastic myeloma may be morphologically indistinguishable from marrow infiltration by immunoblastic lymphoma. Immunohistochemical staining is helpful in making the distinction; immunoblasts show surface staining for CD45 and B-cell antigens such as L26 (CD20), whereas plasmablasts do not express these antigens.[4,7]

PLASMA CELL LEUKAEMIA

The term plasma cell leukaemia may be used to designate a *de novo* leukaemia of neoplastic plasma cells or the terminal phase of multiple myeloma when myeloma cells are present in the peripheral blood in large numbers. Plasma cell leukaemia has been defined by the presence in the circulating blood of at least $2 \times 10^9/l$ plasma cells which also constitute at least 20 per cent of circulating cells.[9] Patients with *de novo* or primary plasma cell leukaemia show clinical features which are common in multiple myeloma such as bone pain, lytic lesions, hypercalcaemia and renal failure but they have a higher incidence of extramedullary lesions and in addition often have hepatomegaly and splenomegaly. The disease is more aggressive than multiple myeloma with a median survival of less than a year. Patients with established multiple myeloma who develop a secondary plasma cell leukaemia have advanced disease which is usually refractory to treatment. Their prognosis is likewise poor.

Peripheral blood

The blood film shows large numbers of circulating neoplastic plasma cells, the morphology of which varies between cases from cells resembling normal plasma cells to primitive, blastic cells showing only minimal evidence of plasma cell differentiation. Anaemia is almost invariable and neutropenia and thrombocytopenia are common. Increased rouleaux formation and increased background staining are usual; in patients with plasma cell leukaemia as the terminal phase of multiple myeloma these abnormalities are often striking since the paraprotein level is commonly high.

Bone marrow cytology

The bone marrow is heavily infiltrated with neoplastic cells showing the same morphological features as those in the peripheral blood. Normal haemopoietic elements are reduced.

Bone marrow histology

There is a diffuse infiltrate of plasma cells which make up the majority of cells in the marrow.[10,11] In the majority of cases the cytological features are similar to those of multiple myeloma; in a minority of cases the cells are very immature with little morphological evidence of plasma cell differentiation.

BENIGN MONOCLONAL GAMMOPATHY – MONOCLONAL GAMMOPATHY OF UNDETERMINED SIGNIFICANCE (MGUS)

Benign monoclonal gammopathy or monoclonal gammopathy of undetermined significance (MGUS) denotes a condition in which there is proliferation of a clone of plasma cells with production of a paraprotein but without the signs of disease which are characteristic of multiple myeloma and related plasma cell dyscrasias. The paraprotein is usually an immunoglobulin (either IgG, IgA or IgM) but is occasionally a Bence Jones protein. The paraprotein concentration is relatively low (in the case of an IgG paraprotein less than 30 g/l, in the case of an IgA or IgM paraprotein less than 20 g/l) and is usually stable. Since there are no features of disease the diagnosis is necessarily made incidentally. Benign monoclonal gammopathy is common. Paraproteins can be detected in about one per cent of adults under the under the age of 70 and in about three per cent of adults over this age. It is not always possible to make a distinction between multiple myeloma and benign monoclonal gammopathy on the basis of any single feature. It is necessary to assess clinical and haematological features, bone marrow cytology and bone marrow histology in order to make the distinction. A period of observation may also be necessary to establish that the concentration of the paraprotein is stable and no disease features are appearing. It should be noted that although this condition is clinically benign it does represent, in some if not all patients, a neoplastic proliferation; if patients are followed for a prolonged period a significant proportion eventually develop overt evidence of multiple myeloma or a related condition. Over a 20-year period of observation the actuarial risk of developing multiple myeloma, Waldenström's macroglobulinaemia or primary (AL) amyloidosis is approximately 30 per cent.[12]

Peripheral blood

The peripheral blood film may show some increase in rouleaux formation but anaemia does not occur and circulating plasma cells are not present.

Bone marrow cytology

The bone marrow may appear completely normal or there may be an increase of plasma cells; plasma cells do not usually exceed five per cent of nucleated cells but may be up to 10 per cent. The plasma cells are usually morphologically fairly normal but some minor dysplastic features may be noted.

Bone marrow histology

Plasma cell infiltration is usually minimal with focal accumulation around capillaries which is often indistinguishable from a reactive plasmacytosis.[5] Immunohistochemical staining with anti-$\varkappa$ and anti-λ antisera shows $\varkappa:\lambda$ ratios of greater than four in approximately 65 per cent of cases, the majority having ratios between four and 16. In comparison almost all cases of overt myeloma have $\varkappa:\lambda$ ratios of greater than 16, the majority being greater than 100.[13]

WALDENSTRÖM'S MACROGLOBULINAEMIA

The condition described by Waldenström as 'essential hyperglobulinaemia' is a disease characterized by a lymphoplasmacytic dyscrasia with secretion of large amounts of an IgM paraprotein. It is a variant of immunocytoma (see page 145) and is distinguished from other cases of immunocytoma on clinical and biochemical features rather than on cytological or histological criteria. Predominant signs and symptoms are either those characteristic of a lymphoma or are caused by the hyperviscosity of blood consequent on the high concentration of IgM. Hepatomegaly, splenomegaly and lymphadenopathy are common. Clinical features consequent on the high concentration of the paraprotein include anaemia (due to a greatly increased plasma volume), impaired vision, cerebral effects, cardiac failure and a bleeding tendency. In some patients the paraprotein has characteristics of a cold agglutinin or a cryoglobulin and in others it is amyloidogenic. Peripheral neuropathy is common and the paraprotein can sometimes be shown to have antibody activity against neural antigens. The incidence of Waldenström's macroglobulinaemia is about a tenth that of multiple myeloma.

Peripheral blood

There is usually a normocytic normochromic anaemia, increased rouleaux formation and increased background staining. Some patients have thrombocytopenia. When the paraprotein has the characteristics of a cold agglutinin or of a cryoglobulin either red cell agglutinates or a cryoglobulin precipitate may be detected in the blood film. The lymphocyte count may be normal or elevated with the lymphocytes usually being mature small lymphocytes showing some features of differentiation to plasma cells.

Bone marrow cytology

The bone marrow is infiltrated by neoplastic cells which most often have the morphology of small lymphocytes with a variable proportion of cells showing some plasmacytoid features (Figs 6.11 and 6.12). Plasma cells are usually increased. In some patients plasmacytic differentiation is prominent. Intranuclear or intracytoplasmic inclusions which are usually PAS-positive are sometimes present. Macrophages and mast cells (Fig. 6.11) are commonly increased. Lympho-

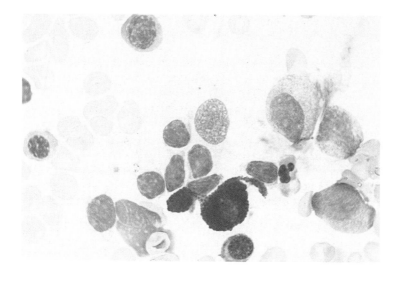

Fig. 6.11 BM aspirate, Waldenström's macroglobulinaemia, showing a mast cell and mature small lymphocytes. MGG × 940.

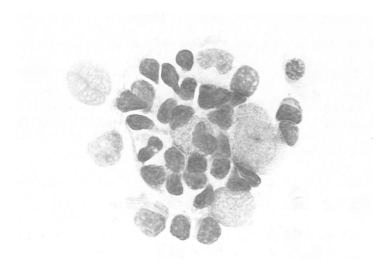

Fig. 6.12 BM aspirate, Waldenström's macroglobulinaemia (same case as Fig. 6.11), showing mature small lymphocytes and one plasmacytoid lymphocyte clustered around a macrophage (reticulum cell). MGG × 940.

plasmacytoid cells may be clustered around macrophages.

Bone marrow histology

The bone marrow histology is not uniform.[14–16] Histological features may be those of a lympho-plasmacytoid or lymphoplasmacytic lymphoma (see page 145). Some patients have an interstitial infiltrate or well-circumscribed nodules of lymph-oid cells, but the majority have either a diffuse infiltration or a mixed nodular-diffuse pattern. A variable proportion of cells show plasmacytoid differentiation or intracytoplasmic or intra-nuclear inclusions (Fig. 6.13). Mature plasma cells are usually increased as are macrophages, mast cells and sometimes eosinophils. Mast cells may be specifically associated with lymphoid infilt-rates. About half of the cases show increased reticulin deposition. The trephine biopsy some-times shows infiltration when the bone marrow aspirate is normal.

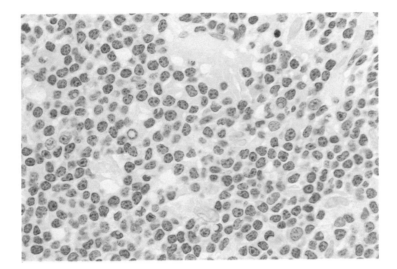

Fig. 6.13 BM trephine biopsy, Waldenström's macroglobulinaemia, showing a diffuse infiltrate of small lymphoid cells, some of which show evidence of plasmacytoid differentiation (Dutcher bodies, 'clock-face' chromatin pattern and/or a Golgi zone). Plastic-embedded, H&E × 377.

Other syndromes associated with secretion of a paraprotein

There are a number of relatively uncommon syndromes associated with the secretion of a paraprotein. In some of these the features of a lymphoproliferative disorder are prominent; in others the clinical and pathological features relate to the characteristics of the paraprotein and only detailed investigation reveals the presence of an abnormal clone of plasma cells, plasmacytoid lymphocytes or lymphocytes.

LIGHT-CHAIN ASSOCIATED (AL) AMYLOIDOSIS

Light-chain associated amyloidosis (AL-type of amyloidosis) is a disease consequent on a plasma cell dyscrasia in which there is production of an amyloidogenic light chain. The features of the disease are usually consequent on the amyloidosis rather than on other features of the plasma cell dyscrasia. Heart failure and renal failure are common manifestations. In a minority of patients light-chain associated amyloidosis is associated with overt multiple myeloma, or with Waldenström's macroglobulinaemia or other immunocytoma (see page 145), but in the majority of patients the plasma cell dyscrasia would be classified as a benign monoclonal gammopathy if

it were not for the amyloidogenic characteristics of the light chains. In a small minority of patients no paraprotein is detectable in serum or urine but in this group also the disease results from a plasma cell dyscrasia, albeit occult. The term primary amyloidosis may be used to describe cases without evidence of multiple myeloma or other overt plasma cell dyscrasia. Amyloid can be formed from either $\varkappa$ or λ light chains, but the majority of cases are λ.

Peripheral blood

The peripheral blood may be normal or may show the features usually associated with multiple myeloma or immunocytoma. Occasionally the features of hyposplenism are present indicating that the spleen is infiltrated by amyloid and has become non-functional.

Bone marrow cytology

The bone marrow aspirate varies from normal through increased plasma cells of normal morphology to overt multiple myeloma or immunocytoma. When the bone marrow aspirate is apparently normal, $\varkappa : \lambda$ imbalance may indicate the presence of an abnormal clone of cells even though the total number of plasma cells is not increased. Very rarely a bone marrow aspirate from a patient with amyloidosis contains either neutrophils which have ingested amyloid[17] or extracellular amyloid deposits.

Bone marrow histology

The bone marrow biopsy may be normal or show increased plasma cells (Fig. 6.14). Sometimes characteristic features of multiple myeloma or immunocytoma are present. In addition, amyloid may be detected either in the walls of small blood vessels (Figs 6.15 to 6.17) or extravascularly. In sections stained with H&E, amyloid is homogeneous and pink (Fig. 6.15). It stains with Congo Red (Fig. 6.16) and following Congo Red staining shows apple-green birefrin-gence on examination with polarized light (Fig. 6.17). It stains metachromatically with crystal violet and methyl violet and fluoresces after staining with thioflavine-T.[18] Light chain associated (AL) amyloid can be distinguished from amyloid of AA type by the abolition of Congo Red staining by prior treatment with potassium permanganate in the latter type.[18] In the majority of cases of light-chain associated amyloid a positive identification can be made with type specific anti-light-chain sera.

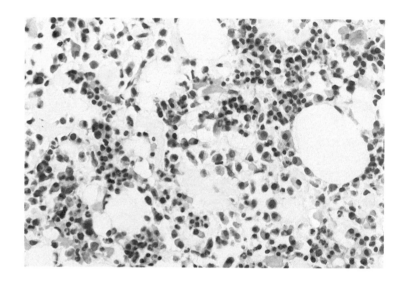

Fig. 6.14 BM trephine biopsy, light-chain associated amyloidosis (AL-type), showing deposition of amorphous eosinophilic material between haemopoietic and fat cells. Note the marked increase in plasma cells in this case. Plastic-embedded, H&E × 377.

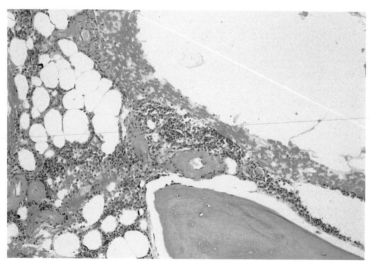

Fig. 6.15 BM trephine biopsy, showing amyloid in the walls of small blood vessels. Paraffin-embedded, H&E × 97.

LIGHT-CHAIN DEPOSITION DISEASE[18-21]

Light-chain deposition disease describes a syndrome of organ damage consequent on the systemic deposition of free light chains. There is an associated plasma cell dyscrasia which may be occult or overt. About 70 per cent of cases have clinical features of a plasma cell dyscrasia, most often multiple myeloma but occasionally solitary plasmacytoma, immunocytoma or other non-Hodgkin's lymphoma. The remaining patients either have features which would usually be interpreted as MGUS (about 15 per cent of cases) or have no serum or urinary paraprotein detectable (also about 15 per cent of cases);[18] those without a detectable paraprotein nevertheless have an occult plasma cell dyscrasia with a clone of cells producing a light chain with a propensity to deposit in and damage tissues. Cases with ϰ light chains are over-represented in relation to cases with λ light chains. In occasional patients a similar syndrome is associated with the systemic deposition of heavy chains in addition to light chains; the term 'monoclonal immunoglobulin deposition disease' has been suggested to include these cases.[21] The predominant organ damage is

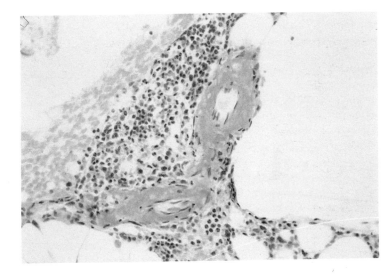

Fig. 6.16 BM trephine biopsy, showing amyloid in the walls of small blood vessels (same case as Fig. 6.15). Paraffin-embedded, Congo Red stain × 390.

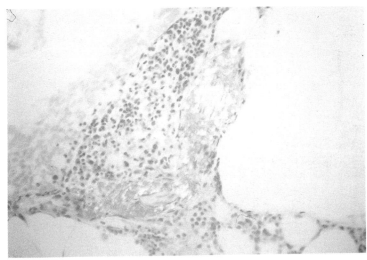

Fig. 6.17 BM trephine biopsy, viewed under polarized light, showing (apple-green) birefringence of the amyloid in the walls of small blood vessels (same case as Fig. 6.15). Paraffin-embedded, Congo Red stain × 390.

renal, with glomerular and tubular deposition causing the nephrotic syndrome, renal failure or both. Occasional patients have presented with the clinical features of hepatic, cardiac or adrenal involvement.

Peripheral blood and bone marrow

There are no specific peripheral blood findings other than those usually associated with renal failure or with multiple myeloma or other plasma cell dyscrasia.

The bone marrow may be apparently normal or show the features of MGUS or of multiple myeloma or a related condition. Some patients who initially have no evidence of multiple myeloma subsequently develop typical features of this disease. In those cases in which the bone marrow is apparently normal it may be possible to demonstrate a monoclonal population of plasma cells. Rarely, light chains are deposited in the bone marrow, either interstitially or in the walls of blood vessels.[18,20] Light-chain deposits are morphologically similar to amyloid deposits on an H&E stain but they do not stain with Congo Red or show birefringence with polarized light, and are negative or react weakly with thioflavine-T; they are PAS-positive and stain blue with a Giemsa stain and Gomori's trichrome stain. The nature of light chain deposits can be confirmed by immunohistochemistry with anti-$\varkappa$ or anti-λ antiserum.

ESSENTIAL CRYOGLOBULINAEMIA

A plasma cell dyscrasia may produce cryoglobulinaemia either when there is secretion of a paraprotein with the characteristics of a cryoglobulin (type I cryoglobulinaemia) or when a paraprotein has antibody activity against another immunoglobulin and the immune complex formed is a cryoglobulin (type II cryoglobulinaemia); in the latter type the paraprotein is usually IgM with antibody activity against polyclonal IgG. In about a quarter of cases cryoglobulinaemia is a manifestation of multiple myeloma or of Waldenström's macroglobulinaemia. In the other three-quarters of patients in whom no overt plasma cell dyscrasia is present the term 'essential cryoglobulinaemia'

is appropriate; in these cases the clone of cells secreting the paraprotein is too small to produce any pathological manifestations other than those due to the characteristics of the cryoglobulin. The clinical features of cryoglobulinaemia may relate to precipitation of the immunoglobulin on chilling or, in the case of type II cryoglobulinaemia, to immune complex formation.

Peripheral blood

In the absence of overt multiple myeloma or Waldenström's macroglobulinaemia, the peripheral blood film is often normal. In a minority of patients a cryoglobulin precipitate is present, usually as a weakly basophilic globular mass, less often as crystals or a fibrillar deposit. Occasionally cryoglobulin precipitates have been ingested by neutrophils or monocytes and are seen as globular, variably basophilic intracytoplasmic inclusions.

Bone marrow cytology and histology

The bone marrow findings are either normal or are those of multiple myeloma, Waldenström's macroglobulinaemia or MGUS.

CHRONIC COLD HAEMAGGLUTININ DISEASE

Chronic cold haemagglutinin disease (CHAD) is a disease characterized by chronic, cold-induced haemolytic anaemia consequent on a lymphoplasmacytic dyscrasia which may be either occult or overt. In patients who do not have clinical or pathological features of a lymphoma at presentation these may subsequently evolve.

Peripheral blood

Unless it has been prepared from warmed blood, the blood film shows red cell agglutinates. If there has been a recent episode of haemolysis a few spherocytes may be present together with polychromatic macrocytes. Some patients have lymphocytosis, with the cells either having the morphology of normal mature lymphocytes or showing some lymphoplasmacytoid features.

Bone marrow cytology and histology

The bone marrow appearances vary from normal to those of an overt immunocytoma.

α HEAVY CHAIN DISEASE

α heavy chain disease is a lymphoplasmacytic dyscrasia, usually affecting predominantly the bowel, associated with the secretion of the heavy chain of IgA into the serum or into the bowel lumen. Some cases evolve into large cell lymphoma of immunoblastic type.

Peripheral blood and bone marrow

The peripheral blood shows no specific abnormality. The bone marrow is usually normal but may be infiltrated by plasma cells.

γ HEAVY CHAIN DISEASE

γ heavy chain disease is a lymphoplasmacytic dyscrasia characterized by lymphadenopathy, hepatomegaly and splenomegaly and by the secretion of the heavy chain of IgG. Some patients have developed amyloidosis, indicating that light chain as well as heavy chain may be secreted.

Peripheral blood

Anaemia, leucopenia and thrombocytopenia are common. In about half of cases there are atypical lymphoplasmacytoid cells and some plasma cells in the peripheral blood. Some cases have eosinophilia.

Bone marrow cytology

The bone marrow is infiltrated by lymphocytes or lymphoplasmacytoid cells.

μ HEAVY CHAIN DISEASE

μ heavy chain disease is a lymphoproliferative disorder characterized by the secretion of the heavy chain of IgM. The majority of patients have had the pathological features of chronic lymphocytic leukaemia. Hepatomegaly and splenomeg-

aly are usual; abdominal lymphadenopathy is more prominent than peripheral lymphadenopathy. Light chain secretion may also occur and may give rise to amyloidosis.

Peripheral blood and bone marrow

The majority of patients show features indistinguishable from those of chronic lymphocytic leukaemia.

THE POEMS SYNDROME[22-24]

The POEMS, or 'Polyneuropathy, Organomegaly, Endocrinopathy, M-protein, Skin changes' syndrome describes a curious constellation of pathological manifestations which has been associated with multiple myeloma (particularly but not exclusively osteosclerotic multiple myeloma), with solitary plasmacytoma, with immunocytoma and with a bone marrow appearance which, but for the many associated pathological features, would be designated MGUS. The syndrome is rare, and occurs at a younger age than is usual in multiple myeloma. The 'polyneuropathy' is both motor and sensory. The 'organomegaly' refers to hepatomegaly, splenomegaly and lymphadenopathy. The pathological features of the enlarged lymph nodes approximate to those of the hyaline-vascular type of Castleman's disease; there is follicular hyperplasia, vascular proliferation and an interfollicular infiltrate of lymphocytes, plasma cells and immunoblasts. The 'endocrinopathy' may include primary gonadal failure, hypothyroidism, Addison's disease and diabetes mellitus. The 'monoclonal gammopathy', present in about three-quarters of patients, is usually an IgGλ or IgAλ paraprotein. 'Skin' manifestations include skin thickening resembling that of scleroderma, oedema, hypertrichosis, hyperpigmentation and Raynaud's phenomenon. Other features of the syndrome include pleural effusion, ascites, papilloedema and finger clubbing.

Peripheral blood and bone marrow

There are no specific peripheral blood features. The bone marrow findings range from normal to those of overt multiple myeloma. About 60 per cent of patients have a significant bone marrow plasmacytosis. In those with multiple myeloma, osteosclerosis is usual but some patients have osteolytic lesions.

ACQUIRED ANGIO-OEDEMA ASSOCIATED WITH PLASMA CELL DYSCRASIA

The majority of cases of acquired angio-oedema described have been associated with a plasma cell dyscrasia or related condition, although some cases have been associated with other B-lineage neoplasms with or without secretion of a para-protein. Associated conditions have included multiple myeloma, immunocytoma or other non-Hodgkin's lymphoma, essential cryoglobu-linaemia, MGUS and chronic lymphocytic leukaemia. The mechanisms of the acquired angio-oedema is C1 inhibitor deficiency con-sequent on excessive consumption; it appears likely that consumption of C1 inhibitor can be due to precipitation of a cryoglobulin, to an im-munological reaction involving the paraprotein or to a reaction of auto-antibodies with neoplastic cells.

Peripheral blood and bone marrow

The peripheral blood and bone marrow findings are those usually associated with multiple myeloma, immunocytoma or other lymphopro-liferative disease. In a minority of cases the bone marrow shows only a slight increase in plasma cells or is normal.

REFERENCES

1 Merlini G, Gobbi PG and Ascari E (1989) The Merlini, Waldenström, Jayakar staging system re-visited. *Eur J Haematol*, **43**, suppl 51, 105–110.

2 Pasqualetti P, Casale R, Collacciani A, Abruzzo BP and Colantonio D (1990) Multiple myeloma: re-lationship between survival and cellular mor-phology. *Am J Hematol*, **33**, 145–147.

3 Greipp PR, Raymond NM, Kyle RA and O'Fallon WM (1985) Multiple myeloma: significance of plasmablastic morphological classification. *Blood*, **65**, 305–310.

4 Carter A, Hocherman I, Linn S, Cohen Y and Tatarsky I (1987) Prognostic significance of plasma cell morphology in multiple myeloma. *Cancer*, **60**, 1060–1065.

5 Bartl R, Frisch B, Diem H, Møndel M and Fateh-Moghadam A (1989) Bone marrow histology and serum β 2 microglobulin in multiple myeloma—a new prognostic strategy. *Eur J Haematol*, **43**, suppl 51, 88–98.

6 Pileri S, Poggi S, Baglioni P, *et al.* (1989) Histology and immunohistology of bone marrow biopsy in multiple myeloma. *Eur J Haematol*, **43**, suppl 51, 52–59.

7 Strand WR, Banks PM and Kyle RA (1984) Anaplastic plasma cell myeloma and immunoblastic lymphoma: clinical, pathologic and immunologic comparison. *Am J Med*, **76**, 861–867.

8 Bartl R, Frisch B, Fateh-Moghadam A, Kettner G, Jaeger K and Sommerfeld W (1986) Histologic classi-fication and staging of multiple myeloma. *Am J Clin Pathol*, **87**, 342–355.

9 Kyle RA, Maldonado JE and Bayrd ED (1974) Plasma cell leukemia. Report on 17 cases. *Arch Intern Med*, **133**, 813–818.

10 Kosmo MA and Gale RP (1987) Plasma cell leukemia. *Semin Hematol*, **24**, 202–208.

11 Bernasconi G, Castelli G, Pagnucco G and Brusa-molino E (1989) Plasma cell leukemia: a report on 15 patients. *Eur J Haematol*, **43**, suppl 51, 76–83.

12 Kyle RA (1989) Monoclonal gammapathy of un-determined significance and smouldering multiple myeloma. *Eur J Haematol*, **43**, suppl 51, 70–75.

13 Peterson LC, Brown BA, Crosson JT and Mladenovic J (1985) Application of the immunoperoxidase tech-nique to bone marrow trephine biopsies in the classi-fication of patients with monoclonal gammopathies. *Am J Clin Pathol*, **85**, 688–693.

14 Rywlin AM, Civantos F, Ortega, RS and Dominguez CJ (1975) Bone marrow histology in monoclonal macroglobulinemia. *Am J Clin Pathol*, **63**, 769–777.

15 Chalazzi G, Bettini R and Pinotti G (1979) Bone marrow patterns and survival in Waldenström's macroglobulinaemia. *Lancet*, **ii**, 965–966.

16 Pangalis GA and Kittas C. Bone marrow involve-ment in chronic lymphocytic leukaemia, small lymphocytic (well differentiated) and lympho-plasmacytic (macroglobulinaemia of Waldenström) non-Hodgkins lymphoma. In: *Chronic Lymphocytic Leukaemia*, Polliack A and Catovsky D (eds). Harwood Academic Publishers, Chur, 1988.

17 Park YK, Trubowitz S and Davis S. Plasma cells in the bone marrow. In: *The Human Bone Marrow: Anatomy, Physiology and Pathophysiology*, volume 2, Trubowitz S and Davis S (eds). CRC Press, Boca Raton, Florida, 1982.

18 Feiner HD (1988) Pathology of dysproteinemia: light chain amyloidosis, non-amyloid immunoglobulin

deposition disease, cryoglobulinemia syndromes and macroglobulinemia of Waldenström. *Hum Pathol*, **11**, 1255–1272.

19 Tubbs RR, Gephardt GN, McMahon JT, Hall PM, Valenzuela R and Vidt DG (1981) Light chain nephropathy. *Am J Med*, **71**, 263–269.

20 Silver MM, Hearn SA, Ritchie S, *et al.* (1986) Renal and systemic light chain deposits and their plasma cell origin identified by immunoelectron microscopy. *Am J Pathol*, **122**, 17–27.

21 Gallo G, Picken M, Buxbaum J and Frangione B (1989) The spectrum of monoclonal immunoglobulin deposition disease associated with immunocytic dyscrasias. *Semin Hematol*, **26**, 234–243.

22 Bardwick PA, Zvaifler NJ, Gill GN, Newman D, Greenway GD and Resnick DC (1980) Plasma cell dyscrasia with polyneuropathy, organomegaly, endocrinopathy, M-protein, and skin changes: the POEMS syndrome. *Medicine*, **59**, 311–322.

23 Moya-Mir MS, Martin-Martin F, Barbadillo R, *et al.* (1980) Plasma cell dyscrasia with polyneuritis and dermato-endocrine alterations. Report of a new case outside Japan. *Postgrad Med J*, **56**, 427–430.

24 Solomons REB and Gibbs DD (1982) Plasma cell dyscrasia with polyneuropathy, organomegaly, endocrinopathy, monoclonal gammopathy and skin changes. *J Roy Soc Med*, **75**, 553–555.

7: Disorders of Erythropoiesis, Granulopoiesis and Thrombopoiesis

In this chapter we shall discuss non-neoplastic haematological disorders, both congenital and acquired, which affect predominantly a single lineage — either erythroid, granulocytic or megakaryocytic. For a more detailed discussion of the peripheral blood features the reader is referred to Bain.[1] In the majority of these conditions diagnosis is based on peripheral blood and bone marrow aspirate features and on supplementary tests. In general a trephine biopsy is of little importance and is not often performed. The changes consequent on infection have been discussed in chapter 2 and will therefore not be dealt with in this chapter.

IRON DEFICIENCY ANAEMIA

Iron deficiency anaemia results from inadequate iron intake, increased loss of iron from the body, or a combination of the two. Peripheral blood features supplemented by biochemical assays are often sufficient for a definitive diagnosis. In more complicated cases a bone marrow aspirate permits a definitive diagnosis. The trephine biopsy is of little importance and, if iron is leached out during decalcification, can be misleading.

Peripheral blood

The peripheral blood shows initially a normocytic, normochromic anaemia and later, when the deficiency is more severe, a hypochromic, microcytic anaemia. Red cells also show anisocytosis, anisochromasia and poikilocytosis, particularly the presence of elliptocytes. Occasional patients show thrombocytosis, thrombocytopenia or the presence of occasional hypersegmented neutrophils.

Bone marrow cytology

Bone marrow cellularity is mildly increased consequent on a moderate degree of erythroid hyperplasia. Erythropoiesis is micronormoblastic with erythroblasts being smaller than normal with scanty or ragged cytoplasm or with cytoplasmic vacuolation (Fig. 7.1). There is a minor

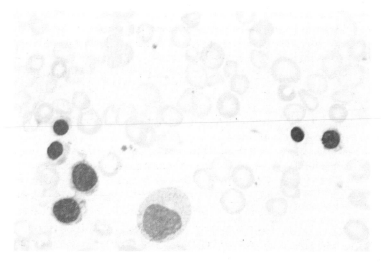

Fig. 7.1 BM aspirate, iron deficiency anaemia, showing erythroblasts with poorly haemoglobinized vacuolated cytoplasm. MGG × 940.

degree of dyserythropoiesis. An iron stain shows siderotic granules to be severely reduced or absent and there is a complete or virtual absence of the iron within macrophages which usually constitutes the body's iron stores (see Fig. 1.36). Since iron is irregularly distributed in the marrow, a number of bone marrow fragments must be available for the performance of an iron stain before it can be concluded that storage iron is lacking. In iron deficiency the bone marrow sometimes shows occasional giant metamyelocytes (see page 212) but otherwise granulopoiesis and thrombopoiesis are usually normal. Individuals whose bone marrows lack storage iron but in whom erythropoiesis is normal should be regarded as iron depleted rather than as iron deficient; a significant proportion of healthy women fall into this group.

Bone marrow histology

Trephine biopsy sections show mild hypercellularity, erythroid hyperplasia and absent iron stores. Iron stores should not be assessed as absent on the basis of paraffin-embedded sections unless it is known that the method of processing employed in the laboratory in question does not lead to leaching out of iron.

SIDEROBLASTIC ANAEMIA

Sideroblastic anaemia as a feature of MDS—refractory anaemia with ring sideroblasts or primary acquired sideroblastic anaemia—has been discussed in chapter 3. Sideroblastic anaemia may also be inherited or may be secondary to exogenous agents such as alcohol, chloramphenicol or certain drugs used in the treatment of tuberculosis. Congenital (inherited) sideroblastic anaemia occurs predominantly but not exclusively in males. Sideroblastic anaemia is most readily diagnosed on a bone marrow aspirate but diagnosis is also possible on good quality trephine biopsy sections.

Peripheral blood

Congenital and secondary sideroblastic anaemias are associated with microcytosis and hypo-chromia, in contrast to the macrocytosis which is usual when sideroblastic erythropoiesis is a feature of MDS. In some patients the peripheral blood film is dimorphic with a mixture of hypochromic microcytes and normochromic normocytes. Congenital sideroblastic anaemia varies in severity from moderate to severe. Secondary sideroblastic anaemia is of mild to moderate severity. In families in which males have sideroblastic anaemia females may show a small population of hypochromic microcytes.

Bone marrow cytology

The bone marrow shows mild hypercellularity and mild erythroid hyperplasia. A proportion of the erythroblasts show micronormoblastic maturation and defective haemoglobinization with ragged or vacuolated cytoplasm. An iron stain shows the presence of abnormal sideroblasts including frequent ring sideroblasts. Iron stores are usually increased.

Bone marrow histology

Trephine biopsy sections show some degree of erythroid hyperplasia. Increased storage iron and ring sideroblasts are detectable in plastic-embedded sections and sometimes in good quality paraffin-embedded sections.

THALASSAEMIA TRAIT AND THALASSAEMIA INTERMEDIA

The various thalassaemic disorders including thalassaemia trait are most readily diagnosed from the peripheral blood features but it is necessary for haematologists and pathologists to be aware of the bone marrow features to avoid misdiagnosis as other conditions. Bone marrow aspiration and trephine biopsy are not of any importance in the diagnosis.

Thalassaemia trait indicates an asymptomatic condition usually consequent on dysfunction of one of the two β genes or lack of one or two of the four α genes. The term thalassaemia intermedia denotes a symptomatic condition, more severe than thalassaemia trait but in which blood transfusion is not generally necessary; the genetic basis is diverse.

Peripheral blood

In β thalassaemia trait and in α thalassaemia trait in which two of the four α genes are lacking the peripheral blood shows microcytosis and sometimes some degree of hypochromia. Some but not all cases of β thalassaemia trait also have basophilic stippling and moderate poikilocytosis including the presence of target cells. In α thalassaemia trait in which only one of the four α genes is lacking the haematological abnormalities are much less and the diagnosis may not be suspected. In thalassaemia intermedia the haematological features are intermediate between those of thalassaemia trait and thalassaemia major.

Bone marrow cytology

In thalassaemia trait the bone marrow aspirate shows moderate erythroid hyperplasia. Erythropoiesis is micronormoblastic and there is moderate dyserythropoiesis including nuclear lobulation and nuclei of irregular shape (Fig. 7.2). An iron stain shows increased siderotic granulation and occasional ring sideroblasts. Storage iron is commonly increased. In thalassaemia intermedia erythroid hyperplasia and dyserythropoiesis are marked; misdiagnosis as myelodysplasia is possible if the diagnosis of thalassaemia is not considered and if it is not appreciated that dysplastic features are confined to the erythroid lineage.

Bone marrow histology

Trephine biopsy sections show erythroid hyperplasia and dyserythropoiesis.

THALASSAEMIA MAJOR

Thalassaemia major indicates a transfusion-dependent thalassaemic condition usually consequent on homozygosity or double heterozygosity for β thalassaemia.

Peripheral blood

The peripheral blood shows striking hypochromia, microcytosis, anisocytosis and poikilocytosis and the presence of basophilic stippling, Pappenheimer bodies and dysplastic circulating erythroblasts.

Bone marrow cytology

The bone marrow shows very marked erythroid hyperplasia, severe erythroid dysplasia and poor haemoglobinization (Fig. 7.3). Some erythroblasts contain cytoplasmic inclusions, seen with difficulty on MGG-stained films, which represent precipitated α chains. There is an increase in macrophages which contain degenerating erythroblasts, cellular debris and haemosiderin. In some patients the increased cell turnover leads to the formation of pseudo-Gaucher cells and sea-blue

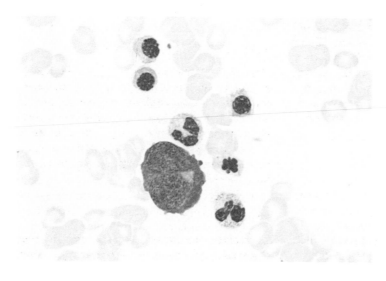

Fig. 7.2 BM aspirate, β-thalassaemia trait, showing erythroid hyperplasia and dyserythropoiesis. There is a binucleated early erythroblast and the late erythroblasts are small and have irregular or lobulated nuclei. MGG × 940.

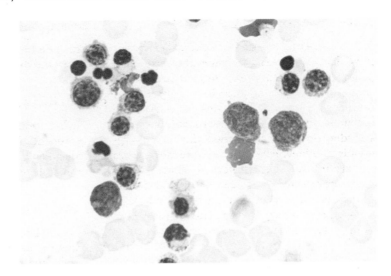

Fig. 7.3 BM aspirate, β-thalassaemia major, showing erythroid hyperplasia and dyserythropoiesis. Several cells contain cytoplasmic inclusions, composed of precipitated alpha chains. MGG × 940.

histiocytes (see pages 234 and 236) may be present. An iron stain shows numerous abnormal sideroblasts and small numbers of ring sideroblasts. Storage iron is considerably increased.

Bone marrow histology

Bone marrow sections show marked erythroid hyperplasia with disappearance of fat spaces. Dyserythropoiesis is also very marked and iron stores are increased.

HAEMOGLOBIN H DISEASE

Haemoglobin H disease is a thalassaemic condition consequent on the lack of three of the four α genes or on a functionally similar defect. There is also decreased red cell life span. Diagnosis rests on peripheral blood features and the results of haemoglobin electrophoresis; bone marrow examination contributes little. Occasionally haemoglobin H disease is an acquired condition, being a feature of MDS.

Peripheral blood

The peripheral blood shows marked hypochromia, microcytosis, anisocytosis and poikilocytosis. Because of the haemolytic component there is also polychromasia and the reticulocyte count is elevated. Demonstration of haemoglobin H

inclusions by the use of an appropriate supravital stain in the peripheral blood is very useful in the confirmation of the diagnosis.

Bone marrow cytology

The bone marrow is hypercellular with marked erythroid hyperplasia and with a defect in haemoglobinization and some dyserythropoietic features.

Bone marrow histology

Bone marrow sections show hypercellularity due to erythroid hyperplasia.

HAEMOLYTIC ANAEMIAS

Haemolytic anaemia may be inherited or acquired. Aetiological factors, pathogenetic mechanisms and morphological features are very varied.[1] Examination of the peripheral blood is of great importance in the diagnosis but examination of the bone marrow adds little, except in detecting complicating megaloblastic anaemia or pure red cell aplasia.

Peripheral blood

Haemolytic anaemias have in common polychromasia and an increased reticulocyte count.

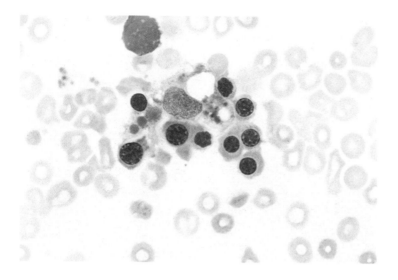

Fig. 7.4 BM aspirate, auto-immune haemolytic anaemia, showing an erythroid island composed of erythroblasts clustered around a debris-laden macrophage. MGG × 940.

Macrocytosis is usual in those patients in whom haemolysis is chronic and severe. Other morphological features are very variable, depending on the precise nature of the condition.[1]

Bone marrow cytology

The bone marrow is hypercellular as a consequence of erythroid hyperplasia (Fig. 7.4). The degree of hyperplasia reflects the extent to which the red cell life span is shortened. In some patients fat cells are totally lost. Haemopoiesis is often macronormoblastic, that is the erythroblasts are increased in size but have nuclear and cytoplasmic characteristics similar to those of normoblasts. In the haemolytic anaemia due to haemoglobin C disease normoblasts have irregular nuclear membranes (Fig. 7.5). Macronormoblastic erythropoiesis should be distinguished from mildly megaloblastic erythropoiesis which may occur in the haemolytic anaemias when there is complicating folic acid deficiency. When haemolysis is extravascular bone marrow macrophages are increased and contain cellular debris. Iron stores are commonly increased, except when there is severe intravascular haemolysis with consequent loss of iron from the body. Siderotic granulation is somewhat increased.

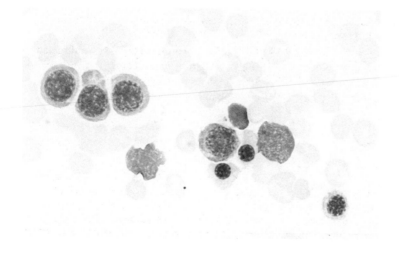

Fig. 7.5 BM aspirate, haemoglobin C disease, showing erythroid hyperplasia and an irregular nuclear outline which is characteristic of this condition. MGG × 940.

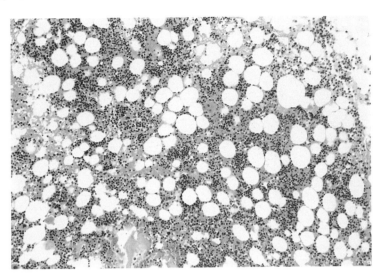

Fig. 7.6 BM trephine biopsy, auto-immune haemolytic anaemia, showing erythroid hyperplasia. Paraffin-embedded, H&E × 97.

Bone marrow histology

The bone marrow is hypercellular with a variable degree of erythroid hyperplasia (Fig. 7.6). The number of erythroid islands is increased and the central macrophage is large and prominent, often staining a dirty greenish colour on MGG because of the presence of increased haemosiderin. An iron stain confirms increased storage iron.

CONGENITAL DYSERYTHROPOIETIC ANAEMIA (CDA)

The congenital dyserythropoietic anaemias (CDA) are a diverse group of inherited conditions all of which are characterized by dysplastic and ineffective erythropoiesis. Three major types of CDA have been recognized but a considerable number of cases not conforming to these categories have also been described. Both peripheral blood and bone marrow aspirate features are important in making the diagnosis, and in type II CDA demonstration of a positive acidified serum lysis test is also required for diagnosis. A trephine biopsy is not of any importance in diagnosis.

Peripheral blood

Specific morphological features vary, dependent on the category of CDA (Table 7.1). All are

Table 7.1 Genetic, peripheral blood and bone marrow features of the congenital dyserythropoietic anaemias

	Type I	Type II (Hempas)*	Type III
Inheritance	Autosomal recessive	Autosomal recessive	Autosomal dominant
Peripheral blood	Mild to moderate anaemia, macrocytosis, marked anisocytosis and poikilocytosis	Mild to severe anaemia, normocytic red cells, moderate anisocytosis and poikilocytosis	Mild anaemia, macrocytosis, marked anisocytosis and poikilocytosis
Bone marrow	Hyperplastic, megaloblastic, moderate binuclearity and internuclear chromatin bridges, nuclear budding and karyorrhexis	Hyperplastic, normoblastic, marked binuclearity and multinuclearity, karyorrhexis	Hyperplastic, megaloblastic, giant erythroblasts with lobulated nuclei or marked multinuclearity—up to a dozen nuclei per cell, karyorrhexis

* Hereditary erythroid multinuclearity with positive acidified serum test.

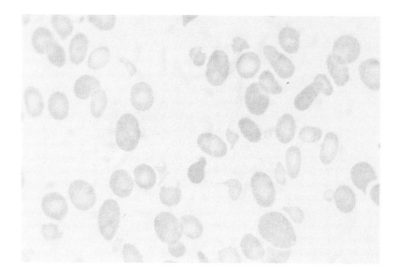

Fig. 7.7 PB, congenital dyserythropoietic anaemia, type I, showing macrocytosis, marked anisocytosis and poikilocytosis. MGG × 940.

characterized by anisocytosis and by poikilocytosis (Fig. 7.7) which often includes the presence of fragments and irregularly contracted cells. Basophilic stippling is common. In all categories the reticulocyte count is not elevated appropriately for the degree of anaemia.

Bone marrow cytology

Bone marrow features characteristic of the different categories of CDA are summarized in Table 7.1 and illustrated in Figs 7.8 to 7.10. In all types there is erythroid hyperplasia and dyserythropoiesis. In type II CDA the increase in cell turnover is such that pseudo-Gaucher cells may be present. Iron stores are commonly increased.

Bone marrow histology

Examination of trephine biopsy sections confirms erythroid hyperplasia and dyserythropoiesis (Fig. 7.11).

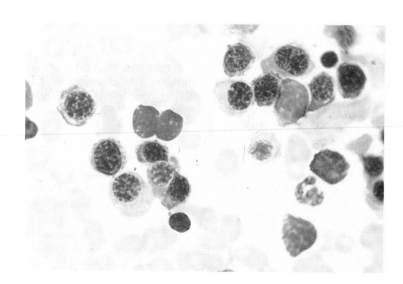

Fig. 7.8 BM aspirate, congenital dyserythropoietic anaemia, type I, showing erythroid hyperplasia and dyserythropoietic features including two pairs of erythroblasts joined by cytoplasmic and nuclear bridges respectively. MGG × 940.

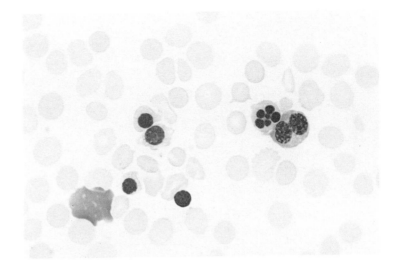

Fig. 7.9 BM aspirate, congenital dyserythropoietic anaemia, type II, showing one binucleate erythroblast and one erythroblast with a multilobulated nucleus. MGG × 940.

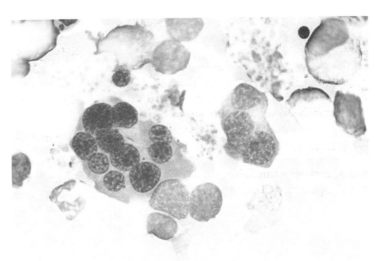

Fig. 7.10 BM aspirate, congenital dyserythropoietic anaemia, type III, showing giant, multinucleated erythroblasts. MGG × 940.

MEGALOBLASTIC ANAEMIA

Megaloblastic anaemia is usually consequent on a deficiency of vitamin B_{12} or folic acid. Less often it is attributable to administration of a drug which interferes with DNA synthesis and rarely to a congenital metabolic defect. The presence of megaloblastic anaemia can usually be suspected from examination of the peripheral blood but examination of a bone marrow aspirate is crucial in the diagnosis. Examination of a trephine biopsy specimen is rarely useful but it is important for pathologists to be able to recognize the histo-logical features of megaloblastic anaemia so that misdiagnosis, particularly as acute leukaemia, does not occur.

Peripheral blood

In most cases there is a macrocytic anaemia with oval macrocytes being particularly characteristic. The mildest cases have macrocytosis without anaemia. Some degree of anisocytosis and poikilocytosis are usual and when anaemia is severe there are striking morphological abnormalities including the presence of tear-drop poikilocytes,

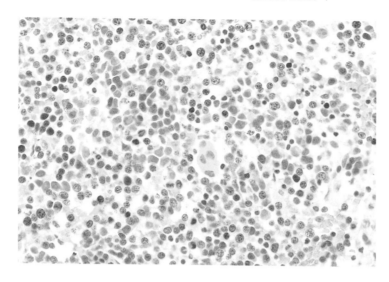

Fig. 7.11 BM clot section, congenital dyserythropoietic anaemia, type I, showing marked erythroid hyperplasia with large numbers of immature erythroid precursors and marked dyserythropoiesis. Paraffin-embedded, H&E × 390.

fragments, basophilic stippling and occasional Howell–Jolly bodies and circulating megaloblasts. Hypersegmented neutrophils are usually present; they are highly suggestive of megaloblastic erythropoiesis although not pathognomonic. They persist for a week or more after commencement of vitamin B_{12} or folic acid therapy. There may also be increased numbers of macropolycytes (tetraploid neutrophils), but this feature is less strongly associated with megaloblastic erythropoiesis. In severe megaloblastic anaemia, leucopenia and thrombocytopenia also occur.

Bone marrow cytology

The bone marrow is hypercellular, often markedly so. Erythropoiesis is hyperplastic and is characterized by the presence of megaloblasts (Fig. 7.12). These are large cells with a chromatin pattern more primitive than is appropriate for the degree of maturation of the cytoplasm. Late megaloblasts may be fully haemoglobinized and lack any cytoplasmic basophilia. They may therefore be described as orthochromatic, a term which is not really appropriate in describing normal erythropoiesis in which the most mature erythroblasts are polychromatic. Erythropoiesis is ineffective so that early erythroid cells are over-represented in comparison with mature cells; macrophages are increased and contain defective red cell pre-

cursors and cellular debris. An iron stain shows abnormally prominent siderotic granules and sometimes occasional ring sideroblasts. Storage iron is usually increased. The mitotic rate is increased and examination of cells in metaphase may show that chromosomes are unusually long.

Granulopoiesis is also hyperplastic, although less so than erythropoiesis. Giant metamyelocytes are usually present (Fig. 7.12). They are twice to three times the size of a normal metamyelocyte and often have nuclei of unusual shapes, E- or Z-shaped rather than U-shaped. Myelocytes and promyelocytes are also increased in size but this abnormality is less obvious and less distinctive than the abnormality of metamyelocytes. When megaloblastic features in erythroblasts are partly or largely masked by co-existing iron deficiency the detection of giant metamyelocytes is diagnostically important.

Megakaryocytes are hypersegmented and have more finely stippled chromatin than normal megakaryocytes.

It is critically important that severe megaloblastic anaemia with 'maturation arrest' is not confused with M6 AML.

Bone marrow histology

There is a variable hypercellularity with loss of fat cells. In some cases this can be so severe that it may resemble the 'packed marrow' appearance

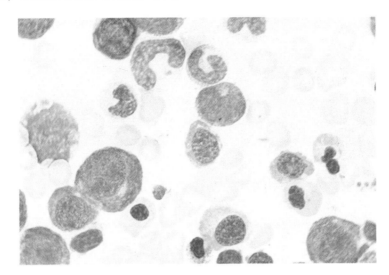

Fig. 7.12 BM aspirate, megaloblastic anaemia, showing hyperplastic megaloblastic erythropoiesis and a giant metamyelocyte. MGG × 940.

seen in acute leukaemia on examination at low power. There is erythroid hyperplasia with predominance of immature precursors (Figs 7.13 and 7.14). The early erythroid cells have large, round to oval, nuclei with one or more basophilic nucleoli which often appear to have rather irregular margins and often abut on the nuclear membrane (Fig. 7.14); there is usually a moderate amount of intensely basophilic cytoplasm. The later erythroid cells show asynchrony of nuclear and cytoplasmic maturation with cells having immature nuclei but haemoglobinized cytoplasm. Granulocytic precursors are increased but may appear relatively inconspicuous in the presence of profound erythroid hyperplasia. Giant metamyelocytes are usually easily seen (Fig. 7.13). Megakaryocytes may be normal or decreased in number. Megaloblastic change in biopsy sections may be mistaken for acute leukaemia by the unwary, particularly if the biopsy is reported without referring to the blood film and marrow aspirate findings and the possibility of megaloblastic anaemia is therefore not considered. Rarely there may have been failure to obtain an aspirate or the presence of immature cells in the peripheral blood in a patient with complicating

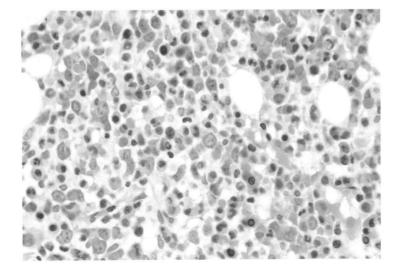

Fig. 7.13 BM trephine biopsy, megaloblastic anaemia, showing marked erythroid hyperplasia with numerous early, intermediate and late megaloblasts. Giant metamyelocytes are also present. Paraffin-embedded, H&E × 390.

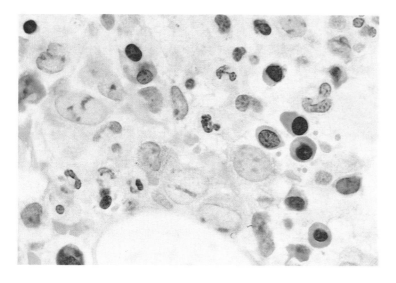

Fig. 7.14 BM trephine biopsy, megaloblastic anaemia, showing several early megaloblasts with prominent, often elongated nucleoli which frequently abut on the nuclear membrane. Numerous late megaloblasts are also seen. Plastic-embedded, H&E × 970.

infection may have given rise to the clinical suspicion of leukaemia; in these circumstances misdiagnosis of leukaemia is more likely.[2] Erythroid islands composed of early megaloblasts are also sometimes mistaken for clusters of carcinoma cells.

ANAEMIA OF CHRONIC DISEASE

The anaemia of chronic disease is characterized by a normocytic, normochromic anaemia or, when more severe, by a hypochromic microcytic anaemia. Such anaemia is secondary to infection, inflammation or malignancy. Diagnosis is based on peripheral blood features and biochemical assays but a bone marrow aspirate is often necessary to exclude the coexistence of a chronic inflammatory disorder and iron deficiency. A bone marrow biopsy does not usually give diagnostically useful information.

Peripheral blood

In addition to the possible occurrence of hypochromia and microcytosis the peripheral blood usually shows increased rouleaux formation and sometimes increased background staining consequent on a reactive increase in various serum proteins. The erythrocyte sedimentation rate is increased.

Bone marrow cytology

The bone marrow is usually of normal cellularity. Erythropoiesis may show no specific abnormality or may be micronormoblastic with defective haemoglobinization. An iron stain shows storage iron to be increased, often markedly so when the condition is very chronic. Erythroblasts show reduced or absent siderotic granulation. The bone marrow often shows non-specific inflammatory changes including increased plasma cells, mast cells and macrophages.

Bone marrow histology

Sections of bone marrow trephine biopsies usually show normal cellularity. There may be increased lymphoid nodules, plasma cells, mast cells and macrophages. An iron stain shows increased storage iron.

SICKLE CELL ANAEMIA AND OTHER SICKLING DISORDERS

Sickle cell anaemia denotes the disease consequent on homozygosity for the β^s genes and the consequent replacement of haemoglobin A by haemoglobin S. Diagnosis of sickle cell anaemia is dependent on peripheral blood features and haemoglobin electrophoresis. Bone marrow aspiration is usually only indicated to detect suspected

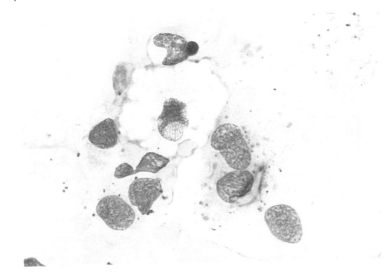

Fig. 7.15 BM aspirate, sickle cell anaemia, showing a foamy macrophage and a macrophage containing a sickled cell. MGG × 940.

complications such as megaloblastic anaemia, pure red cell aplasia or bone marrow necrosis. Trephine biopsy is rarely indicated. The clinical features consequent on sickling of red blood cells can also be consequent on various compound heterozygous states such as sickle cell/haemoglobin C disease and sickle cell/β thalassaemia trait.

Peripheral blood

The peripheral blood shows anaemia, usually with a haemoglobin concentration of 6–10 g/dl. There are variable numbers of sickle cells and in addition target cells, polychromasia and sometimes nucleated red blood cells. In subjects over the age of six months the features of hyposplenism start to appear, particularly Howell–Jolly bodies and Pappenheimer bodies. The neutrophil count may be increased, particularly during episodes of sickling. The blood film in compound heterozygous states is often similar to that of sickle cell anaemia, although patients with sickle cell/haemoglobin C disease may have occasional cells containing haemoglobin C crystals and those with sickle cell/β thalassaemia have microcytosis.

Bone marrow cytology

The bone marrow aspirate shows hypercellularity due to erythroid hyperplasia. Iron stores are often increased and sickle cells are usually present. When there are complicating conditions such as megaloblastic anaemia, pure red cell aplasia or bone marrow necrosis, the appropriate morphological features are superimposed on those of the underlying disease. Bone marrow macrophages may contain occasional sickle cells (Fig. 7.15). Macrophages and various storage cells are sometimes increased (Fig. 7.15) as a consequence of increased cell turnover and episodes of bone marrow infarction. In sickle cell/β thalassaemia erythropoiesis is hyperplastic and micronormoblastic (Fig. 7.16).

Bone marrow histology

Trephine biopsy sections show hypercellularity due to erythroid hyperplasia. During episodes of sickling, sickle cells may be seen within bone marrow sinusoids (Fig. 7.17). Infarcted bone marrow and bone may be present in patients who are experiencing a sickling crisis and foamy macrophages and small fibrotic scars may mark the sites of previous bone marrow infarction.

PURE RED CELL APLASIA

Pure red cell aplasia may be either constitutional or acquired and either acute or chronic. Constitutional pure red cell aplasia, also known as the Blackfan–Diamond syndrome, is a chronic

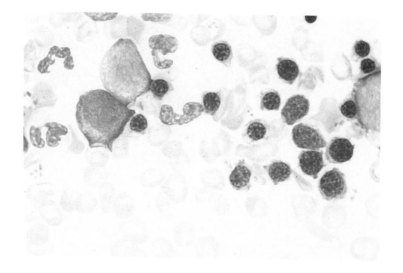

Fig. 7.16 BM aspirate, sickle cell/β-thalassaemia compound heterozygosity, showing erythroid hyperplasia, scanty erythroblast cytoplasm and defective haemoglobinization; several sickle cells are present. MGG ×940.

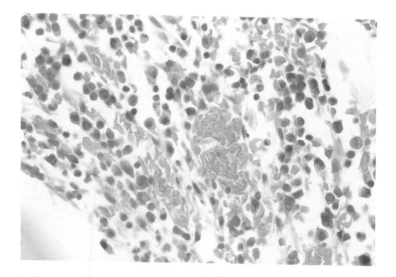

Fig. 7.17 BM trephine biopsy, sickle cell anaemia, showing sinusoids distended by irreversibly sickled erythrocytes. Plastic-embedded, H&E ×377.

condition which usually becomes manifest during the first year of life; it is probably consequent on an inherited stem cell defect and is responsive to corticosteroids. A small percentage of patients with the Blackfan–Diamond syndrome subsequently develop acute myeloid leukaemia. Infants, usually but not always over one year in age, may also suffer from acute pure red cell aplasia designated transient erythroblastopenia of childhood;[3,4] in this condition the aplasia which is probably consequent on infection by an as yet unidentified virus lasts only a matter of months and does not require specific treatment. In older

children and adults the most commonly recognized cause of acute aplasia is parvovirus infection; the aplasia is usually of brief duration and therefore causes symptomatic anaemia only in subjects with a pre-existing red cell defect associated with a shortened red cell life span. In adults chronic aplasia is commonly immunological in origin and may be associated with a thymoma or with auto-immune disease. Marked erythroid hypoplasia may also be a feature of protein-calorie deprivation (kwashiorkor), be induced by hypothermia,[5] occur as part of a hypersensitivity reaction to a drug, or be the dominant feature of MDS.

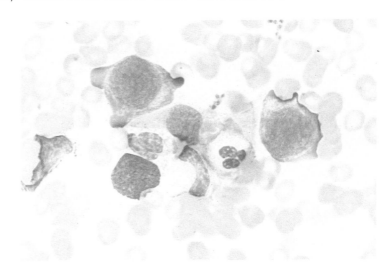

Fig. 7.18 BM aspirate, chronic idiopathic pure red cell aplasia, showing increased proerythroblasts and a lack of maturing erythroblasts. MGG × 940.

Peripheral blood

The peripheral blood shows no specific abnormality. There is a complete absence of polychromatic cells and the reticulocyte count is zero or virtually zero. Associated features differ according to the cause of the red cell aplasia. Macrocytosis is usual in the Blackfan–Diamond syndrome and the red cells have some characteristics similar to those of fetal red cells; occasionally there is mild neutropenia and the platelet count may be somewhat elevated.[3] In transient erythroblastopenia of childhood the red cells are of normal size and lack fetal characteristics; neutropenia, which may be moderately severe, occurs in about a quarter of cases and thrombocytosis in about a third.[3,4] Since symptomatic anaemia following parvovirus-induced aplasia is largely confined to patients with an underlying red cell defect, the blood film usually shows features of an associated disease, most often hereditary spherocytosis or sickle cell anaemia. In such cases the absence of polychromasia despite marked anaemia is diagnostically important and should lead to a reticulocyte count being performed. Neutrophil and platelet counts are only occasionally reduced in patients with parvovirus-induced red cell aplasia. Patients with red cell aplasia associated with thymoma or with auto-immune disease sometimes also have neutropenia or thrombocytopenia. In patients with red cell aplasia as the dominant feature of MDS it is sometimes possible to detect dysplastic features in other lineages.

Bone marrow cytology

Bone marrow cellularity is usually somewhat reduced. There is a striking reduction of maturing erythroid cells. Proerythroblasts are present in normal numbers and sometimes they may be increased (Fig. 7.18). Other lineages are normal. In parvovirus-induced aplasia giant proerythroblasts with prominent nucleoli are often noted. Iron stores are commonly increased since the iron normally in erythroid cells has been deposited in the stores. Since MDS may present as red cell aplasia it is important to examine other lineages carefully for dysplastic features.

Bone marrow histology

The overall bone marrow cellularity is somewhat reduced. There is a striking lack of erythroid islands and of maturing erythroblasts (Fig. 7.19). Large proerythroblasts with strongly basophilic cytoplasm are readily apparent. In parvovirus infection the giant proerythroblasts may show intranuclear eosinophilic degeneration with peripheral condensation of chromatin[6] (Fig. 7.20).

AGRANULOCYTOSIS

Agranulocytosis is an acute, severe, reversible lack of circulating neutrophils consequent on an idiosyncratic reaction to a drug or chemical. At least some cases are consequent on development of antibodies against the causative drug with

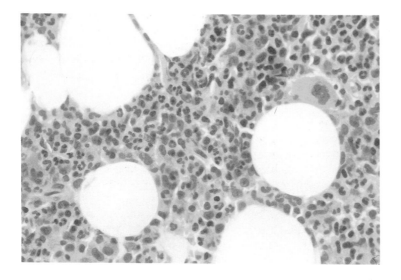

Fig. 7.19 BM trephine biopsy, pure red cell aplasia, showing absence of erythroblastic islands and late erythroblasts; only occasional early and intermediate erythroblasts are present. Parrafin-embedded, H&E × 390.

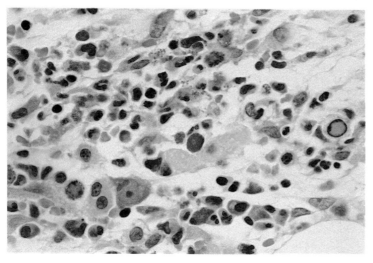

Fig. 7.20 BM trephine biopsy, parvovirus-induced pure red cell aplasia, showing giant proerythroblasts with nuclear degeneration characterized by a central eosinophilic mass and peripheral chromatin condensation. Plastic-embedded, H&E × 480.

destruction of neutrophils resulting from the interaction of the antibody and the drug. However, some cases may result from abnormal metabolism of a drug so that toxic levels result when normal doses are administered. Clinical features are due to sepsis consequent on the neutropenia.

Peripheral blood

The neutrophil count is greatly reduced, usually to less than $0.5 \times 10^9/l$. Residual neutrophils may be morphologically normal but often they show toxic changes consequent on superimposed

sepsis. During recovery there is an outpouring of immature granulocytes into the peripheral blood, constituting a leukaemoid reaction.

Bone marrow cytology

The bone marrow aspirate shows a marked reduction of mature neutrophils. Sometimes myelocytes are also greatly reduced. In severe cases with superimposed sepsis the majority of cells of granulocytic lineage may be promyelocytes with very heavy granulation. This appearance has been confused with hypergranular promyelocytic leukaemia. A useful point allowing differentiation of the two conditions is the prominent Golgi zone and the lack of Auer rods and giant granules in the promyelocytes of agranulocytosis.

Bone marrow histology

Bone marrow sections show a lack of mature granulocytes and often superimposed changes consequent on infection.

IDIOPATHIC HYPEREOSINOPHILIC SYNDROME

The idiopathic hypereosinophilic syndrome is a condition of unknown aetiology characterized by sustained hypereosinophilia and damage to tissues, usually including the heart and central nervous system, by eosinophil products. The clinical features are due to this tissue damage. The idiopathic hypereosinophilic syndrome has been arbitrarily defined as requiring the eosinophil count to be greater than $1.5 \times 10^9/l$ for greater than 6 months and for tissue damage to have occurred.[7] Diagnosis of the idiopathic hypereosinophilic syndrome is mainly dependent on peripheral blood and clinical features and on the exclusion of other diagnoses. A bone marrow aspirate and trephine biopsy are only of importance in excluding eosinophilic leukaemia and lymphoma, the latter being an important cause of reactive eosinophilia. Some cases of idiopathic hypereosinophilic syndrome represent a myeloproliferative disorder and subsequently transform to AML despite initially having no specific evidence of the nature of the underlying disorder.

Peripheral blood

The eosinophil count is considerably elevated and eosinophils usually show some degree of hypogranularity and cytoplasmic vacuolation; completely agranular eosinophils are sometimes present. Eosinophil nuclei may be non-segmented or hypersegmented or occasionally ring-shaped. Neutrophils may show heavy granulation. In contrast to eosinophilic leukaemia, there are usually only occasional if any granulocyte precursors in the peripheral blood. There may be a mild anaemia and thrombocytopenia with red cells showing anisocytosis and poikilocytosis. Nucleated red cells are sometimes present.

Bone marrow cytology

The bone marrow shows an increase of eosinophils and their precursors (Fig. 7.21). Some eosinophil myelocytes show granules with basophilic staining characteristics but this feature is much less striking than in AML of M4Eo type (see page 76). There is no increase in blast cells.

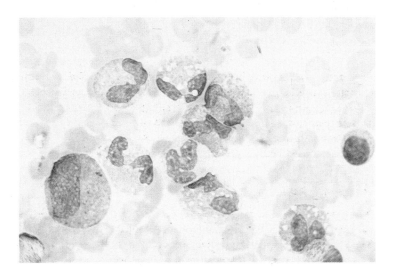

Fig. 7.21 BM aspirate, idiopathic hypereosinophilic syndrome, showing eosinophil hyperplasia; note partial degranulation of eosinophils. MGG × 940.

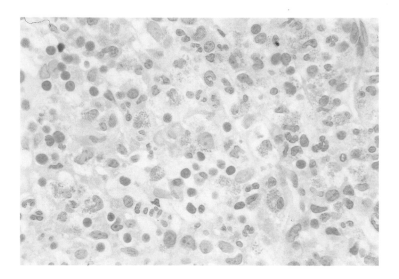

Fig. 7.22 BM trephine biopsy, idiopathic hypereosinophilic syndrome, showing marked granulocytic hyperplasia and increased numbers of immature eosinophil precursors. Plastic-embedded, H&E × 390.

Bone marrow histology

Eosinophils and their precursors are increased (Fig. 7.22). It is important to exclude marrow infiltration by lymphoma since this may be easily overlooked.

CHEDIAK–HIGASHI SYNDROME

The Chediak–Higashi syndrome is a fatal inherited condition characterized by a defect in formation of lysosomes in multiple cell lineages. Patients suffer from albinism, neurological abnormalities and recurrent infections. Haematologically abnormalities are most apparent in the granulocyte series although anaemia and thrombocytopenia also occur.

Peripheral blood

All granulocyte lineages show striking abnormalities. Granules are very large and also have abnormal staining characteristics. Lymphocytes and monocytes may also have abnormally prominent granules. With disease progression there is development of anaemia, neutropenia and thrombocytopenia.

Bone marrow cytology

Granulocyte precursors as well as granulocytes show giant granules with unusual staining charac-

teristics (Fig. 7.23). A secondary haemophagocytic syndrome may occur; it is likely to be consequent on immune deficiency and superimposed infection.

CONGENITAL THROMBOCYTOPENIAS

Congenital thrombocytopenia may be inherited or may be secondary to intra-uterine infection, mutagen exposure or platelet destruction by maternal anti-platelet antibodies.

Peripheral blood

Morphological features are dependent on which specific defect is responsible for thrombocytopenia.[1] In inherited thrombocytopenia the platelets may be of normal size, increased in size as in Bernard–Soulier syndrome or decreased in size as in the Wiskott–Aldrich syndrome. In the grey platelet syndrome they are increased in size and lack the normal azurophilic granules. In the May–Hegglin anomaly and in several other rare inherited defects thrombocytopenia and giant platelets are associated with weakly basophilic cytoplasmic inclusions in neutrophils. When thrombocytopenia is secondary to intra-uterine platelet destruction or damage to megakaryocytes the platelets are usually normal in size and morphology.

Other lineages are generally normal but infants

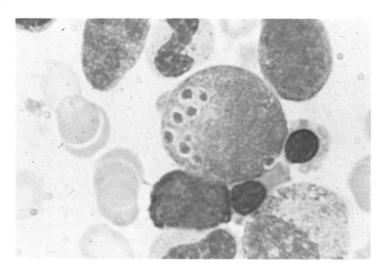

Fig. 7.23 BM aspirate, Chediak–Higashi syndrome, showing granulocyte precursors with giant granules. MGG × 1175.

with the thrombocytopenia-absent radii (TAR) syndrome have been noted to be prone to leukaemoid reactions.

Bone marrow cytology

In inherited thrombocytopenia megakaryocytes are sometimes present in normal numbers, as in Bernard–Soulier syndrome and are sometimes severely reduced in number as in constitutional amegakaryocytic thrombocytopenia. When thrombocytopenia is consequent on intra-uterine damage to megakaryocytes these cells are usually reduced in number. In the TAR syndrome megakaryocytes are greatly reduced in number and are small with poorly lobulated nuclei. When platelets have been destroyed by exposure to maternal anti-platelet antibodies megakaryocytes are present in normal numbers or are increased.

Bone marrow histology

A bone marrow biopsy is not often needed in determining the cause of congenital thrombocytopenia but it can be useful in permitting an accurate assessment of megakaryocyte numbers and morphology. In the grey platelet syndrome there may be associated myelofibrosis, probably consequent on intramedullary release by megakaryocytes of granular contents capable of stimulating fibroblasts.

ACQUIRED THROMBOCYTOPENIAS

Isolated acquired thrombocytopenia is commonly due to peripheral destruction of platelets, either (i) by anti-platelet antibodies, or (ii) by drug-dependent antibodies or (iii) by immune complexes which may attach to platelets both in auto-immune diseases and during or after viral infections, including infection by HIV. Thrombocytopenia may also be consequent on platelet consumption as in thrombotic thrombocytopenic purpura or in disseminated intravascular coagulation. Less often acquired thrombocytopenia is due to megakaryocytic hypoplasia, such as that induced by thiazide diuretics, or a failure of megakaryocytes to produce platelets, as in some patients with MDS who present with isolated thrombocytopenia.

Peripheral blood

When thrombocytopenia is consequent on a sustained increase in the peripheral destruction or consumption of platelets there is usually an increase in platelet size with some giant platelets being present. When thrombocytopenia is due to failure of production, as in sepsis or during chemotherapy, the platelets are small. When thrombocytopenia is due to MDS, platelets often show increased variation in size, and hypogranular or agranular platelets may be present.

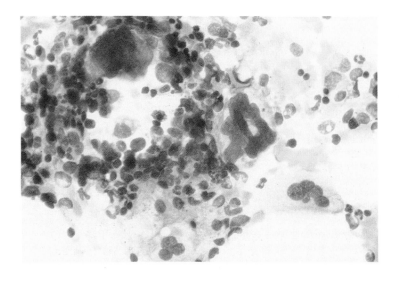

Fig. 7.24 BM aspirate, auto-immune thrombocytopenic purpura, showing five megakaryocytes of varying size and ploidy levels. MGG × 377.

Bone marrow cytology

When thrombocytopenia which is consequent on peripheral destruction or consumption has developed acutely, the bone marrow may show no relevant abnormality but megakaryocytes are noted to be present in normal numbers. With sustained thrombocytopenia there is an increase in megakaryocyte numbers (Fig. 7.24) and a reduction in average size. There is often very little morphological evidence of platelet pro-duction despite the increased platelet production which can be demonstrated by isotopic studies.

When thrombocytopenia is consequent on in-effective thrombopoiesis, for example in the my-elodysplastic syndromes, megakaryocytes may be present in normal or increased numbers and may show dysplastic features. In acquired megakaryo-cytic hypoplasia, for example that due to adverse effects of drugs, megakaryocytes are usually morphologically normal although reduced in number.

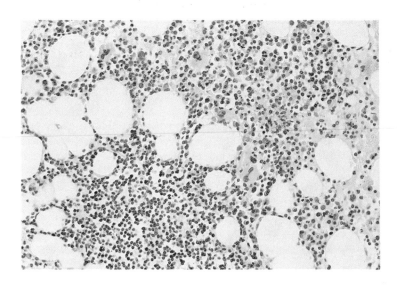

Fig. 7.25 BM trephine biopsy, auto-immune thrombocytopenic purpura, showing a lymphoid nodule and haemopoietic marrow containing increased numbers of megakaryocytes. H&E × 188.

Bone marrow histology

Trephine biopsy is not usually necessary in the investigation of suspected immune thrombocytopenia but is useful in confirming megakaryocytic hypoplasia and in investigating suspected myelodysplasia.

In idiopathic (auto-immune) thrombocytopenia the bone marrow is normocellular with increased numbers of megakaryocytes (Fig. 7.25). Mean megakaryocyte diameter is decreased. There is increased variation in size so that although small megakaryocytes predominate there are also increased numbers of giant forms. There is no abnormal localization of megakaryocytes and clusters are not usually seen.[8]

REACTIVE THROMBOCYTOSIS

The platelet count may increase in response to infection, inflammation and malignant disease. In reactive thrombocytosis it is very rare for the platelet count to exceed $1000 \times 10^9/l$.

Peripheral blood

In contrast to the myeloproliferative disorders, there is no increase in platelet size when thrombocytosis is reactive. The blood film may show other reactive changes including leucocytosis and neutrophilia but the presence of basophilia suggests a myeloproliferative disorder.

Bone marrow cytology

The bone marrow aspirate shows increased numbers of megakaryocytes of normal morphology.

Bone marrow histology

Megakaryocyte numbers are increased. The average megakaryocyte diameter is increased in comparison with normal and there is increased variation in size. There is no clustering or abnormality of distribution.[8]

REFERENCES

1 Bain BJ. *Blood Cells: A Practical Guide.* Gower, London, 1989.
2 Dokal IS, Cox TC and Galton DAG (1990) Vitamin B_{12} and folate deficiency presenting as leukaemia. *BMJ*, **300**, 1263–1264.
3 Glader BE (1987) Diagnosis and management of red cell aplasia in children. *Hematol Oncol Clin North Amer*, **1**, 431–447.
4 Foot ABM, Potter MN, Ropner JE, Wallington TB and Oakhill A (1990) Transient erythroblastopenia of childhood with CD10, TdT, and cytoplasmic μ lymphocyte positivity in bone marrow. *J Clin Pathol*, **43**, 857–859.
5 O'Brien H, Amess JAL and Mollin DL (1982) Recurrent thrombocytopenia, erythroid hypoplasia and sideroblastic anaemia associated with hypothermia. *Br J Haematol*, **51**, 451–456.
6 Cohen H, Walker H, Delhanty JDA, Lucas SB and Huehns ER (1991) Congenital spherocytosis, B19 parvovirus infection and inherited interstitial deletion of the short arm of chromosome 8. *Br J Haematol*, **78**, 251–257.
7 Chusid MJ, Dale DC, West BC and Wolff SM (1975) The hypereosinophilic syndrome. *Medicine*, **54**, 1–27.
8 Thiele J and Fischer R (1991) Megakaryocytopoiesis in haematological disorders: diagnostic features of bone marrow biopsies. *Virchows Archiv (A)* **418**, 87–97.

8: Miscellaneous Disorders

THE EFFECT OF ANTI-CANCER CHEMOTHERAPY

The majority of anti-cancer and immunosuppressive chemotherapeutic agents are damaging to the bone marrow. Most cause hypoplasia, some cause megaloblastosis and some have other more specific effects. The nature of the bone marrow damage depends on dose and duration of therapy. A drug may, for example, cause erythroid hyperplasia and megaloblastic erythropoiesis at a low dose and severe hypoplasia at a higher dose.

Peripheral blood

The most prominent effect of anti-cancer chemotherapy is pancytopenia. This is usual with all the commonly employed agents, the exceptions being vincristine and bleomycin. Neutropenia and thrombocytopenia are apparent well in advance of anaemia. Some degree of anisocytosis and poikilocytosis together with basophilic stippling and Howell–Jolly bodies occur as a consequence of the dyserythropoiesis induced by chemotherapeutic agents. When a megaloblastic change is induced, formation of Howell–Jolly bodies is more marked and macrocytosis is common. Dysplastic changes, including abnormalities of nuclear shape and nuclear inclusions within the cytoplasm, may also be apparent in neutrophils. Platelets are small but do not show any specific morphological abnormality.

Vincristine is unusual in occasionally causing thrombocytosis, although not when it is given in combination with other drugs which are highly toxic to the bone marrow.

Occasionally chemotherapy is followed by the development of microangiopathic haemolytic anaemia. This appears to be particularly a feature of therapy with mitomycin C.

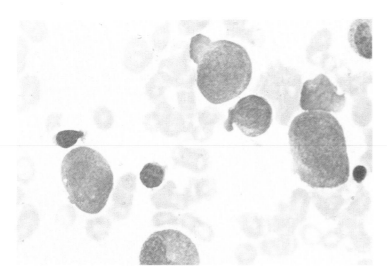

Fig. 8.1 BM aspirate from a patient with severe methotrexate toxicity showing 'maturation arrest'; two promyelocytes and one proerythroblast are seen but maturing cells were severely diminished. MGG × 940.

Bone marrow cytology

The bone marrow aspirate shows a variable degree of hypoplasia. If bone marrow aspiration is performed after an episode of severe hypoplasia early regeneration may produce appearances misinterpreted as 'maturation arrest' (Fig. 8.1). Erythropoiesis is dysplastic, often strikingly so. Drugs which cause megaloblastosis include methotrexate, cyclophosphamide, daunorubicin, adriamycin, cytosine arabinoside, hydroxyurea and azathioprine. The megaloblastosis induced by anti-cancer chemotherapeutic agents, with the exception of folate antagonists, differs from that due to vitamin B_{12} or folate deficiency in that dyserythropoiesis is very striking and hypersegmented neutrophils and giant metamyelocytes are not usually a feature. Depending on drug dose, megaloblastosis may be associated with erythroid hyperplasia (Fig. 8.2) or hypoplasia. Other drugs cause dysplastic features without megaloblastosis. Erythroid dysplasia may be striking, both with megaloblastic and with normoblastic erythropoiesis. Vincristine and other spindle poisons cause mitotic arrest in quite a high proportion of erythroblasts; this is detected if a bone marrow aspirate is done one to two days after the administration of chemotherapy (Fig. 8.3).

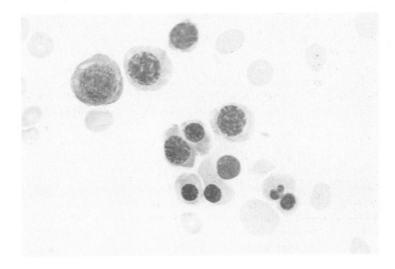

Fig. 8.2 BM aspirate, from a patient taking hydroxyurea for psoriasis, showing erythroid hyperplasia, mild megaloblastosis and one dyserythropoietic cell. MGG × 940.

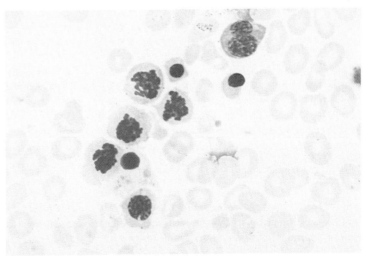

Fig. 8.3 BM aspirate, performed about 24 hours after administration of vincristine, showing a binucleate erythroblast and four erythroblasts arrested in mitosis. MGG × 940.

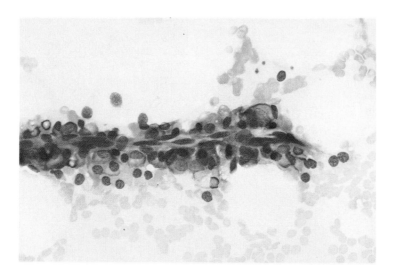

Fig. 8.4 BM aspirate, post-chemotherapy (for AML), showing plasma cells surrounding a capillary in a severely hypoplastic bone marrow. MGG × 377.

Bone marrow histology

Cells exposed to chemotherapeutic agents show karyorrhexis followed by karyolysis. Dead cells degenerate to granular eosinophilic debris. With intensive chemotherapy, depletion of haemopoietic cells is severe and stromal elements become prominent. There are dilated sinusoids containing red cells and fibrin,[1] and sometimes residual lymphocytes and plasma cells, the latter particularly along small blood vessels. Red cells may be extravasated from dilated sinusoids.

In the majority of patients treated with intensive chemotherapy for acute leukaemia[1,2] the marrow is almost completely emptied of haemopoietic cells, particularly when therapy is of the type used in AML. Minor degrees of serous atrophy (gelatinous transformation) (see page 63) sometimes occur. Some patients have collagen deposition, increased osteoblastic activity and focal appositional bone formation.[1] Prominent residual plasma cells (Fig. 8.4) are more a feature of AML than of ALL.[2] Cellular depletion persists for three to four weeks, to be followed by regeneration of fat cells, which are initially small and multiloculated, then by regeneration haemopoietic cells. Erythroid and megakaryocytic regeneration occurs before granulocytic regeneration (Figs 8.5 and 8.6). In the early stages of regeneration clusters of haemopoietic precursors made up of cells from a single lineage (Fig. 8.5) are often seen.

IRRADIATION

Irradiation of a significant proportion of the bone marrow causes a fall in the neutrophil and platelet counts. Extensive irradiation causes pancytopenia. Monitoring of blood counts is therefore carried out during radiotherapy.

Peripheral blood

The blood film may show neutropenia, thrombocytopenia and the features of anaemia.

Bone marrow cytology

The initial change in irradiated bone marrow is pyknosis and karyorrhexis of haemopoietic cells followed by disappearance of haemopoietic and fat cells and replacement by areas of gelatinous transformation. Subsequently, at the site of irradiation there is hypoplastic marrow with haemopoietic cells being replaced by fat. Extensive high-dose irradiation of the bone marrow is followed by aplastic anaemia.

Bone marrow histology

Initially, there may be necrosis of the bone marrow within the field which has received high-dose radiation. Subsequently gelatinous transformation may occur. Later, there is permanent

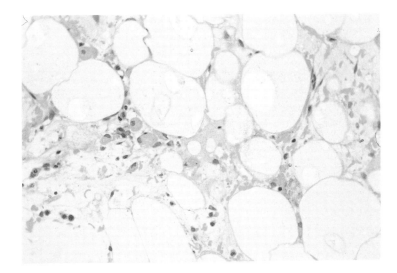

Fig. 8.5 BM trephine biopsy, regeneration post-chemotherapy, showing decreased cellularity, oedema and a cluster of immature regenerating megakaryocytes. Plastic-embedded, H&E × 195.

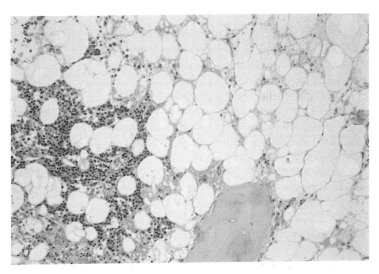

Fig. 8.6 BM trephine biopsy, regeneration post-chemotherapy, showing an area of marked hypocellularity and a large poorly formed erythroid island. Paraffin-embedded, H&E × 97.

replacement of haemopoietic marrow by fat or fibrous tissue.

APLASTIC ANAEMIA

Aplastic anaemia is a heterogeneous disorder characterized by pancytopenia and a hypocellular marrow without any apparent underlying neoplastic process. The name, although well established, is somewhat misleading since all haemopoietic lineages are involved. Aplastic anaemia is rare. In Europe and North America the incidence is of the order of 5–10/1 000 000/year but in various other parts of the world, for example in Asia, the disease is considerably more common. Although some cases are inherited and develop in infancy or childhood, the incidence, in general, increases with age.

The commonest inherited form of aplastic anaemia is Fanconi's anaemia. This is an autosomal recessive condition in which sufferers have defective DNA repair mechanisms. The pancytopenia usually develops between the ages of five and 10 years. Without bone marrow transplantation many patients die from infection or bleeding but approximately 20 per cent develop acute myeloid leukaemia.[3] Other inherited disorders which may progress to aplastic anaemia include dyskeratosis congenita, the Shwachman–Diamond syndrome and amegakaryocytic thrombocytopenia without physical defects.[4]

Known causes of acquired aplastic anaemia include viral hepatitis and exposure to irradiation, drugs (such as chloramphenicol) and chemicals (such as benzene). In many cases the cause is not apparent.

The relationship of aplastic anaemia to hypocellular MDS is problematical since neoplastic clones arise in some cases of aplastic anaemia and may be predictive of subsequent MDS and AML. It may be that hypocellular MDS represents an intermediate stage of evolution of typical aplastic anaemia to MDS[4] or to AML. Aplastic anaemia can also progress through typical hypercellular MDS to AML.[5] Of long-term survivors of aplastic anaemia the number who develop MDS and AML may be as high as 10 per cent.[6] The relationship of aplastic anaemia to paroxysmal nocturnal haemoglobinuria is discussed below.

The diagnosis of aplastic anaemia may be suspected on peripheral blood and bone marrow aspirate findings but a trephine biopsy is essential for diagnosis. This is because of the difficulty in aspiration which is often experienced and the variable degree of hypoplasia in different areas of the marrow. A trephine biopsy is particularly important in distinguishing aplastic anaemia from hypoplastic MDS and from other conditions which lead to a bone marrow aspirate being hypocellular. If bone marrow examination does not confirm a strong clinical suspicion of aplastic anaemia repeat examination at another site is indicated since the bone marrow may be affected in an uneven manner.

Peripheral blood

Severe cases are characterized by pancytopenia and a low reticulocyte count. The lymphocyte count is also low. The anaemia may be normocytic or macrocytic and poikilocytes may be present. Neutrophils often have dark red granules and high alkaline phosphatase activity, even in the absence of any apparent infection. Platelets are of normal size, in contrast to the large platelets which are common when thrombocytopenia is due to increased platelet destruction.

Bone marrow cytology

The bone marrow may be difficult to aspirate with the result being a 'dry tap' or 'blood tap'. In the majority of patients a hypocellular aspirate is obtained with the fragments being composed largely of fat (Fig. 8.7) and the cell trails also being hypocellular. Different lineages are affected to a variable extent so that the M : E ratio may be increased, normal or decreased. Dyserythropoiesis

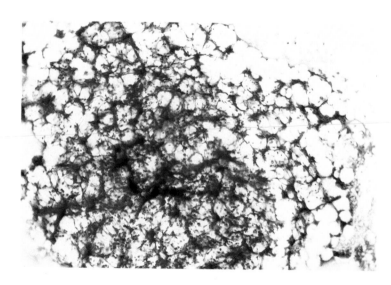

Fig. 8.7 BM aspirate, aplastic anaemia, showing a severely hypoplastic fragment. MGG × 94.

may be seen. Ring sideroblasts are not a feature but otherwise the changes seen can be similar to those observed in the myelodysplastic syndromes.[7,8] Dysplastic changes in granulocytes are less common and pseudo-Pelger neutrophils are not a feature. There is no disproportionate increase in immature granulocyte precursors. Megakaryocytes are often so infrequent in the aspirate that it is difficult to assess their morphology.

In a minority of patients the aspirate is normocellular or even hypercellular.[7,8] Examination of trephine biopsies from such patients shows that such 'hot spots' coexist with extensive areas of hypoplastic marrow.

The bone marrow aspirate shows at least a relative increase in lymphocytes and sometimes an absolute increase. There may also be increased numbers of plasma cells, macrophages and mast cells. Foamy macrophages are sometimes present and macrophage iron is increased.

Bone marrow histology

Trephine biopsy has a major role in the diagnosis of aplastic anaemia. The bone marrow is usually hypocellular with a marked reduction of haemopoietic cells (Figs 8.8 to 8.10). Myeloid cells are mainly replaced by fat but there is a variable inflammatory infiltrate composed of lymphocytes, plasma cells, macrophages, mast cells and sometimes eosinophils[9] (Fig. 8.9). Necrotic cells and cellular debris may be present. Walls of sinusoids may be disrupted and there may be oedema and haemorrhage. In some patients the inflammatory infiltrate is so heavy that the marked reduction of haemopoietic cells is not immediately apparent. Sinusoids are reduced but arterioles and capillaries are normal or increased.[10] Residual erythroid cells show dysplastic features.[9] Iron stores are increased.

A minority of cases have some areas of normal or increased cellularity. Such cellular areas are commonly adjacent to sinusoids[10] and are composed of erythroid cells, all at the same stage of development and showing dysplastic features.[8] This finding is more common in Fanconi's anaemia (Fig. 8.10).

Reticulin shows little if any increase. Various abnormalities of bone have been reported. Some studies have found osteoporosis and others increased osteoblastic and osteoclastic activity and irregular remodelling of bone.[9]

When aplastic anaemia remits, for example following therapy with anti-thymocyte or anti-lymphocyte globulin, dysplastic features are very evident[11,12] and the inflammatory infiltrate often persists.[12]

In the differential diagnosis of hypoplastic MDS and aplastic anaemia the most important feature is the presence of clusters of blasts which are indicative of the former diagnosis. Other features

Fig. 8.8 BM trephine biopsy, aplastic anaemia, showing marked hypocellularity. Plastic-embedded, H&E × 39.

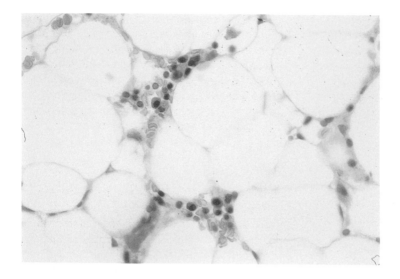

Fig. 8.9 BM trephine biopsy, aplastic anaemia, showing a marked reduction in haemopoietic precursors; many of the remaining cells are plasma cells. Plastic-embedded, H&E × 390.

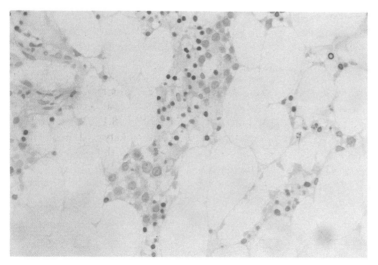

Fig. 8.10 BM trephine biopsy, Fanconi's anaemia, showing large, poorly formed erythroblastic islands containing increased numbers of early erythroblasts. Plastic-embedded, H&E × 188.

which have been found, to some extent, to be predictive of progression to AML and which can therefore be considered to favour a diagnosis of hypocellular MDS are: (i) trilineage atypia, particularly megakaryocyte atypia (ii) increased numbers or clustering of megakaryocytes, and (iii) reticulin fibrosis.[5] In Fanconi's anaemia the development of trilineage dysplasia and reticulin fibrosis may herald transformation to AML. Otherwise there is little relationship between histological features and prognosis. Assessment of cellularity has not been found particularly useful in this regard and an initial suggestion that

the extent of the inflammatory infiltrate was of prognostic importance[9] was not substantiated in three large series of patients treated either with antithymocyte globulin or by bone marrow transplantation.[12,13]

OTHER CAUSES OF BONE MARROW APLASIA AND HYPOPLASIA

Reversible aplasia follows intensive cytotoxic chemotherapy. Transient bone marrow aplasia may precede ALL with the leukaemia supervening some months after remission of the aplasia. In subjects unable to mount a normal immune response to the EB virus, primary infection by the virus may cause bone marrow aplasia. Bone marrow aplasia is also one of the features of graft-versus-host disease (see below).

Other causes of bone marrow hypoplasia include starvation, anorexia nervosa, severe hypothyroidism and copper deficiency.

PAROXYSMAL NOCTURNAL HAEMOGLOBINURIA

Paroxysmal nocturnal haemoglobinuria (PNH) is a heterogeneous disease, the essential feature of which is abnormal complement sensitivity of red cells. This leads, *in vitro*, to lysis of cells when serum is acidified and, *in vivo*, to intravascular haemolysis which is often nocturnal. PNH is a clonal disorder consequent on a somatic mutation in a multipotent myeloid stem cell. In the majority of cases, cells of the abnormal clone coexist with normal polyclonal haemopoietic cells; in a minority the PNH clone constitutes virtually all haemopoietic tissue.[14] About a quarter of cases of PNH evolve to aplastic anaemia.[4] Conversely, five to 10 per cent of patients with aplastic anaemia acquire a PNH clone during the course of their illness, often with associated clinical improvement.[4,14] In a small percentage of cases of PNH there is evolution to acute myeloid leukaemia. The specific PNH defect of red cells

leading to a positive acid lysis has also been observed, occasionally, in patients with other clonal disorders of haemopoiesis including MDS (sideroblastic anaemia and RAEB) and myeloproliferative disorders (myelofibrosis and unclassified MPD). Recovery of PNH can occur with the abnormal clone disappearing and being replaced by normal polyclonal haemopoietic cells.

Peripheral blood

PNH is characterized by some degree of chronic haemolysis with episodes of more severe haemolysis. Red cells do not show any morphological abnormalities other than polychromasia associated with an elevated reticulocyte count. Some patients have neutropenia, thrombocytopenia or both. Neutrophil alkaline phosphatase activity is typically low or absent.

Bone marrow cytology

The most characteristic bone marrow abnormality is hypercellularity due at least in part to erythroid hyperplasia (Fig. 8.11); there is often also granulocytic and megakaryocytic hyperplasia. However, in some patients the specific red cell abnormality of PNH occurs in a patient with bone marrow hypoplasia. Mast cells may be increased.

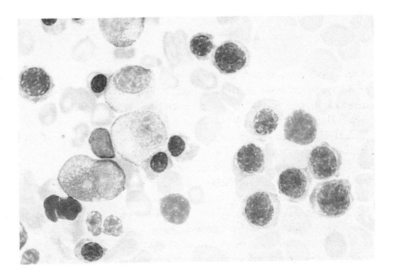

Fig. 8.11 BM aspirate, paroxysmal nocturnal haemoglobinuria, showing erythroid hyperplasia and somewhat abnormal chromatin pattern. MGG × 940.

Bone marrow histology

A trephine biopsy may show hyperplasia or hypoplasia.

BONE MARROW TRANSPLANTATION

Since bone marrow transplantation necessitates prior immunosuppression and often also ablative chemotherapy the haematological features of bone marrow aplasia precede the signs of bone marrow engraftment. Bone marrow transplantation may be complicated by rejection, by graft-versus-host disease, by sepsis or by EBV-triggered lymphoproliferative disease so that patients show the effects of a variety of pathological processes.[15] A bone marrow biopsy is generally more informative than the peripheral blood or bone marrow aspirate.

Peripheral blood

Initially there is a period of two to three weeks of severe pancytopenia, followed by a gradual rise of white cell and platelet counts as engraftment occurs. If there is failure of engraftment or if rejection occurs there is a failure of counts to rise or a subsequent fall. If patients develop EBV-triggered lymphoproliferative disease following transplantation the peripheral blood film may be leucoerythroblastic and show atypical immature lymphoid cells.

Bone marrow cytology

The bone marrow aspirate is initially severely hypoplastic. Subsequently haemopoietic cells gradually reappear. Dysplastic features may be present. In the months following transplantation an appreciable increase may occur in cells which morphologically and immunophenotypically resemble lymphoblasts of L1 ALL;[16] with prolonged follow-up these are no longer apparent. If rejection occurs the abnormalities noted include lymphocytosis, plasmacytosis, increased macrophages and increased iron stores.[15] EBV-triggered lymphoproliferative disease is associated with bone marrow infiltration by highly atypical immature lymphoid cells including bizarre plasmacytoid lymphocytes.

Bone marrow histology[15,17-19]

During the first two weeks cellularity is very low. Thereafter clusters of proliferating cells appear at a variable rate (Fig. 8.12). In the early stages of engraftment the foci of regenerating cells commonly contain cells of only one lineage, and cells may be all at the same stage of development. The topography may be abnormal so that foci

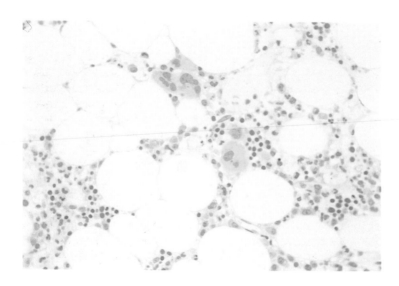

Fig. 8.12 BM trephine biopsy, regeneration following bone marrow transplantation; note cluster of megakaryocytes. Plastic-embedded, H&E × 195.

of granulopoiesis are sometimes present in the intertrabecular area rather than in a paratrabecular position. Megakaryocytes are often clustered. Haemopoietic cells may be dysplastic. Commonly there are stromal changes such as oedema, the presence of foamy macrophages, formation of small granulomas, sinusoidal ectasia and extravasation of red cells into the interstitium; these are probably a result of damage caused by the ablative therapy employed prior to grafting and are more marked in patients transplanted for leukaemia. There may also be lymphoid foci, sometimes with associated eosinophils. If rejection occurs the trephine biopsy may show oedema and fat necrosis, in addition to the features apparent in the aspirate which have been mentioned above. When bone marrow transplantation is complicated by EBV-triggered lymphoproliferative disease an infiltrate by atypical immature lymphocytes is apparent. Rarely immunoblastic lymphoma has supervened.

GRAFT-VERSUS-HOST DISEASE

Graft-versus-host disease (GVHD) usually results from transfer of viable histo-incompatible lymphocytes from a donor into an immunosuppressed host. It may also occur in immunologically normal hosts when lymphocytes are from a donor who is homozygous for an HLA haplotype identical to one of the host's haplotypes; the host is then unable to recognize the recipient's lymphocytes as foreign and so cannot destroy them whereas the tranfused lymphocytes are capable of recognizing and attacking host tissues. GVHD in immunologically normal hosts has most often resulted from transfusions from closely related family members.

The bone marrow features of GVHD differ depending on whether bone marrow has been transplanted or not. When viable lymphocytes only have been transferred the host's bone marrow will be among the tissues which are immunologically attacked and bone marrow aplasia results. In patients who have received donor bone marrow containing viable lymphocytes other tissues are attacked but since the bone marrow is donor in origin it will not be recognized as foreign by donor lymphocytes. The haemopoietic marrow may, however, be indirectly damaged by the immunological reaction between donor cells and host cells including the bone marrow stroma.

It has been suggested that Omenn's syndrome, a condition of infants characterized by combined immunodeficiency and signs suggestive of GVHD, may represent GVHD consequent on transplacental passage of lymphocytes.[20]

Peripheral blood

In patients who have received histo-incompatible donor lymphocytes the consequent bone marrow hypoplasia is reflected in peripheral blood pancytopenia. In bone marrow transplant recipients there are no specific peripheral blood features which indicate the occurrence of GVHD but there is a delay in the appearance of signs of engraftment.

Bone marrow cytology

The bone marrow aspirate is usually hypocellular.

Bone marrow histology

When donor lymphocytes have been transferred without donor bone marrow histological sections of trephine biopsies show aplasia. In GVHD in the setting of bone marrow transplantation histological abnormalities seen include a decrease in haemopoietic cells, increased macrophages, erythrophagocytosis, oedema and perivenous lymphoid infiltrates.[17]

Storage diseases and storage cells in the bone marrow[21-25]

In various inherited diseases the deficiency of an enzyme leads to accumulation of a metabolite in body cells, often in macrophages. The morphologically abnormal bone marrow macrophages containing an excess of the relevant metabolite are referred to as storage cells. Storage cells may also result from an abnormal load of a metabolite such that the enzymes of normal cells are unable to cope. Both bone marrow aspirates and trephine biopsies are useful in the detection of storage diseases. Peripheral blood cells may show related abnormalities.[21,26]

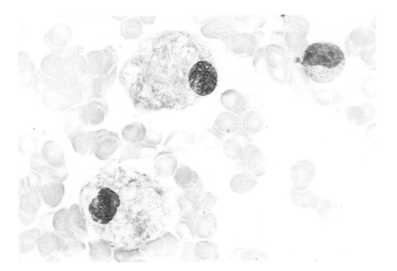

Fig. 8.13 BM aspirate, Gaucher's disease, showing two Gaucher's cells. MGG × 377.

GAUCHER'S DISEASE

Gaucher's disease (hereditary glucosyl ceramide lipidosis) is an inherited condition in which glucocerebrosides accumulate in macrophages including those in the liver, spleen and bone marrow. Although Gaucher's disease can be readily diagnosed by bone marrow aspiration and by trephine biopsy it has been pointed out that this is unnecessary when assays for the relevant enzyme, β-glucocerebrosidase, are available.[27] Gaucher's disease can be transferred to the host by bone marrow transplantation.[28]

Peripheral blood

There are usually no specific peripheral blood features although very occasionally Gaucher's cells may be seen in the peripheral blood, particularly after splenectomy. Pancytopenia develops slowly, as a consequence of hypersplenism. The monocytes of patients with Gaucher's disease are positive for tartrate-resistant acid phosphatase (TRAP) activity whereas normal monocytes are not.[28]

Bone marrow cytology

Gaucher cells are large, round or oval cells with a small, usually eccentric nucleus and voluminous weakly basophilic cytoplasm with a wrinkled or fibrillar or 'onion-skin' pattern (Fig. 8.13). The cells stain with SBB and PAS. They are TRAP-positive and may be positive for iron, particularly in older children and adults. Patients with Gaucher's disease may also have an increase in foamy macrophages and in cells which resemble typical Gaucher cells but also contain more strongly basophilic granules.

Bone marrow histology

Gaucher's cells may be isolated or appear in clumps or sheets, sometimes replacing large areas of the marrow (Fig. 8.14). The cells have abundant pale-staining cytoplasm with a texture that has been likened to watered silk or crumpled tissue paper. There may be an increase in reticulin and collagen deposition.[25]

PSEUDO-GAUCHER CELLS

Cells resembling Gaucher cells but not identical to them on ultrastructural examination[22] are seen in the bone marrow in a variety of haematological conditions[23,24] in which they result from an abnormal load of glucocerebroside presented to macrophages. They are seen in chronic granulocytic leukaemia (Fig. 8.15) acute leukaemia, thalassaemia major and congenital dyserythropoietic anaemia and have been recognized in occasional patients with Hodgkin's disease, non-Hodgkin's lymphoma and a variety of other con-

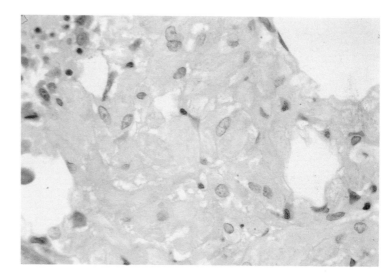

Fig. 8.14 BM trephine biopsy, Gaucher's disease, showing a sheet of large macrophages with characteristic 'watered silk' texture to their cytoplasm. Plastic-embedded, H&E × 390.

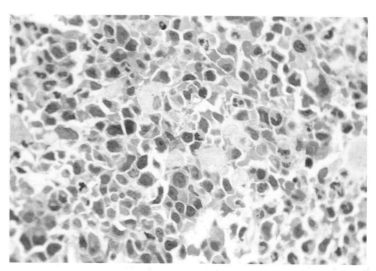

Fig. 8.15 BM trephine biopsy, chronic granulocytic leukaemia, showing granulocytic hyperplasia and several pseudo-Gaucher cells. Plastic-embedded, H&E × 390.

ditions.[23,29] Morphologically similar cells have been seen in multiple myeloma and in lymphoplasmacytoid lymphoma but the macrophages in these cases may contain material derived from immunoglobulin rather than glucocerebroside.[29] Cells considered to resemble Gaucher cells have also been reported in the bone marrow of a patient with atypical mycobacterial infection complicating AIDS;[30] in this case it appears that the abnormal morphology was consequent on large numbers of mycobacteria packing the macrophage cytoplasm rather than on storage of a breakdown product.

NEIMAN–PICK DISEASE

Neiman–Pick disease is an inherited condition (sphingomyelin lipidosis) characterized by the presence of foamy lipid-containing macrophages in the bone marrow and other tissues.

Peripheral blood

Lipid-containing monocytes and lymphocytes may be present in the peripheral blood. Anaemia and various cytopenias may occur as a consequence of hypersplenism.

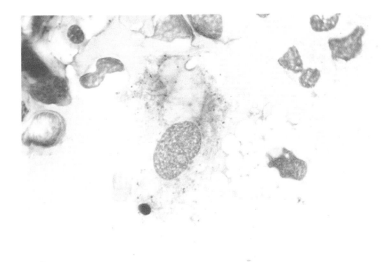

Fig. 8.16 BM aspirate, sickle cell anaemia, showing a foamy macrophage and a sea-blue histiocyte containing a clump of red cells. MGG × 940.

Bone marrow cytology

The foamy macrophages of Nieman–Pick disease are large cells (exceeding 50 μm in diameter) with a nucleus which is usually central. They stain pale blue with Romanowsky stains and variably with PAS and lipid stains. There are also increased numbers of sea-blue histiocytes (see below), possibly reflecting slow conversion of sphingomyelin to ceroid.[23]

Bone marrow histology

The foam cells appear yellow-green on Giemsa and light brown on an H&E stain; they are PAS-positive and usually positive for iron.[25]

OTHER CAUSES OF FOAMY MACROPHAGES[24]

Other metabolic defects which can lead to the presence of increased numbers of foamy macrophages in the bone marrow include hypercholesterolaemia, hyperchylomicronaemia, Wolman's disease, late-onset cholesteryl ester storage disease, Fabry's disease, neuronal lipofuscinosis (Batten's disease) and Tangier disease. In Fabry's disease the storage cells have small globular inclusions which are weakly basophilic on a Romanowsky stain and lightly eosinophilic on H&E; they are PAS-negative and SBB-positive.[31]

Foam cells are also increased as a result of damage to fat cells (Fig. 8.16) including trauma, fat necrosis, bone marrow infarction, infection, pancreatitis and previous performance of a bone marrow biopsy at the same site. Acquired diseases which have been associated with an increase of foamy macrophages include histiocytosis X (Hand–Schüller–Christian disease, Letterer–Siwe disease and eosinophilic granuloma), bone marrow metastases (Fig. 8.17) and a variety of other conditions.[23] Foam cells have been noted in subjects who have, in the past, received polyvinyl pyrrolidine as a plasma expander; in this instance the foam cells are strongly PAS-positive.[32]

MACROPHAGES CONTAINING CHOLESTEROL CRYSTALS

Bone marrow macrophages may contain cholesterol crystals in various hyperlipidaemic conditions, both congenital and acquired. Such conditions include alpha-lipoprotein deficiency, hyperbeta-lipoproteinaemia, poorly controlled diabetes mellitus and hypothyroidism.[33] The cholesterol crystals are soluble and thus appear as negative images within the macrophages.

SEA-BLUE HISTIOCYTOSIS

Sea-blue histiocytosis[34] is an inherited condition

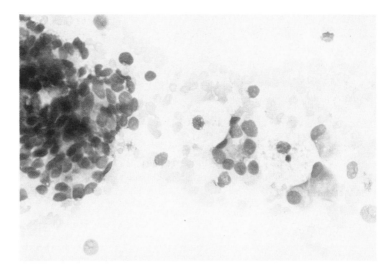

Fig. 8.17 BM aspirate, carcinoma of prostate, showing a clump of carcinoma cells, dispersed carcinoma cells, two osteoblasts and two foamy macrophages. MGG × 377.

characterized by the presence of 'sea-blue histiocytes' — distinctive macrophages containing ceroid or lipofuscin — in the bone marrow, liver, spleen and other organs. The designation of the disease derives from the staining characteristics of the storage cells on a Romanowsky stain. On unstained smears ceroid is brown.

Bone marrow cytology

Sea-blue histiocytes stain blue or blue-green on a Romanowsky stain. They are SBB-, PAS- and oil-red-O-positive and are sometimes positive for iron.

Bone marrow histology

Sea-blue histiocytes are brownish-yellow on an H&E stain and blue on a Giemsa stain. They are PAS-positive and positive for iron. They are acid-fast and exhibit auto-fluorescence.

OTHER CAUSES OF SEA-BLUE HISTIOCYTES

Increased numbers of sea-blue histiocytes are seen in the bone marrow in a great variety of conditions[34] including many of the conditions in which pseudo-Gaucher cells are present or foamy macrophages are increased (Figs 8.16 and 8.18).

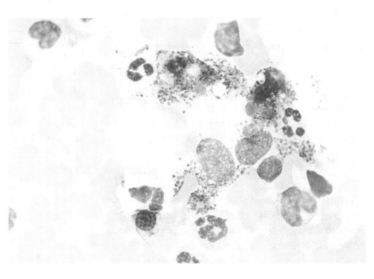

Fig. 8.18 BM aspirate, sea-blue histiocytes in a patient with auto-immune thrombocytopenic purpura. MGG × 940.

CYSTINOSIS

Peripheral blood

There are no specific abnormalities in the peripheral blood.

Bone marrow cytology

Bone marrow histiocytes are packed with almost colourless, refractile crystals of various shapes. They are best seen under polarized light when they are birefringent.

Bone marrow histology

Crystals dissolve out of histological sections leaving a negative image.

MUCOPOLYSACCHARIDOSES

The mucopolysaccharidoses are inherited diseases characterized by the storage of various mucopolysaccharides.[21]

Peripheral blood

Peripheral blood neutrophils may show the Alder–Reilly anomaly.[21,26] Lymphocytes may either be vacuolated or contain abnormal granules which stain metachromatically with toluidine blue.

Bone marrow cytology

Bone marrow macrophages contain abnormal metachromatic granules.[21]

Bone marrow histology

On histological preparations macrophages appear foamy as mucopolysaccharides are water-soluble.

HYPEROXALURIA[35,36]

Hyperoxaluria or oxalosis is a metabolic disorder in which oxalate is deposited in various tissues including the bone, bone marrow, liver, spleen and kidneys. Renal deposition leads to renal failure. The introduction of haemodialysis has pro-

longed life in these patients and has permitted advanced bone marrow lesions to become apparent.

Peripheral blood

There is anaemia as a consequence of renal failure. Hypersplenism also contributes to anaemia and may cause pancytopenia. Deposition of oxalate in the bone marrow further aggravates anaemia and other cytopenias and causes a leuco-erythroblastic blood film.

Bone marrow biopsy

Intertrabecular bone marrow is extensively replaced by needle-like crystals arranged in a radial pattern. There are variable numbers of epithelioid cells and multinucleated cells, including foreign body giant cells, present at the periphery of the crystalline deposits, and engulfing crystals. The surrounding bone marrow shows mild fibrosis.

DEPOSITION OF FOREIGN SUBSTANCES

Foreign substances may be deposited in the bone marrow, principally in bone marrow macrophages. Such substances may be apparent in bone marrow aspirates and in trephine biopsies. There are not usually any associated peripheral blood abnormalities.

In anthracosis there is widespread deposition of anthracotic pigment in body macrophages including those of the bone marrow. Large aggregates of dense black particles are apparent.[37] Silica and anthracotic pigment are often co-deposited. Silica crystals are detected by their birefringence. There may be consequent granuloma formation.

Occasional patients are still seen who have, in the past, been exposed to Thorotrast as a radiographic medium. Thorotrast within macrophages appears as a pale grey refractile material. Bone marrow abnormalities associated with the presence of Thorotrast include hypoplasia, hyperplasia, fibrosis and the development of MDS, acute leukaemia and haemangioendothelioma.[38] The peripheral blood film may be bizarre because of the combined effects of bone marrow fibrosis and Thorotrast-induced splenic atropy.

VASCULAR AND INTRAVASCULAR LESIONS[24,39]

The bone marrow vasculature may be altered as a consequence of bone marrow diseases but in addition the blood vessels within the marrow, particularly arterioles and capillaries, may be involved in a variety of generalized diseases. The peripheral blood film may show related abnormalities but in general the bone marrow aspirate does not give relevant information and a trephine biopsy is necessary to show the lesion.

Peripheral blood

The peripheral blood shows red cell fragments in patients with thrombotic thrombocytopenia purpura or with micro-angiopathic haemolytic anaemia as a consequence of disseminated malignancy. Eosinophilia may be a feature of some types of vasculitis and of cholesterol embolism which may involve the marrow as well as other tissues. Leucocytosis and an elevated erythrocyte sedimentation rate have also been associated with cholesterol embolism. The peripheral blood film may show pancytopenia and leucoerythroblastic features in patients with bone marrow necrosis as a consequence of vascular occlusion.

Bone marrow aspirate

There are no specific abnormalities in the bone marrow aspirate in patients with vascular lesions.

Bone marrow histology

In patients with generalized atherosclerosis the bone marrow arterioles may show arteriosclerotic changes. Embolism of atheromatous material to bone marrow vessels may occur; the embolus may be acellular or composed of hyaline material or cholesterol crystals.[40,41] Bone marrow emboli are present at autopsy in about 10 per cent of patients with generalized cholesterol embolism.[40] Vessels are partly or totally occluded by this material and by the granulomatous tissue which develops as a reaction to it. Any cholesterol crystals appear as empty clefts. Vasculitic lesions are seen in polyarteritis nodosa, with fibrinoid necrosis being a feature. In patients with hypersensitivity reactions to drugs a granulomatous vasculitis may occur. Intravascular and subendothelial hyaline deposits may be seen in bone marrow capillaries in thrombotic thrombocytopenic purpura. In patients with micro-angiopathic haemolytic anaemia as a consequence of disseminated carcinoma, the bone marrow capillaries, like other capillaries, may contain tumour thrombi. In patients with sickle cell disease, sickle cells are usually present in sinusoids. During sickling crises there may also be thrombotic lesions and associated areas of bone marrow necrosis. Sickle cells may also be present in autopsy specimens from patients with sickle cell trait; their presence does not have any particular significance. Thrombi may also be noted in vessels in other patients with bone marrow necrosis.

LANGERHANS' CELL HISTIOCYTOSIS (HISTIOCYTOSIS X)

Langerhans' cell histiocytosis (histiocytosis X) is a heterogeneous disease or group of diseases of uncertain nature characterized by proliferation of Langerhans' cells.[42] Localized and disseminated forms occur. Haematological involvement occurs in the disseminated forms of the disease, which in the past have been referred to by the eponymous terms Letterer–Siwe disease of infants and Hand–Schüller–Christian disease.

Peripheral blood

Pancytopenia occurs as a consequence of hypersplenism as well as bone marrow infiltration.

Bone marrow cytology[33,43]

The bone marrow aspirate may show Langerhans' cells together with a mixed population including eosinophils, monocytes, lipid-laden macrophages, lymphocytes and plasma cells. Haemophagocytosis may occur. Langerhans' cells are large and slightly irregular in shape. The nucleus is somewhat irregular with delicately clumped chromatin and inconspicuous nucleoli. The cytoplasm is weakly basophilic with occasional azurophilic granules.

Bone marrow histology

In those cases with marrow involvement the bone marrow contains clusters or sheets of Langerhans' cells together with eosinophils, monocytes, phagocytic macrophages, lipid-laden macrophages and giant cells. Xanthomatous transformation and fibrosis may occur.[33,43] Langerhans' cells have a characteristic appearance; the nuclei are usually convoluted or twisted and longitudinal grooves may be present. Immunohistochemical staining shows them to express S100 protein, although only a small proportion of cells may stain positively in some cases. Staining with the lectin peanut agglutinin gives a characteristic staining pattern of a cytoplasmic halo with a para-nuclear dot.

REFERENCES

1 Wittels B (1980) Bone marrow biopsy changes following chemotherapy for acute leukemia. *Am J Surg Pathol*, **4**, 135–142.

2 Brody JP, Krause JR and Panchansky L (1985) Bone marrow response to chemotherapy in acute lymphocytic and acute non-lymphocytic leukaemia. *Scand J Haematol*, **35**, 240–245.

3 Gordon-Smith EC and Rutherford T (1989) Fanconi's anaemia — constitutional, familial aplastic anaemia. *Baillière's Clin Haematol*, **2**, 139–152.

4 Marsh JCW and Geary CG (1991) Is aplastic anaemia a pre-leukaemic disorder? *Br J Haematol*, **77**, 447–452.

5 Fohlmeister I, Fischer R, Mödder B, Rister M and Schaefer H-E (1985) Aplastic anaemia and the hypocellular myelodysplastic syndrome: histomorphological, diagnostic, and prognostic features. *J Clin Pathol*, **38**, 1218–1224.

6 de Planque MM, Kluin-Nelemans JC, Van Krieken HJK, *et al.* (1988) Evolution of acquired severe aplastic anaemia to myelodyplasia and subsequent leukaemia. *Br J Haematol*, **70**, 55–62.

7 Frisch B and Lewis SM (1974) The bone marrow in aplastic anaemia: diagnostic and prognostic features. *J Clin Pathol*, **27**, 231–241.

8 Kansu E and Erslev AJ (1976) Aplastic anaemia with 'hot pockets'. *Scand J Haematol*, **17**, 326–334.

9 te Velde J and Haak HL (1977) Histological investigation of methacrylate embedded bone marrow biopsy specimens: correlation with survival after conventional treatment in 15 adult patients. *Br J Haematol*, **35**, 61–69.

10 Burkhardt R, Frisch B and Bartl B (1982) Bone biopsy in haematological disorders. *J Clin Pathol*, **35**, 257–284.

11 Tichelli A, Gratwohl A, Würsh A, Nissen C and Speck B (1988) Late haematological complications in severe aplastic anaemia. *Br J Haematol*, **69**, 413–418.

12 de Planque MM, Van Krieken JHJM, Kluin-Nelemans HC, *et al.* (1989) Bone marrow histopathology of patients with severe aplastic anaemia before treatment and at follow-up. *Br J Haematol*, **72**, 439–444.

13 Sale GE, Rajantie J, Doney K, Appelbaum FR, Storb R and Thomas ED (1987) Does histologic grading of inflammation in bone marrow predict the response of aplastic anaemia patients to antithymocyte globulin therapy? *Br J Haematol*, **67**, 261–266.

14 Rotoli B and Luzzatto L (1989) Paroxysmal nocturnal haemoglobinuria. *Semin Haematol*, **26**, 201–207.

15 Sale GE and Buckner CD (1988) Pathology of bone marrow in transplant recipients. *Hematol Oncol Clin North Amer*, **2**, 735–756.

16 Kobayashi SD, Seki K, Suwa N, *et al.* (1991) The transient appearance of small blastoid cells in the marrow after bone marrow transplantation. *Hematopathology*, **96**, 191–195.

17 Müller-Hermelink HK and Sale GE. Pathological findings in human Bone Marrow transplantation. In: *Pathology of the Bone Marrow*, Lennert K and Hübner K (eds). Gustav Fischer Verlag, Stuttgart, 1984.

18 van den Berg H, Kluin PM, Zwaan FE and Vossen JM (1989) Histopathology of bone marrow reconstitution after bone marrow transplantation. *Histopathology*, **15**, 363–375.

19 van den Berg H, Kluin PH and Vossen JM (1990) Early reconstitution of haematopoiesis after allogeneic bone marrow transplantation: a prospective histopathologic study of bone marrow biopsy specimens. *J Clin Pathol*, **43**, 335–369.

20 Jouan H, Deist F Le and Nezelof C (1987) Omenn's syndrome — pathologic arguments in favour of a graft versus host pathogenesis: a report of nine cases. *Hum Pathol*, **18**, 1011–1108.

21 Brunning RD (1970) Morphological alterations in nucleated blood and marrow cells in genetic disorders. *Hum Pathol*, **1**, 99–124.

22 Hayhoe FGT, Flemans RJ and Cowling DC (1979) Acquired lipidosis of marrow macrophages. *J Clin Pathol*, **32**, 420–428.

23 Savage RA (1984) Specific and not-so-specific histiocytes in bone marrow. *Lab Med*, **15**, 467–471.

24 Bain BJ and Wickramasinghe SN (1986) Pathology of the bone marrow: general considerations. In: *Systemic Pathology*, volume 2, *Blood and Bone Marrow*, Wickramasinghe SN (ed), Symmers W St C (series ed). Churchill Livingstone, Edinburgh, 1986.

25 Lee RE (1988) Histiocytic diseases of the bone marrow. *Hematol Oncol Clin N Amer*, **2**, 657–667.

26 Bain BJ. *Blood Cells: A Practical Guide*. Gower Medical Publishing, London, 1989.

27 Beutler E and Saven A (1990) Misuse of marrow examination in the diagnosis of Gaucher's disease. *Blood*, **76**, 646–648.

28 Beutler E (1988) Gaucher disease. *Blood Reviews*, **2**, 59–70.

29 Papadimitriou JC, Chakravarthy A and Heyman MR (1988) Pseudo-Gaucher cells preceding the appearance of immunoblastic lymphoma. *Am J Clin Pathol*, **90**, 454–458.

30 Solis OG, Belmonte AH, Ramaswamy G and Tchertkoff V (1986) Pseudogaucher cells in *Mycobacterium avium intracellulare* infections in acquired immune deficiency syndrome (AIDS). *Am J Clin Pathol*, **85**, 233–235.

31 Brunning RD. Bone marrow. In: *Ackerman's Surgical Pathology*, 7th edition, volume 2, Rosai J (ed). CV Mosby, St Louis, 1989.

32 Hyun BH, Gulati GL and Ashton JK. *Color Atlas of Clinical Hematology*. Igaku-Shoin, New York, 1986.

33 Frisch B, Lewis SM, Burkhardt R and Bartl R. *Biopsy Pathology of the Bone Marrow*. Chapman and Hall, London, 1985.

34 Varela-Duran J, Roholt PC and Ratliff NB (1980) Sea-blue histiocyte syndrome: a secondary degenerative process of macrophages? *Arch Path Lab Med*, **104**, 30–34.

35 Mathews M, Stauffer M, Cameron EC, Maloney N and Sherrard DJ (1979) Bone biopsy to diagnose hyperoxaluria in patients with renal failure. *Ann Intern Med*, **90**, 777–779.

36 Hricik DE and Hussain R (1984) Pancytopenia and hepatosplenomegaly in oxalosis. *Arch Intern Med*, **184**, 167–168.

37 Miller D (1959) Observations in a case of probable bone marrow anthracosis. *Blood*, **14**, 1350–1353.

38 Jennings RC and Priestley SE (1978) Haemangioendothelioma (Kupffer cell angiosarcoma), myelofibrosis, splenic atrophy, and myeloma paraproteinaemia after parenteral Thorotrast administration. *J Clin Path*, **31**, 1125–1132.

39 Rywlin AM. *Histopathology of the Bone Marrow*. Little Brown, Boston, 1976.

40 Pierce JR, Wren MV and Cousar JB (1978) Cholesterol embolism: diagnosis antemortem by bone marrow biopsy. *Ann Intern Med*, **89**, 937–938.

41 Retan JW and Miller RE (1966) Microembolic complications of atherosclerosis. *Arch Intern Med*, **118**, 534–543.

42 Malone M (1991) The histiocytoses of childhood. *Histopathology*, **19**, 105–119.

43 Favara BE and Jaffe R (1987) Pathology of Langerhans' cell histiocytosis. *Hematol Oncol Clin North Am*, **1**, 75–97.

9: Metastatic Tumour

The bone marrow is one of the more common organs to be involved by tumours that metastasize via the bloodstream. In adults the tumours most often seen are carcinomas of the prostate, breast and lung, although any tumour that gives rise to blood-borne metastases may infiltrate the marrow.[1,2] In children, neuroblastoma, rhabdomyosarcoma, Ewing's sarcoma and retinoblastoma account for the majority of metastases.[3,4] Bone marrow metastases from squamous cell carcinoma, other than that of the lung, and from soft tissue tumours of adults are uncommon.[1]

Infiltration of the marrow may be suspected on the basis of: (i) bone pain (ii) pathological fractures, lytic lesions or sclerotic lesions demonstrated radiologically (iii) unexplained 'hot spots' on isotopic bone scans (iv) hypercalcaemia or elevated serum alkaline phosphatase activity, or (v) unexplained haematological abnormalities. The haematological abnormality most suggestive of marrow infiltration, though not specific for it, is leucoerythroblastic anaemia (see below). Metastases are also occasionally demonstrated when bone marrow examination is carried out for staging purposes in the absence of any features suggestive of bone marrow infiltration. Overall the presence of leucoerythroblastic anaemia is a relatively insensitive indication of infiltration since it is observed in less than half of patients in whom bone marrow metastases can be demonstrated by biopsy.[5-7] Aspirates and trephine biopsies are occasionally positive even when skeletal radiology and isotopic bone scans[5,8] are normal.

Considering the small volume of tissue sampled, both bone marrow aspiration and trephine biopsy are relatively sensitive techniques for detecting bone marrow infiltration. In two autopsy studies which simulated biopsy procedures it was estimated that when osseous metastases were present a bone marrow aspirate would give positive results in 28 per cent of cases[9] and a single trephine biopsy in 35 to 45 per cent.[10] Trephine biopsy is more sensitive than bone marrow aspiration and sensitivity is increased by performing bilateral biopsies or by obtaining a single large biopsy. The sensitivity of aspiration is increased if large numbers of smears are examined and if a clot section is also examined. The detection of tumour cells in a trephine biopsy when none are demonstrable in smears of an aspirate is not uncommon.[2,5,11] Overall about three-quarters of metastases detected by a trephine biopsy are detected by a simultaneous bone marrow aspirate. Such a discrepancy between the biopsy and aspirate findings is usually a result of a desmoplastic stromal reaction to the tumour which renders tumour cells more difficult to aspirate than residual haemopoietic cells. It is also, to some degree, a consequence of the different volumes of tissue sampled. Because of its greater sensitivity, trephine biopsy should always be performed when metastatic malignancy is suspected. However, occasionally tumour cells are seen in aspirate smears when the trephine biopsy is normal[2,5,11] and the two procedures should therefore be regarded as complementary.

Increasingly bone marrow aspiration and trephine biopsy are being performed as staging procedures at the time of diagnosis of a number of solid tumours, principally neuroblastoma in children and carcinomas of the breast and lung in adults. Such investigations are indicated when there is a significant probability of bone marrow metastases and when knowledge of their presence would affect the choice of primary treatment. Biopsy may be indicated, for example, when radical surgery or radiotherapy with curative intent is to be undertaken or when intensive chemotherapy with autologous bone marrow transplantation is being considered.

It can be important to suggest the likely primary site when metastatic lesions are detected in the bone marrow. This is particularly so in the case of adenocarcinoma since, although many such tumours are relatively resistant to therapy, those originating in the breast and prostate may respond to hormonal therapy. Identification of metastatic thyroid carcinoma is likewise important.

The main areas of difficulty in the diagnosis of metastatic tumour in bone marrow are: (i) distinguishing metastatic tumour cells from tumours of haemopoietic cells — for example marrow involvement by high-grade non-Hodgkin's lymphoma or M7 AML (ii) determining the site of origin of metastatic tumour when the primary is unknown, and (iii) detecting small foci of metastatic tumour in biopsies performed as part of tumour staging.

Peripheral blood

Normocytic normochromic anaemia is commonly associated with infiltration of the bone marrow by malignant cells; other cytopenias are less common. In a third to a half of patients with bone marrow infiltration there are nucleated red cells and neutrophil precursors in the blood — designated leucoerythroblastic anaemia when the patient is also anaemic. The presence of leucoerythroblastic anaemia correlates with the degree of reactive bone marrow fibrosis rather than with the extent of malignant infiltration;[6] it is most commonly seen in association with carcinoma of the breast, stomach, prostate and lung. Sometimes bone marrow infiltration is identified in the absence of anaemia or any other abnormality in the peripheral blood.

Significant numbers of circulating malignant cells are rare but may occur in the small cell tumours of childhood, particularly medulloblastoma, neuroblastoma and rhabdomyosarcoma. Circulating neoplastic cells may also be seen in patients with carcinoma, but this is a very rare occurrence.

Patients with metastatic malignant cells in the bone marrow may show peripheral blood abnormalities which are consequent on the malig-

nant disease but are not directly due to the bone marrow infiltration. Such abnormalities can include iron deficiency anaemia, the anaemia of chronic disease, micro-angiopathic haemolytic anaemia, neutrophilia, eosinophilia, thrombocytopenia, thrombocytosis and increased rouleaux formation.

Bone marrow cytology

When bone marrow infiltration has led to reactive myelofibrosis attempts at aspiration may result in a 'dry tap' or a 'blood tap' or a small amount of marrow containing haemopoietic cells, tumour cells or both may be aspirated with difficulty. When there is an associated increase in bone turnover the aspirate may contain a mixture of tumour cells, osteoblasts and osteoclasts (Fig. 9.1). Sometimes the aspirate is wholly or partly necrotic and this observation should lead to the suspicion of malignant infiltration. When a satisfactory aspirate is obtained it may contain large numbers of tumour cells mixed with a variable number of residual haemopoietic cells, or tumour cells may be scanty and found only after a prolonged search. Examination of the tail and edges of the film and examination of many films is important if scanty tumour cells are to be detected. The detection of scattered neoplastic cells in smears of bone marrow aspirates is enhanced by the use of appropriate monoclonal antibodies such as those for cytokeratin, carcinoembryonic antigen, human milk-fat globulin and epithelial membrane antigen.[12,13] Positive reactions with such antibodies allow single neoplastic cells to be identified with more confidence.

Malignant cells are usually considerably larger than any haemopoietic cells other than megakaryocytes. However, in the small cell tumours of childhood the malignant cells may be similar in size to blast cells, and acute leukaemia then enters into the differential diagnosis. Malignant cells are commonly cohesive and therefore occur as tight clumps with or without dispersed cells. Sometimes only irregularly distributed dispersed cells are present. Neoplastic cells are usually pleomorphic with regard to size, shape and nuclear characteristics. Cell outlines may be indistinct or

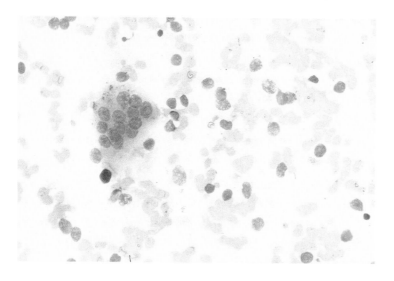

Fig. 9.1 BM aspirate, carcinoma of prostate, showing carcinoma cells and an osteoclast. MGG × 377.

cells may appear smudged. Some cells may be multinucleated. The nuclei are often hyperchromatic and may contain nucleoli. Mitotic figures may be frequent. Carcinoma cells usually have moderately abundant cytoplasm which shows a variable degree of basophilia and may contain vacuoles. Carcinoma cells are sometimes phagocytic. In the small cell tumours of childhood, cytoplasm may be scanty, thus increasing the resemblance to leukaemic cells.

It is not usually possible to predict the tissue of origin from the cytological features of the neoplastic cells in smears of bone marrow aspirates.

In view of this it is important to also examine histological sections of marrow particles, particularly if a trephine biopsy has not been performed. Sections may show features such as gland formation which are helpful in suggesting the tissue of origin. In a small percentage of cases cytological features in smears may suggest the tissue of origin. Melanoma cells may be recognized by the presence of pigment (Fig. 9.2), the nature of which can be confirmed by specific stains (see below). Such stains may be positive even when no pigment is detected in routinely stained films but otherwise the cells of amelanotic melanoma

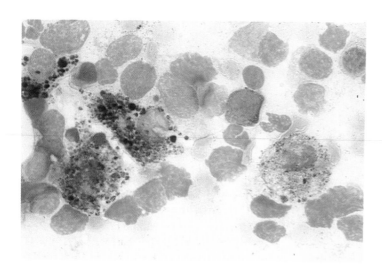

Fig. 9.2 BM aspirate, malignant melanoma, showing melanoma cells containing melanin. MGG × 940.

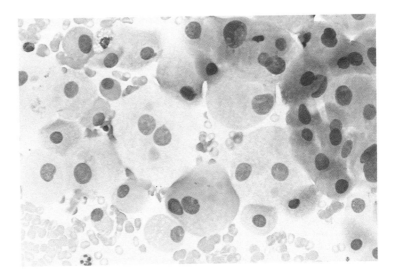

Fig. 9.3 BM aspirate, carcinoma of kidney, showing 'clear cells' with voluminous pale cytoplasm. MGG × 940.

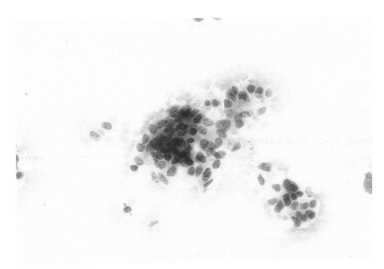

Fig. 9.4 BM aspirate, carcinoid tumour, showing cells with relatively small nuclei and a variable amount of cytoplasm. MGG × 377.

cannot be distinguished from other neoplastic cells. Melanin may also be present in macrophages. Clear cell carcinomas are also distinctive and suggest a renal primary; the cells have a relatively small nucleus and abundant very weakly basophilic cytoplasm (Fig. 9.3). Cells of metastatic carcinoid tumour also have a relatively small nucleus and moderately abundant cytoplasm (Fig. 9.4). In children neuroblastoma (Fig. 9.5) may be identified by the presence of blue-grey fibrillar material extracellularly or by the presence of cells with irregular 'tails'; rosettes of tumour cells are distinctive but are not com-

mon. In metastatic rhabdomyosarcoma (Fig. 9.6) there may be multinucleated giant cells or spindle-shaped binucleated rhabdomyoblasts.[4] Less specific changes, such as foamy or vacuolated cytoplasm or displacement of nuclei by cytoplasmic mucin, may be noted in metastatic adenocarcinoma originating in various primary sites (Fig. 9.7). In squamous cell carcinoma metastatic tumour cells have sometimes been noted, on Romanowsky stains, to have a reddish cytoplasmic margin and with the cytoplasm adjacent to the nucleus being more basophilic.[14] In small cell carcinoma of the lung the cells are smaller

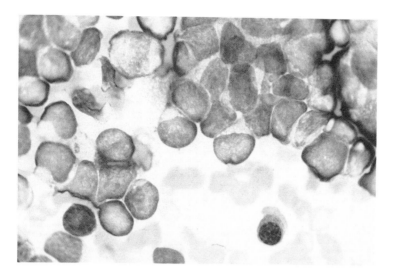

Fig. 9.5 BM aspirate, neuroblastoma, showing neoplastic cells which are relatively small and have a high nucleo-cytoplasmic ratio and a diffuse chromatin pattern. MGG × 940.

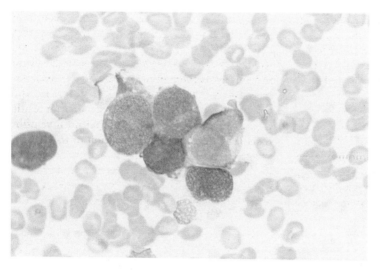

Fig. 9.6 BM aspirate, rhabdomyosarcoma. MGG × 940.

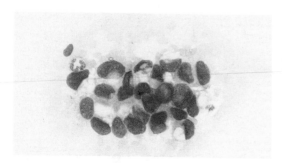

Fig. 9.7 BM aspirate, carcinoma of breast, showing adenocarcinoma cells with secretory globules. MGG × 377.

than those of most carcinomas but are nevertheless still larger than haemopoietic blasts; they have scanty weakly basophilic cytoplasm and their nuclei, which have coarse chromatin and inconspicuous nucleoli, may appear 'moulded' by the nuclei of adjacent tumour cells (Fig. 9.8).

Non-haemopoietic neoplastic cells in a bone marrow aspirate must be distinguished from lymphoma cells and the cells of acute leukaemia. Other cells which are sometimes confused with malignant cells include osteoblasts, osteoclasts, reticulum cells, endothelial cells, atypical megakaryocytes and crushed erythroblasts.

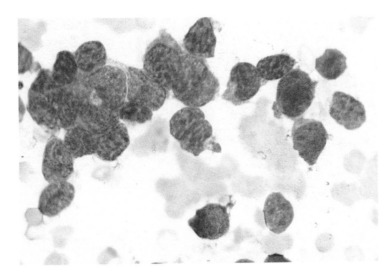

Fig. 9.8 BM aspirate, oat cell carcinoma of lung, showing carcinoma cells with scanty cytoplasm and 'moulding' of cells by adjacent cells. MGG × 940.

When the bone marrow is infiltrated by malignant cells there may be associated non-specific changes including increased plasma cells or mast cells, granulocytic or megakaryocytic hyperplasia, increased macrophages and increased storage iron. Gelatinous degeneration is rare.

Bone marrow histology

Marrow infiltration by metastatic tumour may be focal or diffuse. Reticulin and collagen fibrosis are commonly present and are most marked in those cases with greater degrees of marrow infiltration. Marked fibrosis is most common in carcinomas of the breast, stomach, prostate and lung.[6,15,16] The proportion of tumour cells to stroma is variable, and in cases with severe myelofibrosis there may be associated osteosclerosis (Figs 9.9 and 9.10). Failure to recognize the tumour cells within the fibrous stroma can result in a mistaken diagnosis of idiopathic myelofibrosis. The degree of differentiation of metastatic tumour is very variable and as a result it is often impossible to be certain of the site of the primary tumour on purely morphological grounds. Frequently metastases are undifferentiated and the

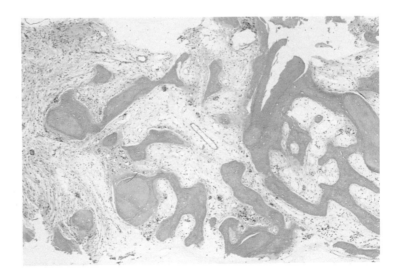

Fig. 9.9 BM trephine biopsy, carcinoma of the breast, showing osteosclerosis and replacement of the marrow by dense fibrous tissue containing tumour cells. Paraffin-embedded, H&E × 39.

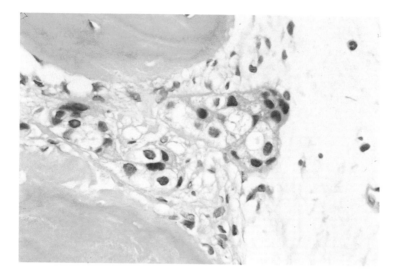

Fig. 9.10 BM trephine biopsy, carcinoma of the breast (same case as Fig. 9.9), showing a group of tumour cells with hyperchromatic nuclei and vacuolated cytoplasm. Paraffin-embedded, H&E × 390.

differential diagnosis includes poorly differenti-ated carcinoma, high-grade non-Hodgkin's lymph-oma and malignant melanoma. In such cases immunohistochemical staining for leucocyte common antigen (CD45), epithelial markers (cytokeratin and epithelial membrane antigen) (Figs 9.11 to 9.13) and S100 protein (expressed in most malignant melanomas)[12,17] is invaluable. In poorly differentiated carcinomas it is not usually possible to determine the site of origin of the tumour. In tumours showing differentiation it may be possible to determine the type of car-cinoma and suggest the likely site of origin — for

example, in metastatic squamous carcinoma, the lung is the most likely primary site.

Metastatic adenocarcinoma (Fig. 9.14) can be diagnosed on the basis of the formation of glands and/or the presence of mucin (best detected using a combined diastase-treated PAS/Alcian blue stain). Metastatic adenocarcinoma may arise from primary tumours in the gastro-intestinal tract, breast, prostate, ovary, endometrium, pancreas and many other sites. The two primary sites whose identification is most important because of their sensitivity to hormonal therapy are breast and prostate. Metastatic prostatic carcinoma may

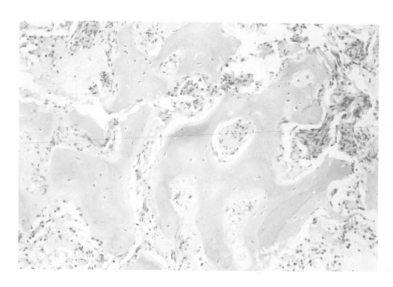

Fig. 9.11 BM trephine biopsy, poorly differentiated prostatic carcinoma, showing osteosclerosis and replacement of the marrow by dense fibrous tissue containing tumour cells. Paraffin-embedded, H&E × 97.

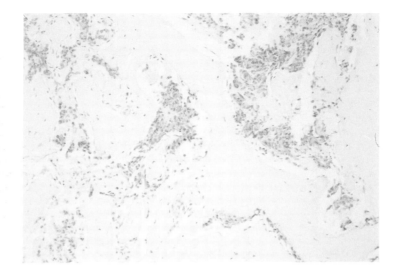

Fig. 9.12 BM trephine biopsy, poorly differentiated prostatic carcinoma, showing expression of cytokeratin by tumour cells (same case as Fig. 9.11). Paraffin-embedded, Peroxidase-anti-peroxidase, anti-cytokeratin monoclonal antibody × 97.

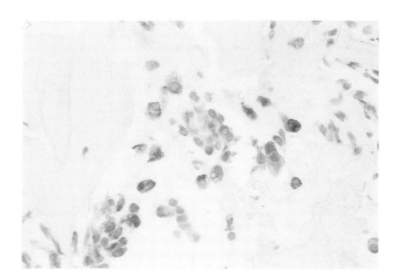

Fig. 9.13 BM trephine biopsy, as for Fig. 9.12, × 390.

be identified by immunohistochemical staining with antibodies that react with prostatic-specific antigen.[18] Since these antibodies may also react with some colonic tumours[19] the use of parallel staining with anti-prostatic-specific acid phosphatase has been recommended. Identification of breast carcinoma is usually based on its resemblance to primary breast cancer (Fig. 9.15). Immunohistochemical staining is not usually helpful although, of the markers available, alpha-lactalbumin which is found in most primary breast cancers appears to be relatively specific.[20]

Clear cell carcinomas have large amounts of clear cytoplasm due to the presence of abundant glycogen or lipid; mucin stains are negative. Likely primary sites of metastatic clear cell carcinoma include kidney, ovary, and lung. Metastatic follicular carcinoma of the thyroid may be suspected on morphological grounds if follicles containing colloid are seen. Immunohistochemical staining for thyroglobulin is useful in confirming the thyroid origin of a tumour.

Metastatic small cell carcinoma of the lung commonly involves the bone marrow (see below).

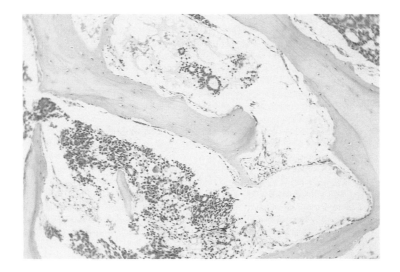

Fig. 9.14 BM trephine biopsy, well-differentiated prostatic carcinoma, showing a tumour composed of small well-defined glandular structures. Plastic-embedded, H&E × 97.

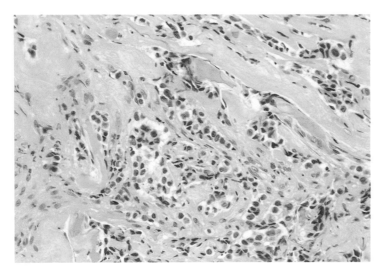

Fig. 9.15 BM trephine biopsy, carcinoma of the breast, showing tumour cells with hyperchromatic nuclei arranged in cords and strands in a dense fibrous (desmoplastic) stroma. Paraffin-embedded, H&E × 390.

The cells are small with intensely hyperchromatic nuclei and scant cytoplasm (Fig. 9.16); necrosis is common and there is often smearing of nuclei which can render interpretation difficult. Morphological variants of small cell carcinoma in which the cells are slightly larger and have either a fusiform or polygonal shape are also seen. The principal differential diagnosis of metastatic small cell carcinoma is that of non-Hodgkin's lymphoma. Small cell carcinoma is positive for cytokeratin on immunohistochemical staining. Other tumours showing neuroendocrine differentiation such as carcinoid tumours (Fig. 9.17)

and medullary carcinoma of the thyroid may metastasize to the bone marrow. Immunohistochemical staining for chromogranin identifies neuroendocrine differentiation in these tumours.[21] In addition medullary carcinomas of the thyroid stain positively for calcitonin.

Malignant melanoma is found in the bone marrow in approximately five per cent of patients with disseminated disease.[22] If melanin is present in the tumour cells (Fig. 9.18) or associated macrophages, the diagnosis is relatively easy, although the nature of any pigment present should be confirmed by either a Masson–Fontana or a

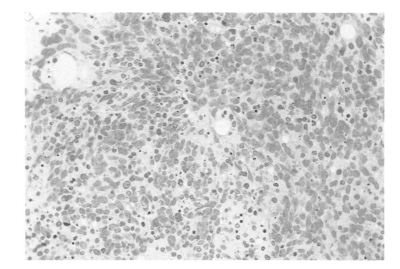

Fig. 9.16 BM trephine biopsy, oat cell carcinoma of the bronchus, showing a sheet of small cells with hyperchromatic ovoid nuclei and scanty cytoplasm; in places there is nuclear 'moulding'. Plastic-embedded, H&E × 390.

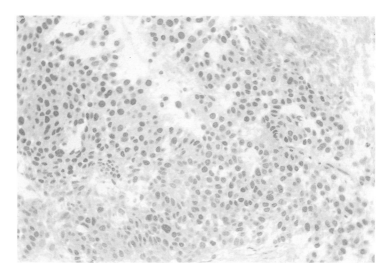

Fig. 9.17 BM trephine biopsy, carcinoid tumour (unknown primary site), showing relatively uniform cells with ovoid hyperchromatic nuclei and eosinophilic cytoplasm; in some areas the cells are arranged in trabeculae. Plastic-embedded, H&E × 390.

Schmorl stain for melanin. However, not infrequently, metastatic malignant melanoma is amelanotic. Malignant melanoma should be suspected if metastatic tumour is composed of polygonal or spindle cells with prominent nucleoli. Immunohistochemical staining for S100 protein is usually positive.[17]

The differential diagnosis of metastatic spindle cell tumour within the marrow includes carcinoma showing spindle cell differentiation, malignant melanoma and soft tissue sarcomas. Soft tissue sarcomas rarely metastasize to the marrow and when they do the primary tumour is

usually readily apparent. Spindle cell carcinomas and melanomas express cytokeratin and S100 protein respectively on immunohistochemical staining.

Many of the malignant tumours that occur in childhood are composed of small cells with relatively uniform round nuclei. The differential diagnosis of bone marrow infiltration by such cells in a child includes non-Hodgkin's lymphoma (usually lymphoblastic or Burkitt's lymphoma), metastatic neuroblastoma, rhabdomyosarcoma, retinoblastoma or Ewing's sarcoma. In order to make a specific diagnosis the clinical features,

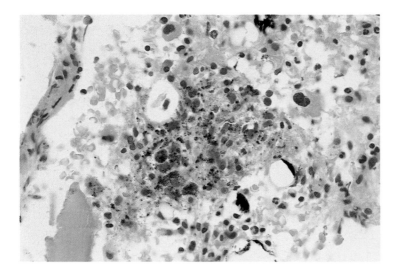

Fig. 9.18 BM trephine biopsy, malignant melanoma, showing a focal tumour infiltrate composed of cells containing large amounts of melanin; the tumour cells have hyperchromatic nuclei, and some have prominent nucleoli. (It should be noted that it is unusual to see large amounts of melanin in metastatic malignant melanoma.) Paraffin-embedded, H&E × 390.

morphological findings and histochemical and immunohistochemical staining characteristics all need to be considered. The marrow findings in lymphoblastic and Burkitt's lymphoma are described on pages 159 and 177; both express leucocyte common antigen (CD45). Neuroblastoma is the most common malignant solid tumour in children and often metastasizes to the bone marrow. The majority of cases occur in children under four years of age. The cells forming the tumour are slightly larger than small lymphocytes with regular, round hyperchromatic nuclei and little cytoplasm[23] (Fig. 9.19). Rosettes are

present in a minority of cases; these consist of tumour cells arranged around central fibrillary material which is pink on an H&E stain. The cells of neuroblastoma may show focal PAS-positivity although this is usually less marked than that seen in rhabdomyoblastoma and Ewing's sarcoma. Neuroblastoma is usually positive for neurone-specific enolase on immunocyto-chemical staining. Rhabdomyosarcoma metastasizes to the bone marrow in approximately 16 per cent of cases.[1] Several histological variants are recognized: (i) embryonal, which may be further subdivided into myxoid, spindle cell or

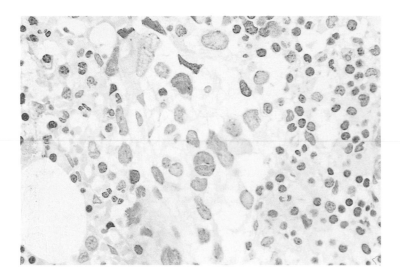

Fig. 9.19 BM trephine biopsy, neuroblastoma, showing a focal area of infiltration; note the fibrillar, faintly eosinophilic material between the tumour cells. Plastic-embedded, H&E × 390.

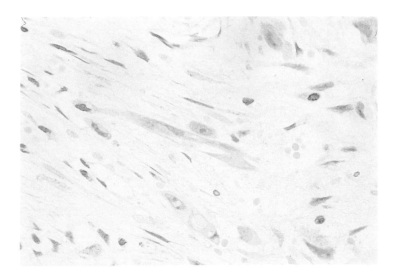

Fig. 9.20 BM trephine biopsy, rhabdomyosarcoma, showing elongated cells with plentiful eosinophilic cytoplasm (rhabdomyoblasts). Plastic-embedded, H&E × 390.

round cell patterns[23] (ii) alveolar, which is characterized by a pattern of irregular spaces lined by tumour cells,[24] and (iii) pleomorphic which is very rare and not usually seen in children. Diagnosis depends on the recognition of skeletal muscle differentiation. Rhabdomyoblasts have abundant pink granular cytoplasm which may contain cross-striations and may be oval, spindle, tadpole or strap shaped (Fig. 9.20). The number of rhabdomyoblasts is variable; in some tumours the majority of cells are undifferentiated round or spindle cells. Immunohistochemical staining for desmin is usually positive, although staining for

myoglobin, which is said to be more specific, is variable.[23] Ewing's sarcoma is a malignant tumour that may arise in bone or soft tissue. Most patients are in the second decade of life and approximately 35 per cent of cases develop bone marrow metastases.[1] The tumour cells are approximately twice the size of small lymphocytes and have round to oval vesicular nuclei (Fig. 9.21). There is usually PAS-positive cytoplasmic staining for glycogen which may be finely dispersed or in the form of large blocks of positively staining material (Fig. 9.22). The PAS staining is often decreased by formalin fixation.

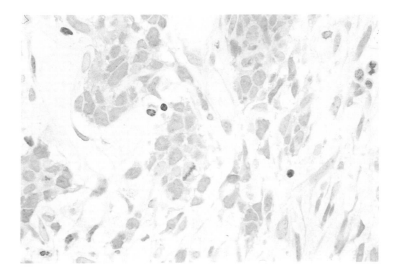

Fig. 9.21 BM trephine biopsy, Ewing's sarcoma, showing irregular groups of cells in a fibrous stroma; the cells have ovoid nuclei with indistinct nucleoli and scanty cytoplasm. Plastic-embedded, H&E × 390.

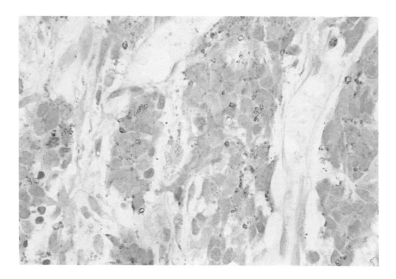

Fig. 9.22 BM trephine biopsy, Ewing's sarcoma, showing large granules of glycogen in the cytoplasm. Plastic-embedded, PAS × 390.

The role of bone marrow examination in the staging of solid tumours

Examination of the bone marrow by aspiration and trephine biopsy is an established part of the staging of neuroblastoma in children in most large centres. The bone marrow biopsy is positive in approximately half of all patients at the time of initial diagnosis, most of whom have evidence of metastatic spread at other sites.[25] Discordance between marrow aspirate and biopsy findings is common; the biopsy alone is positive in 20 per cent of cases whereas the tumour is seen in the aspirate smears when the biopsy appears normal in seven per cent. Taking bilateral bone marrow aspirates and trephine biopsies from the iliac crests increases the sensitivity of the staging procedure by approximately 10 per cent. Careful examination of smears and biopsy sections is necessary because infiltration is often focal. In cases in which the marrow appearances are suspicious but not diagnostic of marrow infiltration, immuno-cytochemical staining of aspirate smears or frozen sections of trephine biopsies with antibodies against neuroectodermal tissue (UJ13A and UJ127.11) may be of value in confirming marrow involvement.[26-28] Immunohistochemical staining of paraffin-embedded sections of trephine biopsies with antibodies to neurone-specific enolase does not increase the sensitivity of marrow biopsy as a means of detecting tumour cells.[28]

The assessment of marrow infiltration is more difficult in patients who have been treated with chemotherapy. It has been suggested that the appearances in post-treatment marrow biopsies be divided into four grades: grade 1, normal (or hypocellular) marrow; grade 2, marrow with reticulin fibrosis as the only abnormality; grade 3, distorted architecture with collagen fibrosis; grade 4, marrow with obvious tumour cells with or without other abnormalities.[29]

In adults examination of the bone marrow is not a routine staging procedure for most solid tumours and although it has been advocated for small cell carcinoma of the lung and breast cancer it is by no means universal even in these tumours. In small cell carcinoma of the lung the bone marrow biopsy is positive in 25-30 per cent of cases;[7,30,31] the aspirate is only slightly less sensitive at detecting marrow involvement. It has been suggested that bone marrow examination is indicated in patients with small cell carcinoma of the lung in order to identify patients who may be suitable for attempted curative therapy.[32] However some studies have shown no difference in survival between cases with and without marrow involvement,[7,32] and the value of routine bone marrow examination has therefore been questioned.[7]

Several studies have evaluated the use of marrow aspiration and biopsy in the staging of breast cancer. Detection of subclinical metastatic disease may be useful in identifying patients with apparently localized disease who may benefit from adjuvant chemotherapy. The bone marrow biopsy is positive in 25–55 per cent of patients with positive isotope bone scans, but only four to 10 per cent of patients with negative isotope bone scans have tumour present on bone marrow biopsy.[5,33] At the time of first recurrence 23 per cent of all patients have positive bone marrow biopsies. In an attempt to increase the sensitivity of bone marrow examination as a staging procedure some studies have used routine immunocytochemical staining to identify micrometastases that would not be detected by conventional techniques. The method used has involved aspirating bone marrow from multiple (up to eight) sites under general anaesthesia at the time of initial surgery, pooling the material and preparing several smears. Tumour cells are then detected by staining with antibodies that react with epithelial membrane antigen (EMA),[34,35] cytokeratin[36] or a cocktail containing both antibodies.[37] Micrometastases are present in 27–35 per cent of cases at the time of diagnosis and there is a correlation between their presence and the size of the primary tumour.[35,37] The presence of bone marrow micrometastases is a predictor of early relapse in bone. Despite this, routine immunocytochemical staining to detect micrometastases has not as yet come into widespread use.

REFERENCES

1 Anner RM and Drewinko B (1977) Frequency and significance of bone marrow involvement by metastatic solid tumours. *Cancer*, **39**, 1337–1344.

2 Singh G, Krause JR and Breitfeld V (1977) Bone marrow examination for metastatic tumour. *Cancer*, **40**, 2317–2321.

3 Finkelstein JZ, Ekert H, Isaacs H and Higgins G (1970) Bone marrow metastases in children with solid tumours. *Am J Dis Child*, **119**, 49–52.

4 Delta BG and Pinkel D (1964) Bone marrow aspiration in children with malignant tumours. *J Paediat*, **64**, 542–546.

5 Ingle JN, Tormey DC, and Tan HK (1978) The bone marrow examination in breast cancer. *Cancer*, **41**, 670–674.

6 Rubins JR (1983) The role of myelofibrosis in malignant myelosclerosis. *Cancer*, **51**, 308–311.

7 Tritz DB, Doll DC, Ringenberg S, *et al.* (1989) Bone marrow examination in small cell lung cancer. *Cancer*, **63**, 763–766.

8 Becker FO and Schwartz TB (1973) Normal fluoride 18 bone scans in metastatic bone disease. *JAMA*, **225**, 628–629.

9 Suprun H and Rywlin AM (1976) Metastatic carcinoma in histologic sections of aspirated bone marrow: a comparative autopsy study. *South Med J*, **69**, 438–439.

10 Lang W, Stauch G, Soudah B and Georgii A. The effectiveness of Bone Marrow punctures for staging carcinomas of the breast and lung. In: *Pathology of the Bone Marrow*, Lennert K (ed). Gustav Fischer Verlag, Stuttgart, 1984.

11 Savage RA, Hoffman GC and Shaker K (1978) Diagnostic problems involved in detection of metastatic neoplasms by bone-marrow aspirate compared with needle biopsy. *Am J Clin Pathol*, **70**, 623–627.

12 Gatter KC, Abdulaziz Z, Beverley P, *et al.* (1982) Use of monoclonal antibodies for the histopathological diagnosis of human malignancy. *J Clin Pathol*, **35**, 1253–1267.

13 Athanasou NA, Quinn J, Heryet A, Woods CG and McGee J O'D (1987) The effect of decalcification on cellular antigens. *J Clin Pathol*, **40**, 874–878.

14 Jonsson LL and Rundles RW (1951) Tumour metastases in bone marrow. *Blood*, **6**, 16–25.

15 Kiely JM and Silverstein MN (1969) Metastatic carcinoma simulating agnogenic myeloid metaplasia. *Cancer*, **24**, 1041–1044.

16 Spector JI and Levine PH (1973) Carcinomatous bone marrow invasion simulating acute myelofibrosis. *Am J Med Sci*, **266**, 145–148.

17 Gatter KC, Ralfkiaer E, Skinner J, *et al.* (1985) An immunohistochemical study of malignant melanoma and its differential diagnosis from other malignant tumours. *J Clin Pathol*, **38**, 1353–1357.

18 Nadji M, Tabei SZ, Castro A, *et al.* (1984) Prostatic-specific antigen. An immunohistologic marker for prostatic neoplasms. *Cancer*, **48**, 1229–1239.

19 Wilbur DC, Krenzer K and Bonfiglio TA (1987) Prostatic specific antigen staining in carcinomas of non-prostatic origin. *Am J Clin Pathol*, **88**, 530.

20 Lee AK, De Lellis RA, Rosen PP, *et al.* (1984) Alpha-lactalbumin as an immunohistochemical marker for breast carcinomas. *Am J Surg Pathol*, **8**, 93–100.

21 Lloyd RV, Cano M, Rosa P, Hille A and Huttner WB (1988) Distribution of chromogranin A and secretogranin I (chromogranin B) in neuroendocrine cells and tumour. *Am J Pathol*, **130**, 296–304.

22 Savage RA, Lucas PV and Hoffman GC (1978) Melanoma in marrow aspirates (letter). *Am J Clin Pathol*, **79**, 268–269.

23 Variend S (1985) Small cell tumours in childhood: a review. *J Pathol*, **145**, 1–27.

24 Enzinger FM and Shiraki M (1969) Alveolar rhabdomyosarcoma; an analysis of 110 cases. *Cancer*, **24**,
18−31.

25 Franklin IM and Pritchard J (1983) Detection of bone
marrow invasion by neuroblastoma is improved by
sampling at two sites with aspirates and biopsies.
J Clin Pathol, **36**, 1215−1218.

26 Rogers DW, Treleavan JG, Kemshead JT and
Pritchard J (1989) Monoclonal antibodies for detect-
ing bone marrow invasion by neuroblastoma. *J Clin
Pathol*, **42**, 422−426.

27 Carey PJ, Thomas L, Buckle G and Reid MM (1990)
Immunocytochemical examination of bone marrow
in disseminated neuroblastoma. *J Clin Pathol*, **43**,
9−12.

28 Reid MM, Wallis JP, McGuckin AG, Pearson ADJ
and Malcolm AJ (1991) Routine histological compared with immunohistological examination of bone
marrow trephine biopsy specimens in disseminated
neuroblastoma. *J Clin Pathol*, **44**, 485−486.

29 Reid MM and Hamilton PJ (1988) Histology of
neuroblastoma involving bone marrow: the problem
of detecting residual tumour after initiation of
chemotherapy. *Br J Haematol*, **69**, 487−490.

30 Lawrence JB, Eleff M, Behm FG and Johnston CL
(1984) Bone marrow examination in small cell carcinoma of the lung. *Cancer*, **53**, 2188−2190.

31 Levitan N, Byrne RE, Bromer RH, *et al.* (1985) The
value of the bone scan and bone marrow biopsy in
staging small cell lung cancer. *Cancer*, **56**, 652−654.

32 Kelly BW, Morris JF, Harwood BP and Bruya TE
(1984) Methods and prognostic value of bone marrow
examination in small cell carcinoma of the lung.
Cancer, **53**, 99−102.

33 Landys K (1982) Prognostic value of bone marrow
biopsy in breast cancer. *Cancer*, **49**, 513−518.

34 Mansi JL, Berger U, Easton D, *et al.* (1987) Micrometastases in bone marrow in patients with breast
cancer: evaluation as an early predictor of bone
metastases. *BMJ*, **295**, 1093−1096.

35 Berger U, Bettelheim R, Mansi JL, Easton D,
Coombes RC and Neville AM (1988) The relationship between micrometastases in the bone marrow,
histopathologic features of the primary tumor in
breast cancer and prognosis. *Am J Clin Pathol*, **90**,
1−6.

36 Ellis G, Ferguson M, Yamanaka E, Livingston RB
and Gown AM (1989) Monoclonal antibodies for
detection of occult carcinoma cells in bone marrow
of breast cancer patients. *Cancer*, **63**, 2509−2514.

37 Untch M, Harbeck N and Eiemann W (1988) Micrometastases in bone marrow in patients with breast
cancer. *BMJ*, **296**, 290.

10: Diseases of Bone

Trephine biopsies, particularly trans-cortical biopsies, are useful in assessing bone pathology. Diseases of bone are also not infrequently encountered when examining bone marrow trephine biopsies taken for the investigation of haematological disease. The normal structure of bone is described in chapter 1 (page 1). Before discussing the more important diseases of bone that can be diagnosed on trephine biopsy it is necessary to consider briefly some aspects of the normal physiology of bone.

Bone is in a constant state of turnover in adult life, by a process of remodelling during which resorption and formation are balanced in order to maintain the total skeletal mass. Microscopic portions of the trabecular and cortical bone surface are resorbed by osteoclasts which form small resorption bays (Howship's lacunae). Bone formation starts soon after resorption ceases, with the deposition of unmineralized matrix (osteoid) in layers (lamellae) by osteoblasts. After a time lag of 10–15 days (the osteoid maturation time) the osteoid becomes mineralized along an advancing front (the mineralization front), starting at the base of the previous resorption bay (the cement line).[1]

For the study of metabolic bone disease undecalcified sections of bone are essential. Osteoid seams, that is layers of non-calcified bone on the surface of trabeculae, are a feature of normal bone. In H&E-stained sections they appear paler and pinker than calcified bone but they can be recognized more easily in sections stained for calcium with alizarin red or von Kossa's silver stain. The mineralization front appears as a metachromatic granular line in toluidine blue stained sections.

Morphometry of bone

Morphometric methods are commonly used in the diagnosis of diseases of bone. These may be divided into static and dynamic measurements. Static measurements include: (i) the proportion of trabecular surface which is resting, resorbing or covered by osteoid (by a perimeter intersect technique) (ii) the thickness of osteoid seams, and (iii) the proportion of the section occupied by mineralized bone, osteoid, woven bone, lamellar bone or fibrous tissue (by a point-counting technique). Dynamic studies may be performed using a tetracycline labelling technique. When a single dose of tetracycline is administered it becomes incorporated at the mineralization front; this can be visualized as a single line in undecalcified sections examined under ultra-violet light. By giving two doses of tetracycline at known intervals and measuring the distance between the two lines of incorporation it is possible to measure the mean rate of mineralization.

OSTEOPOROSIS

Osteoporosis is defined as a decreased amount of bone per unit volume. There is no decrease in the external dimensions of the bone which is histologically normal, but there is a reduction in the amount of trabecular bone per unit volume of cancellous bone and there may also be thinning of the cortex (Fig. 10.1). The disorder is common in the elderly, in whom it causes considerable morbidity as a result of increased susceptibility to fractures. Osteoporosis is more common in women, and its frequency increases progressively after the menopause. The cause is not known, but

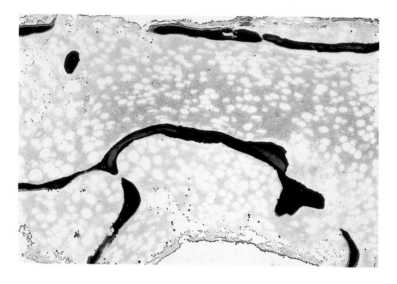

Fig. 10.1 BM trephine biopsy, osteoporosis, showing a decrease in the total amount of bone with thinning of trabeculae. Paraffin-embedded (non-decalcified), Tripp and MacKay stain × 39.

the mechanism is thought to be increased osteoclastic resorption in conjunction with a reduced rate of bone formation.[2] In a minority of cases osteoporosis is secondary to other disease such as Cushing's syndrome, thyrotoxicosis, hypopituitarism, malnutrition, malabsorption, and chronic heparin or corticosteroid administration. Diffuse osteoporosis is also sometimes associated with multiple myeloma, aplastic anaemia, chronic granulocytic leukaemia, systemic mastocytosis and polycythaemia rubra vera. Localized osteoporosis can occur following immobilization of a limb.

Plain radiographs of the vertebral column are usually only abnormal in advanced disease and are an unreliable means of diagnosing osteoporosis. An assessment of the severity of osteoporosis can be made using biopsies from the iliac crest.[3] The trabeculae are thinned and are reduced to slender strands, often with complete transection, but they are otherwise normal and there is no increase in osteoid seams. Rather, osteoid seams and the number of osteoblasts tend to be reduced. Accurate assessment of the severity of osteoporosis requires the use of static morphometric measurements. Iliac trabecular bone normally occupies approximately 23 per cent (SD ± 3 per cent) of the measured area in adults under 50 years of age, but this falls to 16 per cent (SD ± 6 per cent) in elderly individuals.[4] When the

amount of trabecular bone falls below 11 per cent (SD ± 3 per cent) vertebral fractures tend to occur.[1]

Recently reliable non-invasive techniques for the measurement of bone mass at the sites most prone to fracture have become available; these include dual proton absorptiometry, quantitative CT, and dual-energy X-ray absorptiometry.[5] It seems likely these techniques will render iliac crest biopsy unnecessary for the diagnosis of osteoporosis.

The peripheral blood is normal in osteoporosis; the bone marrow is essentially normal, although increased numbers of mast cells have been reported.[6] There may, however, be an appearance of hypocellularity since the loss of bone leads to an increased percentage of the marrow cavity being occupied by fat cells.

OSTEOMALACIA

Osteomalacia literally means softening of the bones. It is a consequence of a failure of mineralization of the bone matrix resulting in abnormally wide osteoid seams around the bone trabeculae (Fig. 10.2). Numerous causes of osteomalacia have been described, but the majority of cases are consequent on a deficiency of vitamin D, due in turn to reduced intake, inadequate exposure to sunlight, or to abnormalities of absorption or metabolism of the vitamin (as in renal disease). Rarely,

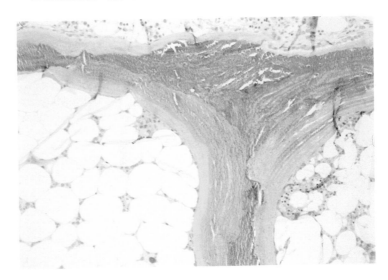

Fig. 10.2 BM trephine biopsy, osteomalacia, showing wide osteoid seams on the surface of the bone trabecula. Plastic-embedded. H&E × 97.

osteomalacia is caused by a hereditary end-organ resistance to vitamin D and its metabolites. In adults, severe osteomalacia predisposes to fractures. In children, in whom the epiphyses have not yet closed, the clinical picture is that of rickets, with its characteristic skeletal deformities.

In normal adults approximately 0.5 per cent of the whole bone area (that is, bone plus marrow) is made up of osteoid, which covers 13 per cent (SD ± 7 per cent) of the trabecular bone surface. A mineralization front is seen in more than 60 per cent of the surface osteoid. Under polarized light, normal osteoid seams are seen to be composed of between one and four lamellae.[1] In osteomalacia there is an increase in both total osteoid and the area of trabecular surface covered by osteoid; the osteoid seams are greater than five lamellae in thickness, and the mineralization front is decreased. Double tetracycline labelling shows a reduction in the mineralization rate (normal mean value 0.7 µm per day). The bone marrow is usually normal.

The peripheral blood and bone marrow aspirate are usually normal in osteomalacia but children with severe vitamin D deficiency rickets have been reported to develop a hypocellular bone marrow with fibrosis, thrombocytopenia and a leucoerythroblastic anaemia associated with extramedullary erythropoiesis.[7]

HYPERPARATHYROIDISM

Skeletal changes occur in both primary and secondary hyperparathyroidism. The extent of the changes depends on the severity and duration of the underlying disease. Primary hyperparathyroidism is usually the result of a parathyroid adenoma; primary hyperplasia is a less common cause. Very rarely there is an underlying parathyroid carcinoma. Secondary hyperparathyroidism is usually a consequence of renal disease; less commonly the underlying cause is intestinal malabsorption. Parathormone acts on bone to increase resorption, although it is unclear whether this is a result of increased osteoclastic or decreased osteoblastic activity.[2]

The skeletal changes in hyperparathyroidism follow a predictable sequence. The earliest change is the presence of excess osteoid seams around the bone trabeculae, an appearance that closely resembles osteomalacia. Later, osteoclasts are activated and there is increased bone resorption. Howship's lacunae and osteoclasts are prominent and there is fibrosis of the paratrabecular marrow. This appearance is known as osteitis fibrosa. The Howship's lacunae may be filled by large bizarre osteoclasts and, as the lacunae enlarge, trabeculae may be transected. Fibrosis increases and fibrous tissue eventually fills some intertrabecular spaces completely. There is a moderate increase in the vascularity of the marrow. At this stage macroscopic cysts may be visible (osteitis fibrosa cystica). Haemosiderin-laden macrophages are frequently seen within the fibrous tissue consequent on microhaemorrhages; foreign body type giant cells may also be present. This final stage is sometimes referred to as osteitis fibrosa cystica.

Only a minority of patients with hyperparathyroidism have significant bone disease and because of earlier diagnosis and treatment severe manifestations (osteitis fibrosa cystica) are rarely seen nowadays.

There are no specific peripheral blood or bone marrow aspirate abnormalities associated with primary hyperparathyroidism, although mild anaemia may occur.[8]

RENAL OSTEODYSTROPHY

The majority of patients with chronic renal failure have some abnormality of bone structure. The manifestations are complex and include combinations of bone disease due to secondary hyperparathyroidism (80−90 per cent of cases), osteomalacia (20−40 per cent of cases) and osteosclerosis (around 30 per cent of cases).[1,9] The most severe changes are seen in those patients with chronic renal failure who are maintained on dialysis. There is marked geographical variation in the nature of renal osteodystrophy with hyperparathyroid bone disease predominating in the United States and osteomalacia in the United Kingdom. In adults the symptoms are rarely severe. Secondary hyperparathyroidism in renal failure is consequent on hypocalcaemia which is in turn caused by a combination of reduced hydroxylation of vitamin D and phosphate retention by the kidney. The major cause of renal osteomalacia is the toxic action of aluminium derived from the dialysate. The geographical variations in the incidence are related to the concentration of aluminium in the water used for dialysis. The use of de-ionized water for dialysis has resulted in a fall in the incidence of osteomalacia in some centres.[1]

Histologically the changes are those previously described in hyperparathyroidism (osteitis fibrosa), often combined with those of osteomalacia (Fig. 10.3). The most severe changes of osteitis fibrosa cystica are seen only rarely. Osteosclerosis, due to increased formation of woven bone, may be widespread throughout the skeleton. With advanced renal osteodystrophy the bone marrow may be hypocellular and extensively fibrosed with proliferation of vessels, particularly arterioles. Patients with renal osteodystrophy have been noted to have mononuclear cells within the haemopoietic marrow which are positive for tartrate-resistant acid phosphatase; these cells are probably osteoclast precursors.[10]

There may also be abnormal deposition of aluminium or iron. Aluminium deposition occurs

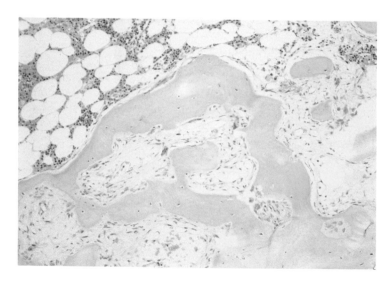

Fig. 10.3 BM trephine biopsy, renal osteodystrophy, showing irregular bone trabeculae with prominent resorption bays (Howship's lacunae) and replacement of haemopoietic marrow by fibrous tissue. Paraffin-embedded, H&E × 97.

at the osteoid/mineralized bone junction. It is detected as a red/purple line on an Irwin stain of an undecalcified biopsy[11] and provides evidence of exposure to an excessive aluminium concentration in the dialysate. Aluminium may also be detected inside bone marrow cells, possibly macrophages.[12] In dialysis patients who are iron-overloaded, iron may also be deposited at the mineralization front;[13] iron deposition may be aetiologically related to osteomalacia.

Renal osteodystrophy may contribute to the anaemia of chronic renal failure, and also cause leucopenia and thrombocytopenia.[14] There are no specific associated morphological abnormalities in the peripheral blood or bone marrow aspirate although a 'dry tap' may occur.

PAGET'S DISEASE OF BONE

Paget's disease of bone is a disease of unknown aetiology characterized by increased osteoclastic resorption of bone followed by uncoordinated formation of disordered reactive bone. The disease is uncommon before the age of 40 and becomes progressively more common with increasing age. In approximately 15 per cent of cases the disease is confined to a single bone (monostotic) but in the majority of cases several bones are involved, most commonly the vertebral column, pelvis, femur, skull and sacrum. The clinical features are pain due to microfractures, and neurological symptoms, consequent on damage to nerves as they pass through the foramina in the skull and vertebrae. Rarely there is high-output cardiac failure as a result of the highly vascular lesions acting as arterio-venous shunts. The development of an osteosarcoma is an uncommon but well-established complication of Paget's disease.

In the initial stages of the disease increased bone resorption is the dominant feature. The trabeculae have a scalloped appearance due to increased numbers of resorption bays containing very large, bizarre osteoclasts with numerous nuclei (Fig. 10.4). The increased resorption of bone is followed by the deposition of disordered woven bone. Osteoblasts are increased. At this stage the marrow cavity is partly occupied by loose connective tissue; there is increased vascularity with arterioles and capillaries being particularly increased. Eventually new bone formation becomes the dominant feature and lamellar bone is laid down causing thickening of the bone trabeculae. However the lamellar bone is laid down in an uncoordinated haphazard fashion. The irregular cement lines which appear more basophilic than the surrounding bone form a characteristic mosaic pattern that is the hallmark of Paget's disease (Fig. 10.5). Each of the cement lines represents a surface where bone resorption has been followed by bone deposition. The trabeculae eventually become massively thickened and encroach upon the marrow cavity.

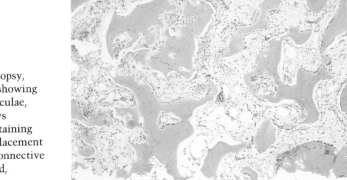

Fig. 10.4 BM trephine biopsy, Paget's disease of bone, showing thickening of bone trabeculae, numerous resorption bays (Howship's lacunae) containing large osteoclasts and replacement of marrow by vascular connective tissue. Paraffin-embedded, H&E × 39.

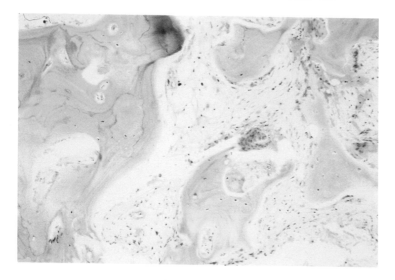

Fig. 10.5 BM trephine biopsy, Paget's disease of bone (same case as Fig. 10.4), showing thickening of bone trabeculae with a typical mosaic pattern of cement lines and large bizarre osteoclasts. Paraffin-embedded, Giemsa × 97.

Severe Paget's disease may have an associated mild anaemia. The bone marrow aspirate does not show any specific abnormality, but increased osteoblasts and osteoclasts are sometimes seen.

It should be noted that prolonged bleeding, consequent on the greatly increased vascularity, has been reported following trephine biopsy in a patient with Paget's disease.[15]

OSTEOSCLEROSIS

Osteosclerosis is used to describe a group of conditions in which there is an increase in the amount of bone per unit volume, usually consequent on increased bone formation. Osteosclerosis is most often seen in conjunction with severe bone marrow fibrosis either in a myeloproliferative disorder or in metastatic carcinoma. Osteosclerosis occasionally occurs in multiple myeloma, but osteolytic lesions are much more characteristic. It is also associated with a plasma cell dyscrasia in the POEMS syndrome (see page 201). Osteosclerosis may occur without a primary bone marrow disease in the congenital condition designated osteopetrosis (see below) and also, rarely, in adults in the absence of any associated disease (Fig. 10.6). The cause of isolated osteosclerosis in adults is unknown.

In the myeloproliferative disorders (see Fig. 4.23) the term osteomyelosclerosis[16] is sometimes used. The new bone may be either bone formed on the endosteal surface of the trabeculae leading to marked trabecular thickening, or irregular spicules of metaplastic woven bone within the fibrous tissue. The strands of woven bone may intersect the intertrabecular spaces and in severe cases the medullary cavity is almost completely obliterated. Some conversion of woven bone to mature bone occurs.

Metastases from various types of carcinoma may cause dense bone marrow fibrosis and osteosclerosis but the commonest associations are with carcinomas of the breast and prostate (see Figs 9.9 and 9.11). When osteosclerosis is due to metastatic carcinoma malignant cells can be detected within the fibrous tissue. The bone changes do not differ from those associated with the myeloproliferative diseases.

In idiopathic osteosclerosis the bone trabeculae are increased in thickness by mature lamellar bone.

In osteomyelosclerosis the peripheral blood and bone marrow changes are those of the underlying disease. In osteosclerosis associated with metastatic carcinoma a leucoerythroblastic anaemia is usual and there is sometimes also thrombocytopenia or leucopenia; a bone marrow aspirate may be impossible or the aspirate may contain tumour cells or increased osteoblasts and osteoclasts. In idiopathic osteosclerosis the peripheral blood and the bone marrow aspirate are normal.

In osteosclerosis the bone may be so hard that

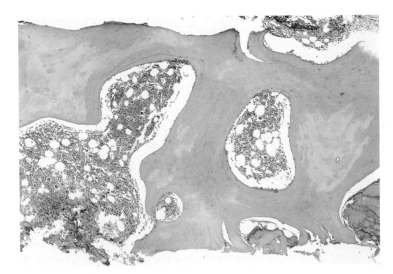

Fig. 10.6 BM trephine biopsy, idiopathic osteosclerosis, showing marked thickening of bone trabeculae by mature lamellar bone. The intervening marrow is normal. Paraffin-embedded, H&E × 39.

penetration of the bone is impossible or needles bend or break. Open biopsy may then be necessary for diagnosis.

OSTEOPETROSIS (ALBERS–SCHONBERG DISEASE)

Osteopetrosis, also known as marble bone disease and Albers–Schonberg disease, is a hereditary metabolic disease consequent on a defect in osteoclast function.[17,18] Osteoclasts may be increased, decreased or present in normal numbers but are always qualitatively abnormal. The result is osteosclerosis with gradual obliteration of the marrow cavity, both by bony encroachment and associated fibrosis. Although the bone density is increased the bone is more fragile than normal. Osteopetrosis occurs in an autosomal recessive form, that manifests itself either *in utero* or during infancy, and as an autosomal dominant form in adults. The autosomal recessive form is a severe disease with symptoms of marrow failure due to obliteration of the marrow cavity; the autosomal dominant form has much milder clinical manifestations with an increased predisposition to fractures. Histologically the trabeculae are thickened by increased amounts of mature lamellar bone.

In the severe infantile form of osteopetrosis there is increasingly severe leucoerythroblastic anaemia and thrombocytopenia associated with extramedullary haemopoiesis. In the milder adult form of the disease there is only mild anaemia.

OSTEOGENESIS IMPERFECTA

Osteogenesis imperfecta comprises a group of related hereditary diseases due to abnormalities in the synthesis of type I collagen. Several different biochemical defects have been identified, all of which are associated with increased fragility of the skeleton and a tendency to fractures. Other manifestations include blue sclera, laxity of joints, and abnormalities of dentition. The most severe variant (type II) has an autosomal recessive inheritance and is fatal in the perinatal period. Several other variants have been described that are compatible with survival into adult life; these usually have an autosomal dominant inheritance. Histologically there is thinning of the cortex and trabeculae. In some cases there is loss of the normal lamellar structure of the bone.[19]

The peripheral blood and bone marrow aspirate are normal.

REFERENCES

1 Ellis HA. Metabolic bone disease. In: *Recent Advances in Histopathology* 11, Anthony PP and Macsween RNM (eds). Churchill Livingstone, Edinburgh, 1981.

2 Raisz LG (1988) Local and systemic factors in the

pathogenesis of osteoporosis. *N Eng J Med*, **318**, 818–828.

3 Beck JS and Nordin BEC (1960) Histological assessment of osteoporosis by iliac crest biopsy. *J Pathol Bacteriol*, **80**, 391–397.

4 Ellis HA and Peart KM (1972) Quantitative observations on mineralised and non-mineralised bone in the iliac crest. *J Clin Pathol*, **25**, 277–286.

5 Fogelman I and Blake G. How to measure osteoporosis. In: *Osteoporosis*, Smith R (ed). Royal College of Physicians, London, 1990.

6 Frame B and Nixon RK (1968) Bone marrow mast cells in osteoporosis of aging. *N Eng J Med*, **279**, 626–30.

7 Yetgin S and Ozsoylu S (1982) Myeloid metaplasia in vitamin D deficiency rickets. *Scand J Haematol*, **28**, 180–185.

8 Zingraff J, Drueke T, Marie P, Man NK, Jungers P and Border P (1978) Anaemia and secondary hyperparathyroidism. *Arch Intern Med*, **138**, 1650–1652.

9 Teitelbaum SL (1984) Renal osteodystrophy. *Hum Pathol*, **15**, 306–323.

10 Kaye M and Henderson J (1988) Nature of mononuclear cells positive for acid phosphatase activity in bone marrow of patients with renal osteodystrophy. *J Clin Pathol*, **41**, 277–279.

11 McClure J, Fazzalari NL, Fassett RG and Pugsley DG (1983) Bone histoquantitative findings and histochemical staining reactions for aluminium in chronic renal failure patients treated with haemodialysis fluids containing high and low concentrations of aluminium. *J Clin Pathol*, **36**, 1281–1287.

12 Kaye M (1983) Bone marrow aluminium storage in renal failure. *J Clin Pathol*, **36**, 1288–1291.

13 Pierides AM and Myli MP (1984) Iron and aluminium osteomalacia in haemodialysis patients. *New Engl J Med*, **310**, 323.

14 Weinberg SG, Lubin A, Weiner SN, Deorus MP, Ghose MK and Kopelman SN (1977) Myelofibrosis in renal osteodystrophy. *Am J Med*, **63**, 755–776.

15 Ben-Chetrit E, Flusser D and Assaf Y (1984) Severe bleeding complicating percutaneous bone marrow biopsy. *Arch Intern Med*, **144**, 2284.

16 Burkhardt R, Frisch B and Bartl R (1982) Bone biopsy in haematological disorders. *J Clin Pathol*, **35**, 257–284.

17 Shapiro F (1980) Human osteopetrosis. Histologic, ultrastructural and biochemical study. *J Bone Joint Surg*, **62A**, 384.

18 Case records of the Massachussets General Hospital (1982) case 37. *New Engl J Med*, **307**, 735–743.

19 Falvo KA and Bullough PG (1973) Osteogenesis imperfecta: a histometric analysis. *J Bone Joint Surg*, **55A**, 275–286.

Index

- 700   520   480
190   620   450   70
      +150 +121
            101